The Future of Nursing

LEADING CHANGE, ADVANCING HEALTH

Committee on the Robert Wood Johnson Foundation
Initiative on the Future of Nursing, at the Institute of Medicine

INSTITUTE OF MEDICINE
OF THE NATIONAL ACADEMIES

THE NATIONAL ACADEMIES PRESS
Washington, D.C.
www.nap.edu

THE NATIONAL ACADEMIES PRESS   500 Fifth Street, N.W.   **Washington, DC 20001**

NOTICE: The project that is the subject of this report was approved by the Governing Board of the National Research Council, whose members are drawn from the councils of the National Academy of Sciences, the National Academy of Engineering, and the Institute of Medicine. The members of the committee responsible for the report were chosen for their special competences and with regard for appropriate balance.

This study was supported by Contract No. 65815 between the National Academy of Sciences and the Robert Wood Johnson Foundation. Any opinions, findings, conclusions, or recommendations expressed in this publication are those of the author(s) and do not necessarily reflect the view of the organizations or agencies that provided support for this project.

Library of Congress Cataloging-in-Publication Data

Committee on the Robert Wood Johnson Foundation Initiative on the Future of Nursing, at the Institute of Medicine.
   The future of nursing : leading change, advancing health / Committee on the Robert Wood Johnson Foundation Initiative on the Future of Nursing, at the Institute of Medicine.
      p. ; cm.
   Includes bibliographical references and index.
   ISBN 978-0-309-15823-7 (hardcover) — ISBN 978-0-309-15824-4 (pdf) 1. Nursing—Practice—United States. 2. Nursing—United States. 3. Leadership—United States. I. Robert Wood Johnson Foundation. II. Institute of Medicine (U.S.) III. Title.
   [DNLM: 1. Nursing—trends—United States. 2. Education, Nursing—United States. 3. Health Policy—United States. 4. Leadership—United States. 5. Nurse's Role—United States. WY 16 AA1]
   RT86.7.C65 2011
   610.73—dc22
                                    2010052816

Additional copies of this report are available from the National Academies Press, 500 Fifth Street, N.W., Lockbox 285, Washington, DC 20055; (800) 624-6242 or (202) 334-3313 (in the Washington metropolitan area); Internet, http://www.nap.edu.

For more information about the Institute of Medicine, visit the IOM home page at: **www.iom.edu.**

First Printing, February 2011
Second Printing, May 2011
Third Printing, December 2011
Fourth Printing, February 2012

Cover credit: Photos reprinted with permission from Tom Semkow; Gregory Benson; Lisa Hollis, Cedars-Sinai Medical Center; and Sam Kittner/kittner.com.

The serpent has been a symbol of long life, healing, and knowledge among almost all cultures and religions since the beginning of recorded history. The serpent adopted as a logotype by the Institute of Medicine is a relief carving from ancient Greece, now held by the Staatliche Museen in Berlin.

Suggested citation: IOM (Institute of Medicine). 2011. *The Future of Nursing: Leading Change, Advancing Health.* Washington, DC: The National Academies Press.

"Knowing is not enough; we must apply.
Willing is not enough; we must do."
—Goethe

INSTITUTE OF MEDICINE

OF THE NATIONAL ACADEMIES

Advising the Nation. Improving Health.

THE NATIONAL ACADEMIES
Advisers to the Nation on Science, Engineering, and Medicine

The **National Academy of Sciences** is a private, nonprofit, self-perpetuating society of distinguished scholars engaged in scientific and engineering research, dedicated to the furtherance of science and technology and to their use for the general welfare. Upon the authority of the charter granted to it by the Congress in 1863, the Academy has a mandate that requires it to advise the federal government on scientific and technical matters. Dr. Ralph J. Cicerone is president of the National Academy of Sciences.

The **National Academy of Engineering** was established in 1964, under the charter of the National Academy of Sciences, as a parallel organization of outstanding engineers. It is autonomous in its administration and in the selection of its members, sharing with the National Academy of Sciences the responsibility for advising the federal government. The National Academy of Engineering also sponsors engineering programs aimed at meeting national needs, encourages education and research, and recognizes the superior achievements of engineers. Dr. Charles M. Vest is president of the National Academy of Engineering.

The **Institute of Medicine** was established in 1970 by the National Academy of Sciences to secure the services of eminent members of appropriate professions in the examination of policy matters pertaining to the health of the public. The Institute acts under the responsibility given to the National Academy of Sciences by its congressional charter to be an adviser to the federal government and, upon its own initiative, to identify issues of medical care, research, and education. Dr. Harvey V. Fineberg is president of the Institute of Medicine.

The **National Research Council** was organized by the National Academy of Sciences in 1916 to associate the broad community of science and technology with the Academy's purposes of furthering knowledge and advising the federal government. Functioning in accordance with general policies determined by the Academy, the Council has become the principal operating agency of both the National Academy of Sciences and the National Academy of Engineering in providing services to the government, the public, and the scientific and engineering communities. The Council is administered jointly by both Academies and the Institute of Medicine. Dr. Ralph J. Cicerone and Dr. Charles M. Vest are chair and vice chair, respectively, of the National Research Council.

www.national-academies.org

Project Staff

SUSAN HASSMILLER, Study Director
ADRIENNE STITH BUTLER, Senior Program Officer
ANDREA M. SCHULTZ, Associate Program Officer
KATHARINE BOTHNER, Research Associate
THELMA L. COX, Administrative Assistant
TONIA E. DICKERSON, Senior Program Assistant
GINA IVEY, Communications Director
LORI MELICHAR, Research Director
JULIE FAIRMAN, Distinguished Nurse Scholar-in-Residence
JUDITH A. SALERNO, Executive Officer, IOM

Consultants

CHRISTINE GORMAN, Technical Writer
RONA BRIERE, Consultant Editor

Reviewers

This report has been reviewed in draft form by individuals chosen for their diverse perspectives and technical expertise, in accordance with procedures approved by the National Research Council's Report Review Committee. The purpose of this independent review is to provide candid and critical comments that will assist the institution in making its published report as sound as possible and to ensure that the report meets institutional standards for objectivity, evidence, and responsiveness to the study charge. The review comments and draft manuscript remain confidential to protect the integrity of the deliberative process. We wish to thank the following individuals for their review of this report:

John Benson, Jr., University of Nebraska Medical Center
Bobbie Berkowitz, University of Washington
George Boggs, American Association of Community Colleges
Marilyn P. Chow, Kaiser Permanente
Jordan J. Cohen, The George Washington University
Nancy W. Dickey, Texas A&M Health Science Center
Tine Hansen-Turton, National Nursing Centers Consortium and Public Health Management Corporation
Ann Hendrich, Ascension Health
Beverly Malone, National League for Nursing
Edward O'Neil, Center for the Health Professions, University of California, San Francisco
Robert L. Phillips, Jr., Robert Graham Center
Joy Reed, North Carolina Department of Health and Human Services
Thomas Ricketts, University of North Carolina School of Public Health

Vinod Sahney, Institute for Healthcare Improvement
Charlotte Yeh, AARP Services Incorporated
Heather Young, Betty Irene Moore School of Nursing, University of
California, Davis

Although the reviewers listed above have provided many constructive comments and suggestions, they were not asked to endorse the conclusions or recommendations nor did they see the final draft of the report before its release. The review of this report was overseen by **Kristine Gebbie,** School of Nursing, Hunter College City University of New York and **Mark R. Cullen,** Stanford University. Appointed by the National Research Council and Institute of Medicine, they were responsible for making certain that an independent examination of this report was carried out in accordance with institutional procedures and that all review comments were carefully considered. Responsibility for the final content of this report rests entirely with the authoring committee and the institution.

Foreword

The founding documents of the Institute of Medicine (IOM) call for experts to discuss, debate, and examine possible solutions for the multitude of complex health concerns that face the United States and the world. Equally important is the timely implementation of those solutions in a way that improves health. The United States is at an important crossroads as health care reforms are being carried out and the system begins to change. The possibility of strengthening the largest component of the health care workforce—nurses—to become partners and leaders in improving the delivery of care and the health care system as a whole inspired the IOM to partner with the Robert Wood Johnson Foundation (RWJF) in creating the RWJF Initiative on the Future of Nursing, at the IOM. In this partnership, the IOM and RWJF were in agreement that accessible, high-quality care cannot be achieved without exceptional nursing care and leadership. By working together, the two organizations sought to bring more credibility and visibility to the topic than either could by working alone. The organizations merged staff and resources in an unprecedented partnership to explore challenges central to the future of the nursing profession.

To support this collaborative effort, the IOM welcomed staff from RWJF, as loaned employees, to provide specific content expertise in nursing, research, and communications. Combining staff from two different organizations was an experiment that integrated best practices from both organizations and inspired us to think in fresh ways about how we conduct our work. We are indebted to RWJF for the leadership, support, and partnership that made this endeavor possible.

I am deeply grateful to the committee—led by Donna Shalala, committee chair and former Secretary of the Department of Health and Human Services, and Linda Burnes Bolton, committee vice chair—and to the staff, especially Susan

Hassmiller, Adrienne Stith Butler, Andrea Schultz, and Katharine Bothner, who produced this report. Their work will serve as a blueprint for how the nursing profession can transform itself into an ever more potent and relevant force for lasting solutions to enhance the quality and value of U.S. health care in ways that will meet the future health needs of diverse populations. The report calls on nurses, individually and as a profession, to embrace changes needed to promote health, prevent illness, and care for people in all settings across the lifespan. The nursing profession cannot make these changes on its own, however. The report calls for multisector support and interprofessional collaboration. In this sense, it calls on all health professionals and health care decision makers to work with nurses to make the changes needed for a more accessible, cost-effective, and high-quality health care system.

Since its foundation 40 years ago, the IOM has produced many reports echoing the theme of high-quality, safe, effective, evidence-based, and patient-centered care. The present report expands on this theme by addressing the critical role of nursing. It demonstrates that achieving a successful health care system in the future rests on the future of nursing.

Harvey V. Fineberg, M.D., Ph.D.
President, Institute of Medicine

Preface

This report is being published at a time of great opportunity in health care. Legislation passed in March 2010 will provide insurance coverage for 32 million more Americans. The implications of this new demand on the nation's health care system are significant. How can the system accommodate the increased demand while improving the quality of health care services provided to the American public?

Nursing represents the largest sector of the health professions, with more than 3 million registered nurses in the United States. The question presented to the committee that produced this report was: What roles can nursing assume to address the increasing demand for safe, high-quality, and effective health care services? In the near term, the new health care laws identify great challenges in the management of chronic conditions, primary care (including care coordination and transitional care), prevention and wellness, and the prevention of adverse events (such as hospital-acquired infections). The demand for better provision of mental health services, school health services, long-term care, and palliative care (including end-of-life care) is increasing as well. Whether improvements in all these areas of care will slow the rate of growth in health care expenditures remains to be seen; however, experts believe they will result in better health outcomes.

What nursing brings to the future is a steadfast commitment to patient care, improved safety and quality, and better outcomes. Most of the near-term challenges identified in the health care reform legislation speak to traditional and current strengths of the nursing profession in such areas as care coordination, health promotion, and quality improvement. How well nurses are trained and do their jobs is inextricably tied to most health care quality measures that have been targeted for improvement over the past few years. Thus for nursing, health care reform provides an opportunity for the profession to meet the demand for safe, high-quality, patient-centered, and equitable health care services. We believe nurses have key roles to play as team members and leaders for a reformed and better-integrated, patient-centered health care system.

This report begins with the assumption that nursing can fill such new and expanded roles in a redesigned health care system. To take advantage of these opportunities, however, nurses must be allowed to practice in accordance with their professional training, and the education they receive must better prepare them to deliver patient-centered, equitable, safe, high-quality health care services. Additionally, they must engage with physicians and other health care professionals to deliver efficient and effective care and assume leadership roles in the redesign of the health care system. In particular, we believe that preparation of an expanded workforce, necessary to serve the millions who will now have access to health insurance for the first time, will require changes in nursing scopes of practice, advances in the education of nurses across all levels, improvements in the practice of nursing across the continuum of care, transformation in the utilization of nurses across settings, and leadership at all levels so nurses can be deployed effectively and appropriately as partners in the health care team.

In 2008, the Robert Wood Johnson Foundation (RWJF) approached the Institute of Medicine (IOM) to propose a partnership between the two organizations to assess and respond to the need to transform the nursing profession to meet these challenges. The resulting collaborative partnership created a unique blend of organizational expertise and content expertise, drawing on the IOM's mission to serve as adviser to the nation to improve health and RWJF's long-standing commitment to ensuring that the nursing workforce has the necessary capacity, in terms of numbers, skills, and competence, to meet the present and future health care needs of the public. Recognizing that the nursing profession faces the challenges outlined above, RWJF and the IOM established a 2-year Initiative on the Future of Nursing. The cornerstone of the initiative is the work of this IOM committee. The Committee on the Robert Wood Johnson Foundation Initiative on the Future of Nursing, at the Institute of Medicine was tasked with producing a report containing recommendations for an action-oriented blueprint for the future of nursing, including changes in public and institutional policies at the national, state, and local levels. The specific charge to the committee is presented in Box P-1.

The committee held five meetings that included three technical workshops, which were designed to gather information on topics related to the study charge. In addition to these meetings, the committee hosted three public forums on the fu-

---

BOX P-1
Committee Charge

An ad hoc committee will examine the capacity of the nursing workforce to meet the demands of a reformed health care and public health system. It will develop a set of bold national recommendations, including ones that address the delivery of nursing services in a shortage environment and the capacity of the nursing education system. In its report, the committee will define a clear agenda and blueprint for action including changes in public and institutional policies at the national, state, and local levels. Its recommendations would address a range of system changes, including innovative ways to solve the nursing shortage in the United States.

The committee may examine and produce recommendations related to the following issues, with the goal of identifying vital roles for nurses in designing and implementing a more effective and efficient health care system:

- Reconceptualizing the role of nurses within the context of the entire workforce, the shortage, societal issues, and current and future technology;
- Expanding nursing faculty, increasing the capacity of nursing schools, and redesigning nursing education to assure that it can produce an adequate number of well-prepared nurses able to meet current and future health care demands;
- Examining innovative solutions related to care delivery and health professional education by focusing on nursing and the delivery of nursing services; and
- Attracting and retaining well-prepared nurses in multiple care settings, including acute, ambulatory, primary care, long-term care, community, and public health.

---

ture of nursing that focused on acute care; care in the community, with emphasis on community health, public health, primary care, and long-term care; and nursing education. Summaries of these forums have been published separately, are available at www.iom.edu/nursing, and are included on the CD-ROM in the back of this report. The committee also conducted a series of site visits in conjunction with each public forum to learn how nurses function in various health care and educational settings. In addition to the workshops, forums, and site visits, the committee collected testimony and welcomed public input throughout the study process, conducted a literature review, and commissioned a series of papers from a research network of esteemed colleagues.

For this committee, the IOM assembled an extraordinary group of professionals, including experts from areas such as business, academia, health care delivery, and health policy. The team brought diverse perspectives to the table that went well outside the nursing profession. Most of the members did not have a degree in nursing and were not involved in nursing education, practice, research, or governance. We are grateful to these committee members and to the exceptionally talented staff of the IOM and RWJF, all of whom worked hard with enthusiasm, great skill, flexibility, clarity, and drive.

Donna E. Shalala, Ph.D., FAAN
Chair

Linda Burnes Bolton, Dr.P.H., R.N., FAAN
Vice Chair

Acknowledgments

To begin, the committee would like to thank the sponsor of this study. Funds for the committee's work were provided by the Robert Wood Johnson Foundation (RWJF).

Numerous individuals and organizations made important contributions to the study process and this report. The committee wishes to express its gratitude for each of these contributions, although space does not permit identifying all of them here. Appendix A lists the individuals who provided valuable information at the committee's open workshops and its three forums on the future of nursing. In conjunction with each of the forums, the committee also visited several clinical sites to gather information on the role of nurses in various settings; these visits helped the committee understand the experiences of nurses and other health professionals and administrators. The committee greatly appreciates the time and information provided by all of these individuals.

The committee also gratefully acknowledges the contributions of the many individuals who provided data and research support. The RWJF Nursing Research Network, led by Lori Melichar and coordinated by Patricia (Polly) Pittman with the assistance of Emily Bass of AcademyHealth, created a series of research products that synthesized, translated, and disseminated information to inform the committee's deliberations. Research products from this network were managed by Linda Aiken, University of Pennsylvania; Peter Buerhaus, Vanderbilt University; Christine Kovner, New York University; and Joanne Spetz, University of California, San Francisco.

The committee would like to thank as well the authors whose commissioned papers added to the evidence base for the study: Barbara L. Nichols, Catherine R. Davis, and Donna R. Richardson of the Commission on Graduates of Foreign

Nursing Schools International; Barbara J. Safriet, Lewis and Clark Law School; Julie Sochalski, University of Pennsylvania School of Nursing, and Jonathan Weiner, Johns Hopkins University Bloomberg School of Public Health; Linda Cronenwett of the University of North Carolina at Chapel Hill School of Nursing, Christine A. Tanner of Oregon Health & Science University School of Nursing, Catherine L. Gilliss of Duke University School of Nursing, Kathleen Dracup of the University of California, San Francisco School of Nursing, Donald M. Berwick, Institute for Healthcare Improvement, Virginia Tilden, University of Nebraska Medical Center College of Nursing, and Linda H. Aiken of the University of Pennsylvania School of Nursing; and Linda Norlander, Group Health Home Care and Hospice. The committee also thanks the following fellows of the RWJF Executive Nurse Leadership Program: Susan Birch, Jody Chrastek, Erin Denholm, Karen Drenkard, Lynne M. Dunphy, Christina Esperat, Kathryn Fiandt, Jill Fuller, Catherine Garner, Mary Ellen Glasgow, Tine Hansen-Turton, Loretta Heuer, Cynda Hylton Rushton, Jane Kirschling, Richard C. MacIntyre, Rosalie O. Mainous, Gloria McNeal, Wanda Montalvo, Teri A. Murray, Mary E. Newell, Victoria Niederhauser, Suzanne Prevost, Maxine Proskurowski, Cynthia Teel, Donna Torrisi, and Marykay Vandriel.

Finally, the committee acknowledges the following individuals who provided additional data, reports, and support to the committee: Kathy Apple, National Council of State Boards of Nursing; William Baer and Lauren Peay, Arnold & Porter, LLP; Geraldine "Polly" Bednash and the staff of the American Association of Colleges of Nursing; Richard Blizzard, the Gallup Organization; Julie Dashiell, RWJF; Tine Hansen-Turton, National Nursing Center Consortium; Charlene Hanson, Georgia Southern University; Paul C. Light, New York University; Beverly Malone and the staff of the National League for Nursing; Diana Mason and Joy Jacobson, Hunter College, City University of New York; Mark B. McClellan, The Brookings Institution; Mary D. Naylor, University of Pennsylvania; Julienne M. Palbusa, The National Academies; Ciaran S. Phibbs, Veterans Affairs Medical Center; Deborah Sampson, Boston College School of Nursing; Shoshanna Sofaer, City University of New York; Kevin M. Stange, University of Michigan; and Ellen-Marie Whelan, Center for American Progress.

Contents

APPENDIXES*

---

*Appendixes F–J are not printed in this report but can be found on the CD-ROM in the back of this book.

Tables, Figures, and Boxes

TABLES

FIGURES

BOXES

---

*This nurse profile was inadvertently omitted from the prepublication version of this report.

Acronyms and Abbreviations*

AACN	American Association of Colleges of Nursing
AAI	Arkansas Aging Initiative
AAMC	Association of American Medical Colleges
AARP	American Association of Retired Persons
ACA	Affordable Care Act
ACO	accountable care organization
ADN	associate's degree in nursing
AIDS	acquired immune deficiency syndrome
AMA	American Medical Association
ANA	American Nurses Association
ANCC	American Nurses Credentialing Center
AONE	American Organization of Nurse Executives
APRN	advanced practice registered nurse
ARRA	American Recovery and Reinvestment Act
BSN	bachelor's of science in nursing
CBO	Congressional Budget Office
CCNE	Commission on Collegiate Nursing Education
CHC	community health center
CMA	California Medical Association
CMS	Centers for Medicare and Medicaid Services

---

*The acronyms and abbreviations used in the Summary and Chapters 1–7 appear in this list.

CNA   certified nursing assistant
CNL   clinical nurse leader
CNM   certified nurse midwife
CNO   chief nursing officer
CNS   clinical nurse specialist
CRNA   certified registered nurse anesthetist
CSA   California Society of Anesthesiologists

DEU   dedicated education unit
DNP   doctor of nursing practice
DRG   diagnosis-related group

EHR   electronic health record

FHBC   Family Health and Birth Center
FQHC   federally qualified health center
FTC   Federal Trade Commission
FTE   full-time equivalent

GAO   Government Accountability Office
GCHSSC   Gulf Coast Health Services Steering Committee

HealthSTAT   Health Students Taking Action Together
HEET   Hospital Employee Education and Training
HHS   Health and Human Services
HIT   health information technology
HIV   human immunodeficiency virus
HNC   Harambee Nursing Center
HRSA   Health Resources and Services Administration

ICU   Intensive Care Unit
IHI   Institute for Healthcare Improvement
INLP   Integrated Nurse Leadership Program
INQRI   Interdisciplinary Nursing Quality Research Initiative
IOM   Institute of Medicine

LIFE   Living Independently for Elders
LPN/LVN   licensed practical nurse/licensed vocational nurse

MD   medical doctor
MedPAC   Medicare Payment Advisory Commission
MSN   master's of science in nursing

NA	nursing assistant
NAQC	Nursing Alliance for Quality Care
NASN	National Association of School Nurses
NCEMNA	National Coalition of Ethnic Minority Nurse Associations
NCLEX-RN	National Council Licensure Examination for Registered Nurses
NCQA	National Committee for Quality Assurance
NCSBN	National Council of State Boards of Nursing
NFP	Nurse–Family Partnership
NHIT	national health care information technology
NHWC	National Health Workforce Commission
NLN	National League for Nursing
NMHC	nurse-managed health clinic
NNCC	National Nursing Centers Consortium
NP	nurse practitioner
NQF	National Quality Forum
NRN	Nursing Research Network
NSNA	National Student Nurses Association
NSSRN	National Sample Survey of Registered Nurses
OCNE	Oregon Consortium for Nursing Education
OHSU	Oregon Health and Science University
OPM	Office of Personnel Management
PACE	Program of All-Inclusive Care for the Elderly
PCMH	Patient-Centered Medical Home™
PhD	doctor of philosophy
RN	registered nurse
RWJF	Robert Wood Johnson Foundation
SAMHSA	Substance Abuse and Mental Health Services Administration
SEIU	Service Employees International Union
SOPP	Scope of Practice Partnership
TCAB	Transforming Care at the Bedside
TCM	Transitional Care Model
TIGER	Technology Informatics Guiding Education Reform
TWU	Texas Woman's University
UAMS	University of Arkansas for Medical Sciences
UHC	University HealthSystem Consortium
UP	University of Portland
UPMC	University of Pittsburgh Medical Center

USF	University of South Florida
UTH	University of Texas Health Science Center at Houston School of Nursing
VA	Department of Veterans Affairs
VANA	Veterans Affairs Nursing Academy
VNACJ	Visiting Nurse Association of Central Jersey
VNSNY	Visiting Nurse Service of New York

Summary[1]

The United States has the opportunity to transform its health care system to provide seamless, affordable, quality care that is accessible to all, patient centered, and evidence based and leads to improved health outcomes. Achieving this transformation will require remodeling many aspects of the health care system. This is especially true for the nursing profession, the largest segment of the health care workforce. This report offers recommendations that collectively serve as a blueprint to (1) ensure that nurses can practice to the full extent of their education and training, (2) improve nursing education, (3) provide opportunities for nurses to assume leadership positions and to serve as full partners in health care redesign and improvement efforts, and (4) improve data collection for workforce planning and policy making.

A VISION FOR HEALTH CARE

In 2010, Congress passed and the President signed into law comprehensive health care legislation. With the enactment of these laws, collectively referred to in this report as the Affordable Care Act (ACA), the United States has an opportunity to transform its health care system to provide higher-quality, safer,

---

[1] This summary does not include references. Citations for the discussion presented in the summary appear in the subsequent report chapters.

1

more affordable, and more accessible care. During the course of its work, the Committee on the Robert Wood Johnson Foundation Initiative on the Future of Nursing, at the Institute of Medicine developed a vision for a transformed health care system. The committee envisions a future system that makes quality care accessible to the diverse populations of the United States, intentionally promotes wellness and disease prevention, reliably improves health outcomes, and provides compassionate care across the lifespan. In this envisioned future, primary care and prevention are central drivers of the health care system. Interprofessional collaboration and coordination are the norm. Payment for health care services rewards value, not volume of services, and quality care is provided at a price that is affordable for both individuals and society. The rate of growth of health care expenditures slows. In all these areas, the health care system consistently demonstrates that it is responsive to individuals' needs and desires through the delivery of truly patient-centered care.

The ACA represents the broadest changes to the health care system since the 1965 creation of the Medicare and Medicaid programs and is expected to provide insurance coverage for an additional 32 million previously uninsured Americans. Although passage of the ACA is historic, realizing the vision outlined above will require a transformation of many aspects of the health care system. This is especially true for the nursing profession, which, with more than 3 million members, represents the largest segment of the health care workforce.

STUDY CHARGE

In 2008, the Robert Wood Johnson Foundation (RWJF) approached the Institute of Medicine (IOM) to propose a partnership to assess and respond to the need to transform the nursing profession. Recognizing that the nursing profession faces several challenges in fulfilling the promise of a reformed health care system and meeting the nation's health needs, RWJF and the IOM established a 2-year Initiative on the Future of Nursing. The cornerstone of the initiative is this committee, which was tasked with producing a report containing recommendations for an action-oriented blueprint for the future of nursing, including changes in public and institutional policies at the national, state, and local levels (Box S-1). Following the report's release, the IOM and RWJF will host a national conference on November 30 and December 1, 2010, to begin a dialogue on how the report's recommendations can be translated into action. The report will also serve as the basis for an extensive implementation phase to be facilitated by RWJF.

THE ROLE OF NURSES IN REALIZING A
TRANSFORMED HEALTH CARE SYSTEM

By virtue of its numbers and adaptive capacity, the nursing profession has the potential to effect wide-reaching changes in the health care system. Nurses'

BOX S-1
Committee Charge

An ad hoc committee will examine the capacity of the nursing workforce to meet the demands of a reformed health care and public health system. It will develop a set of bold national recommendations, including ones that address the delivery of nursing services in a shortage environment and the capacity of the nursing education system. In its report, the committee will define a clear agenda and blueprint for action including changes in public and institutional policies at the national, state, and local levels. Its recommendations would address a range of system changes, including innovative ways to solve the nursing shortage in the United States.

The committee may examine and produce recommendations related to the following issues, with the goal of identifying vital roles for nurses in designing and implementing a more effective and efficient health care system:

- Reconceptualizing the role of nurses within the context of the entire workforce, the shortage, societal issues, and current and future technology;
- Expanding nursing faculty, increasing the capacity of nursing schools, and redesigning nursing education to assure that it can produce an adequate number of well-prepared nurses able to meet current and future health care demands;
- Examining innovative solutions related to care delivery and health professional education by focusing on nursing and the delivery of nursing services; and
- Attracting and retaining well-prepared nurses in multiple care settings, including acute, ambulatory, primary care, long-term care, community, and public health.

---

regular, close proximity to patients and scientific understanding of care processes across the continuum of care give them a unique ability to act as partners with other health professionals and to lead in the improvement and redesign of the health care system and its many practice environments, including hospitals, schools, homes, retail health clinics, long-term care facilities, battlefields, and community and public health centers. Nurses thus are poised to help bridge the gap between coverage and access, to coordinate increasingly complex care for a wide range of patients, to fulfill their potential as primary care providers to the full extent of their education and training, and to enable the full economic value of their contributions across practice settings to be realized. In addition, a promising field of evidence links nursing care to high quality of care for patients, including protecting their safety. Nurses are crucial in preventing medication errors, reducing rates of infection, and even facilitating patients' transition from hospital to home.

Nursing practice covers a broad continuum from health promotion, to disease prevention, to coordination of care, to cure—when possible—and to palliative care when cure is not possible. While this continuum of practice is well matched to the needs of the American population, the nursing profession has its challenges. It is not as diverse as it needs to be—with respect to race, ethnicity, gender, and age—to provide culturally relevant care to all populations. Many members of the profession require more education and preparation to adopt new roles quickly in response to rapidly changing health care settings and an evolving health care system. Restrictions on scope of practice, policy- and reimbursement-related limitations, and professional tensions have undermined the nursing profession's ability to provide and improve both general and advanced care. Producing a health care system that delivers the right care—quality care that is patient centered, accessible, evidence based, and sustainable—at the right time will require transforming the work environment, scope of practice, education, and numbers of America's nurses.

KEY MESSAGES

As a result of its deliberations, the committee formulated four key messages that structure the discussion and recommendations presented in this report:

1. Nurses should practice to the full extent of their education and training.
2. Nurses should achieve higher levels of education and training through an improved education system that promotes seamless academic progression.
3. Nurses should be full partners, with physicians and other health professionals, in redesigning health care in the United States.
4. Effective workforce planning and policy making require better data collection and an improved information infrastructure.

The recommendations offered in this report focus on the critical intersection between the health needs of diverse populations across the lifespan and the actions of the nursing workforce. They are intended to support efforts to improve the health of the U.S. population through the contributions nurses can make to the delivery of care. But they are not necessarily about achieving what is most comfortable, convenient, or easy for the nursing profession.

Key Message #1: Nurses Should Practice to the Full Extent of Their Education and Training (Chapter 3)

Nurses have great potential to lead innovative strategies to improve the health care system. However, a variety of historical, regulatory, and policy barriers have limited nurses' ability to generate widespread transformation. Other barriers include fragmentation of the health care system, high rates of turnover among nurses, difficulties for nurses transitioning from school to practice, and an aging workforce and other demographic challenges. Many of these barriers have developed as a result of structural flaws in the U.S. health care system; others reflect limitations in the present work environment or the capacity and demographic makeup of the nursing workforce itself. Regulatory barriers are particularly problematic.

Regulations defining scope-of-practice limitations vary widely by state. Some are highly detailed, while others contain vague provisions that are open to interpretation. Some states have kept pace with the evolution of the health care system by changing their scope-of-practice regulations to allow nurse practitioners to see patients and prescribe medications without a physician's supervision or collaboration. However, the majority of state laws lag behind in this regard. As a result, what nurse practitioners are able to do once they graduate varies widely for reasons that are related not to their ability, education or training, or safety concerns, but to the political decisions of the state in which they work. Depending on the state, restrictions on the scope of practice of an advanced practice registered nurse may limit or deny altogether the authority to prescribe medications, admit patients to the hospital, assess patient conditions, and order and evaluate tests.

Because many of the problems related to varied scopes of practice are the result of a patchwork of state regulatory regimes, the federal government is especially well situated to promote effective reforms by collecting and disseminating best practices from across the country and incentivizing their adoption. Specifically, the Federal Trade Commission has a long history of targeting anticompetitive conduct in the health care market, including restrictions on the business practices of health care providers, as well as policies that could act as a barrier to the entry of new competitors in the market. As a payer and administrator of health insurance coverage for federal employees, the Office of Personnel Management and the Federal Employees Health Benefits Program have a responsibility to promote and ensure the access of employees/subscribers to the widest choice of competent, cost-effective health care providers. Principles of equity would suggest that this subscriber choice should be promoted by policies ensuring that full, evidence-based practice is permitted to all providers regardless of geographic location. Finally, the Centers for Medicare and Medicaid Services has the responsibility to promulgate rules and policies that promote Medicare and Medicaid beneficiaries' access to appropriate care, and therefore can ensure that its rules and polices reflect the evolving practice abilities of licensed providers.

In addition to barriers related to scope of practice, high turnover rates among newly graduated nurses highlight the need for a greater focus on managing the transition from school to practice. In 2002, the Joint Commission recommended the development of nurse residency programs—planned, comprehensive periods of time during which nursing graduates can acquire the knowledge and skills to deliver safe, quality care that meets defined (organization or professional society) standards of practice. Residency programs are supported predominantly in hospitals and larger health systems, with a focus on acute care. This has been the area of greatest need since most new graduates gain employment in acute care settings, and the proportion of new hires (and nursing staff) that are new graduates is rapidly increasing. It is essential, however, that residency programs outside of acute care settings be developed and evaluated. Much of the evidence supporting the success of residencies has been produced through self-evaluations by the residency programs themselves. For example, one organization, Versant,[2] has demonstrated a profound reduction in turnover rates for new graduate registered nurses—from 35 to 6 percent at 12 months and from 55 to 11 percent at 24 months—compared with new graduate registered nurse control groups hired at a facility prior to implementation of the residency program.

Key Message #2: Nurses Should Achieve Higher Levels of Education and Training Through an Improved Education System That Promotes Seamless Academic Progression (Chapter 4)

Major changes in the U.S. health care system and practice environment will require equally profound changes in the education of nurses both before and after they receive their license. An improved education system is necessary to ensure that the current and future generations of nurses can deliver safe, quality, patient-centered care across all settings, especially in such areas as primary care and community and public health.

Nursing is unique among the health professions in the United States in that it has multiple educational pathways leading to an entry-level license to practice. The qualifications and level of education required for entry into the nursing profession have been widely debated by nurses, nursing organizations, academics, and a host of other stakeholders for more than 40 years. During that time, competencies needed to practice have expanded, especially in the domains of community and public health, geriatrics, leadership, health policy, system improvement and change, research and evidence-based practice, and teamwork and collaboration. These new competencies have placed increased pressures on the education system and its curricula.

Care within hospital and community settings also has become more complex. In hospitals, nurses must make critical decisions associated with care for sicker, frailer patients and work with sophisticated, life-saving technology. Nurses are being called upon to fill primary care roles and to help patients manage chronic illnesses, thereby preventing acute care episodes and disease progression. They

---

[2] Versant is a nonprofit organization that provides, supervises, and evaluates nurse transition-to-practice residency programs for children's and general acute care hospitals. See http://www.versant.org/item.asp?id=35.

are expected to use a variety of technological tools and complex information management systems that require skills in analysis and synthesis to improve the quality and effectiveness of care. Across settings, nurses are being called upon to coordinate care and collaborate with a variety of health professionals, including physicians, social workers, physical and occupational therapists, and pharmacists, most of whom hold master's or doctoral degrees. Shortages of nurses in the positions of primary care providers, faculty, and researchers continue to be a barrier to advancing the profession and improving the delivery of care to patients.

To respond to these demands of an evolving health care system and meet the changing needs of patients, nurses must achieve higher levels of education and training. One step in realizing this goal is for a greater number of nurses to enter the workforce with a baccalaureate degree or progress to this degree early in their career. Moreover, to alleviate shortages of nurse faculty, primary care providers, and researchers, a cadre of qualified nurses needs to be ready to advance to the master's and doctoral levels. Nursing education should therefore include opportunities for seamless transition to higher degree programs—from licensed practical nurse (LPN)/licensed vocational nurse (LVN) degrees, to the associate's degree in nursing (ADN) and bachelor's of science in nursing (BSN), to master's of science in nursing (MSN), and to the PhD and doctor of nursing practice (DNP). Further, nursing education should serve as a platform for continued lifelong learning. Nurses also should be educated with physicians and other health professionals as students and throughout their careers. Finally, as efforts are made to improve the education system, greater emphasis must be placed on increasing the diversity of the workforce, including in the areas of gender and race/ethnicity, as well as ensuring that nurses are able to provide culturally relevant care.

While the capacity of the education system will need to expand, and the focus of curricula will need to be updated to ensure that nurses have the right competencies, a variety of traditional and innovative strategies already are being used across the country to achieve these aims. Examples include the use of technologies such as online education and simulation, consortium programs that create a seamless pathway from the ADN to the BSN, and ADN-to-MSN programs that provide a direct link to graduate education. Collectively, these strategies can be scaled up and refined to effect the needed transformation of nursing education.

Key Message #3: Nurses Should Be Full Partners, with Physicians and Other Health Professionals, in Redesigning Health Care in the United States (Chapter 5)

Strong leadership is critical if the vision of a transformed health care system is to be realized. To play an active role in achieving this vision, the nursing profession must produce leaders throughout the system, from the bedside to the boardroom. These leaders must act as full partners with physicians and other health professionals, and must be accountable for their own contributions to delivering high-quality care while working collaboratively with leaders from other health professions.

Being a full partner transcends all levels of the nursing profession and requires leadership skills and competencies that must be applied within the profession and in collaboration with other health professionals. In care environments, being a full partner involves taking responsibility for identifying problems and areas of waste, devising and implementing a plan for improvement, tracking improvement over time, and making necessary adjustments to realize established goals. Moreover, being a full partner translates more broadly to the health policy arena. To be effective in reconceptualized roles, nurses must see policy as something they can shape rather than something that happens to them. Nurses should have a voice in health policy decision making and be engaged in implementation efforts related to health care reform. Nurses also should serve actively on advisory committees, commissions, and boards where policy decisions are made to advance health systems to improve patient care.

Strong leadership on the part of nurses, physicians, and others will be required to devise and implement the changes necessary to increase quality, access, and value and deliver patient-centered care. While not all nurses begin their career with thoughts of becoming a leader, leadership is fundamental to advancing the profession. To ensure that nurses are ready to assume leadership roles, leadership-related competencies need to be embedded throughout nursing education, leadership development and mentoring programs need to be made available for nurses at all levels, and a culture that promotes and values leadership needs to be fostered. Equally important, all nurses—from students, to bedside and community nurses, to chief nursing officers and members of nursing organizations, to researchers—must take responsibility for their personal and professional growth by developing leadership competencies. They must exercise these competencies in a collaborative environment in all settings, including hospitals, communities, schools, boards, and political and business arenas, both within nursing and across the health professions. And in doing so, they must not only mentor others along the way, but develop partnerships and gain allies both within and beyond the health care environment.

Key Message #4: Effective Workforce Planning and Policy Making Require Better Data Collection and an Improved Information Infrastructure (Chapter 6)

Achieving a transformation of the health care system and the practice environment will require a balance of skills and perspectives among physicians, nurses, and other health professionals. However, strategic health care workforce planning to achieve this balance is hampered by the lack of sufficiently reliable and granular data on, for example, the numbers and types of health professionals currently employed, where they are employed and in what roles, and what types of activities they perform. These data are required to determine regional health care workforce needs and to establish regional targets and plans for appropriately increasing the supply of health professionals. Additionally, understanding of the impact of innovations such as bundled payments, medical homes, accountable care organizations, health information technology, and comparative effectiveness will be incomplete without information on and analysis of the necessary contributions of the various types of health professionals. Data collection and analysis across the health professions will also be essential because of the overlap in scopes of practice for primary care providers such as physicians, physician assistants, and nurse practitioners and the increasing shift toward team-based care. In the specific context of this study, planning for fundamental, wide-ranging changes in the education and deployment of the nursing workforce will require comprehensive data on the numbers and types of nurses currently available and required to meet future needs. Once an infrastructure for collecting and analyzing workforce data is in place, systematic assessment and projection of nursing workforce requirements by role, skill mix, region, and demographics will be needed to inform necessary changes in nursing practice and education.

The ACA mandates the creation of a National Health Care Workforce Commission whose mission is, among other things, to "[develop] and [commission] evaluations of education and training activities to determine whether the demand for health care workers is being met," and to "[identify] barriers to improved coordination at the Federal, State, and local levels and recommend ways to address such barriers."[3] The ACA also authorizes a National Center for Workforce Analysis, as well as state and regional workforce centers, and provides funding for workforce data collection and studies. A priority for these new structures and resources should be systematic monitoring of the supply of health care workers across professions, review of the data and methods needed to develop accurate predictions of future workforce needs, and coordination of the collection of data on the health care workforce at the state and regional levels. To be most useful, the data and information gathered must be timely and publicly accessible.

RECOMMENDATIONS

Recommendation 1: Remove scope-of-practice barriers. *Advanced practice registered nurses should be able to practice to the full extent of their education and training. To achieve this goal, the committee recommends the following actions.*

For the Congress:

- Expand the Medicare program to include coverage of advanced practice registered nurse services that are within the scope of practice under applicable state law, just as physician services are now covered.

---

[3] *Patient Protection and Affordable Care Act*, H.R. 3590 § 5101, 111th Congress.

- Amend the Medicare program to authorize advanced practice registered nurses to perform admission assessments, as well as certification of patients for home health care services and for admission to hospice and skilled nursing facilities.
- Extend the increase in Medicaid reimbursement rates for primary care physicians included in the ACA to advanced practice registered nurses providing similar primary care services.
- Limit federal funding for nursing education programs to only those programs in states that have adopted the National Council of State Boards of Nursing Model Nursing Practice Act and Model Nursing Administrative Rules (Article XVIII, Chapter 18).

For state legislatures:

- Reform scope-of-practice regulations to conform to the National Council of State Boards of Nursing Model Nursing Practice Act and Model Nursing Administrative Rules (Article XVIII, Chapter 18).
- Require third-party payers that participate in fee-for-service payment arrangements to provide direct reimbursement to advanced practice registered nurses who are practicing within their scope of practice under state law.

For the Centers for Medicare and Medicaid Services:

- Amend or clarify the requirements for hospital participation in the Medicare program to ensure that advanced practice registered nurses are eligible for clinical privileges, admitting privileges, and membership on medical staff.

For the Office of Personnel Management:

- Require insurers participating in the Federal Employees Health Benefits Program to include coverage of those services of advanced practice registered nurses that are within their scope of practice under applicable state law.

For the Federal Trade Commission and the Antitrust Division of the Department of Justice:

- Review existing and proposed state regulations concerning advanced practice registered nurses to identify those that have anticompetitive effects without contributing to the health and safety of the public. States with unduly restrictive regulations should be urged to amend them to allow advanced practice registered nurses to provide care to patients in all circumstances in which they are qualified to do so.

Recommendation 2: Expand opportunities for nurses to lead and diffuse collaborative improvement efforts. *Private and public funders, health care organizations, nursing education programs, and nursing associations should expand opportunities for nurses to lead and manage collaborative efforts with physicians and other members of the health care team to conduct research and to redesign and improve practice environments and health systems. These entities should also provide opportunities for nurses to diffuse successful practices.*

To this end:

- The Center for Medicare and Medicaid Innovation should support the development and evaluation of models of payment and care delivery that use nurses in an expanded and leadership capacity to improve health outcomes and reduce costs. Performance measures should be developed and implemented expeditiously where best practices are evident to reflect the contributions of nurses and ensure better-quality care.
- Private and public funders should collaborate, and when possible pool funds, to advance research on models of care and innovative solutions, including technology, that will enable nurses to contribute to improved health and health care.
- Health care organizations should support and help nurses in taking the lead in developing and adopting innovative, patient-centered care models.
- Health care organizations should engage nurses and other front-line staff to work with developers and manufacturers in the design, development, purchase, implementation, and evaluation of medical and health devices and health information technology products.
- Nursing education programs and nursing associations should provide entrepreneurial professional development that will enable nurses to initiate programs and businesses that will contribute to improved health and health care.

Recommendation 3: Implement nurse residency programs. *State boards of nursing, accrediting bodies, the federal government, and health care organizations should take actions to support nurses' completion of a transition-to-practice program (nurse residency) after they have completed a prelicensure or advanced practice degree program or when they are transitioning into new clinical practice areas.*

The following actions should be taken to implement and support nurse residency programs:

- State boards of nursing, in collaboration with accrediting bodies such as the Joint Commission and the Community Health Accreditation Program, should support nurses' completion of a residency program after they have completed a prelicensure or advanced practice degree program or when they are transitioning into new clinical practice areas.
- The Secretary of Health and Human Services should redirect all graduate medical education funding from diploma nursing programs to support the implementation of nurse residency programs in rural and critical access areas.
- Health care organizations, the Health Resources and Services Administration and Centers for Medicare and Medicaid Services, and philanthropic organizations should fund the development and implementation of nurse residency programs across all practice settings.
- Health care organizations that offer nurse residency programs and foundations should evaluate the effectiveness of the residency programs in improving the retention of nurses, expanding competencies, and improving patient outcomes.

Recommendation 4: Increase the proportion of nurses with a baccalaureate degree to 80 percent by 2020. *Academic nurse leaders across all schools of nursing should work together to increase the proportion of nurses with a baccalaureate degree from 50 to 80 percent by 2020. These leaders should partner with education accrediting bodies, private and public funders, and employers to ensure funding, monitor progress, and increase the diversity of students to create a workforce prepared to meet the demands of diverse populations across the lifespan.*

- The Commission on Collegiate Nursing Education, working in collaboration with the National League for Nursing Accrediting Commission, should require all nursing schools to offer defined academic pathways, beyond articulation agreements, that promote seamless access for nurses to higher levels of education.
- Health care organizations should encourage nurses with associate's and diploma degrees to enter baccalaureate nursing programs within 5 years of graduation by offering tuition reimbursement, creating a culture that fosters continuing education, and providing a salary differential and promotion.
- Private and public funders should collaborate, and when possible pool funds, to expand baccalaureate programs to enroll more students by offering scholarships and loan forgiveness, hiring more faculty, expanding clinical instruction through new clinical partnerships, and using technology to augment instruction. These efforts should take into consideration strategies to increase the diversity of the nursing workforce in terms of race/ethnicity, gender, and geographic distribution.

- The U.S. Secretary of Education, other federal agencies including the Health Resources and Services Administration, and state and private funders should expand loans and grants for second-degree nursing students.
- Schools of nursing, in collaboration with other health professional schools, should design and implement early and continuous interprofessional collaboration through joint classroom and clinical training opportunities.
- Academic nurse leaders should partner with health care organizations, leaders from primary and secondary school systems, and other community organizations to recruit and advance diverse nursing students.

Recommendation 5: Double the number of nurses with a doctorate by 2020. *Schools of nursing, with support from private and public funders, academic administrators and university trustees, and accrediting bodies, should double the number of nurses with a doctorate by 2020 to add to the cadre of nurse faculty and researchers, with attention to increasing diversity.*

- The Commission on Collegiate Nursing Education and the National League for Nursing Accrediting Commission should monitor the progress of each accredited nursing school to ensure that at least 10 percent of all baccalaureate graduates matriculate into a master's or doctoral program within 5 years of graduation.
- Private and public funders, including the Health Resources and Services Administration and the Department of Labor, should expand funding for programs offering accelerated graduate degrees for nurses to increase the production of master's and doctoral nurse graduates and to increase the diversity of nurse faculty, scientists, and researchers.
- Academic administrators and university trustees should create salary and benefit packages that are market competitive to recruit and retain highly qualified academic and clinical nurse faculty.

Recommendation 6: Ensure that nurses engage in lifelong learning. *Accrediting bodies, schools of nursing, health care organizations, and continuing competency educators from multiple health professions should collaborate to ensure that nurses and nursing students and faculty continue their education and engage in lifelong learning to gain the competencies needed to provide care for diverse populations across the lifespan.*

- Faculty should partner with health care organizations to develop and prioritize competencies so curricula can be updated regularly to ensure that graduates at all levels are prepared to meet the current and future health needs of the population.
- The Commission on Collegiate Nursing Education and the National

League for Nursing Accrediting Commission should require that all nursing students demonstrate a comprehensive set of clinical performance competencies that encompass the knowledge and skills needed to provide care across settings and the lifespan.

- Academic administrators should require all faculty to participate in continuing professional development and to perform with cutting-edge competence in practice, teaching, and research.
- All health care organizations and schools of nursing should foster a culture of lifelong learning and provide resources for interprofessional continuing competency programs.
- Health care organizations and other organizations that offer continuing competency programs should regularly evaluate their programs for adaptability, flexibility, accessibility, and impact on clinical outcomes and update the programs accordingly.

Recommendation 7: Prepare and enable nurses to lead change to advance health. *Nurses, nursing education programs, and nursing associations should prepare the nursing workforce to assume leadership positions across all levels, while public, private, and governmental health care decision makers should ensure that leadership positions are available to and filled by nurses.*

- Nurses should take responsibility for their personal and professional growth by continuing their education and seeking opportunities to develop and exercise their leadership skills.
- Nursing associations should provide leadership development, mentoring programs, and opportunities to lead for all their members.
- Nursing education programs should integrate leadership theory and business practices across the curriculum, including clinical practice.
- Public, private, and governmental health care decision makers at every level should include representation from nursing on boards, on executive management teams, and in other key leadership positions.

Recommendation 8: Build an infrastructure for the collection and analysis of interprofessional health care workforce data. *The National Health Care Workforce Commission, with oversight from the Government Accountability Office and the Health Resources and Services Administration, should lead a collaborative effort to improve research and the collection and analysis of data on health care workforce requirements. The Workforce Commission and the Health Resources and Services Administration should collaborate with state licensing boards, state nursing workforce centers, and the Department of Labor in this effort to ensure that the data are timely and publicly accessible.*

- The Workforce Commission and the Health Resources and Services Administration should coordinate with state licensing boards, including those for nursing, medicine, dentistry, and pharmacy, to develop and promulgate a standardized minimum data set across states and professions that can be used to assess health care workforce needs by demographics, numbers, skill mix, and geographic distribution.

- The Workforce Commission and the Health Resources and Services Administration should set standards for the collection of the minimum data set by state licensing boards; oversee, coordinate, and house the data; and make the data publicly accessible.
- The Workforce Commission and the Health Resources and Services Administration should retain, but bolster, the Health Resources and Services Administration's registered nurse sample survey by increasing the sample size, fielding the survey every other year, expanding the data collected on advanced practice registered nurses, and releasing survey results more quickly.
- The Workforce Commission and the Health Resources and Services Administration should establish a monitoring system that uses the most current analytic approaches and data from the minimum data set to systematically measure and project nursing workforce requirements by role, skill mix, region, and demographics.
- The Workforce Commission and the Health Resources and Services Administration should coordinate workforce research efforts with the Department of Labor, state and regional educators, employers, and state nursing workforce centers to identify regional health care workforce needs, and establish regional targets and plans for appropriately increasing the supply of health professionals.
- The Government Accountability Office should ensure that the Workforce Commission membership includes adequate nursing expertise.

CONCLUSION

Nurses are already committed to delivering high-quality care under current regulatory, business, and organizational conditions. But the power to change those conditions to deliver better care does not rest primarily with nurses, regardless of how ably led or educated they are; it also lies with governments, businesses, health care institutions, professional organizations and other health professionals, and the insurance industry. The recommendations presented in this report are directed to individual policy makers; national, state, and local government leaders; payers; health care researchers; executives; and professionals—including nurses and others—as well as to larger groups such as licensing bodies, educational institutions, and philanthropic and advocacy organizations, especially those advocating for consumers. Together, these groups have the power to transform the health care system to provide seamless, affordable, quality care that is accessible to all, patient centered, and evidence based and leads to improved health outcomes.

Overview of the Report

This report is organized into three parts. Part I presents the report's key messages and important contextual information for the study. Chapter 1 offers the committee's vision for health care in the United States, explains why nurses have an essential role in realizing this vision and why a fundamental transformation of the nursing profession is needed if they are to fulfill this role, and details four key messages that structure the discussion and recommendations in Parts II and III. As context for the remainder of the report, Chapter 2 describes how the U.S. health care system is evolving and sets forth principles the committee believes should guide that evolution.

Part II details the fundamental transformation of the nursing profession that is needed to achieve the improved health care system described in Chapter 1. This transformation needs to occur in three broad areas: practice (Chapter 3), education (Chapter 4), and leadership (Chapter 5). This part of the report also addresses the crucial need for better data on the health care workforce to inform this transformation and that of the overall health care system (Chapter 6).

Chapters 2 through 6 include a series of case studies and profiles illustrating the work of nurses and innovative models that either were developed by nurses or feature nurses in a leadership role. These case studies and profiles not only provide texture to the report but also offer real-life examples of nurses working in reconceptualized roles and directly affecting the quality, accessibility, and value of health care. Cumulatively, these case studies and profiles offer a glimpse into what the future of nursing could be.

Finally, Part III offers the committee's blueprint for action in the form of recommendations and related research priorities (Chapter 7).

In addition, the report includes 10 appendixes. Appendix A describes the study methods and information sources used to inform the committee's deliberations; Appendix B contains biographical sketches of the committee members; Appendix C offers highlights from the three public forums held by the committee on the future of nursing in the areas of acute care, care in the community, and education; Appendix D contains the consensus model for advanced practice registered nurse (APRN) regulation that is referenced in Chapter 3 and in recommendation 1 in Chapter 7; and Appendix E provides a brief description of undergraduate nursing education in the United States. Appendixes F–J are not printed in this report but can be found on the CD-ROM in the back of this book and contain papers commissioned by the committee on the following topics: matching nursing practice and skills to future needs; transformational models of nursing across different care settings; federal options for maximizing the value of APRNs in providing quality, cost-effective health care; the future of nursing education; and international models of nursing.

Part I

Key Messages and Study Context

1

Key Messages of the Report

The U.S. health care system is characterized by a high degree of fragmentation across many sectors, which raises substantial barriers to providing accessible, quality care at an affordable price. In part, the fragmentation in the system comes from disconnects between public and private services, between providers and patients, between what patients need and how providers are trained, between the health needs of the nation and the services that are offered, and between those with insurance and those without (Stevens, 1999). Communication between providers is difficult, and much care is redundant because there is no way of sharing results.

This report is being published at an opportune time. In 2010, Congress passed and the President signed into law comprehensive health care legislation. These laws, the Patient Protection and Affordable Care Act (Public Law 111-148) and the Health Care and Education Affordability Reconciliation Act (Public Law 111-152), are collectively referred to throughout this report as the Affordable Care Act (ACA). The ACA represents the broadest changes to the health care system since the 1965 creation of the Medicare and Medicaid programs and is expected to provide insurance coverage for an additional 32 million previously uninsured Americans. The need to improve the health care system is becoming increasingly evident as challenges related to both the quality and costs of care persist.

As discussed in the preface, this study was undertaken to explore how the nursing profession can be transformed to help exploit these opportunities and contribute to building a health care system that will meet the demand for safe, quality, patient-centered, accessible, and affordable care. This chapter presents the key messages that emerged from the study committee's deliberations. It begins by describing a vision for a transformed system that can meet the health needs of the U.S. population in the 21st century. The chapter then delineates the roles of nurses in realizing this vision. The third section explains why a fundamental transformation of the nursing profession will be required if nurses are to assume these roles. The final section presents conclusions.

A VISION FOR HEALTH CARE

During the course of its work, the Committee on the Robert Wood Johnson Foundation Initiative on the Future of Nursing, at the Institute of Medicine developed a vision for a transformed health care system, while recognizing the demands and limitations of the current health care system outlined above. The committee envisions a future system that makes quality care accessible to the diverse populations of the United States, intentionally promotes wellness and disease prevention, reliably improves health outcomes, and provides compassionate care across the lifespan. In this envisioned future, primary care and prevention are central drivers of the health care system. Interprofessional collaboration and coordination are the norm. Payment for health care services rewards value, not volume of services, and quality care is provided at a price that is affordable for both individuals and society. The rate of growth of health care expenditures slows. In all these areas, the health care system consistently demonstrates that it is responsive to individuals' needs and desires through the delivery of truly patient-centered care. Annex 1-1 lists the committee's definitions for three core terms related to its vision: health, health care, and the health care system.

THE ROLE OF NURSES IN REALIZING THIS VISION

The ACA provides a call to action for nurses, and several sections of the legislation are directly relevant to their work.[1] For example, sections 5501 through 5509 are aimed at substantially strengthening the provision of primary care—a need generally recognized by health professionals and policy experts; section 2717 calls for "ensuring the quality of care"; and section 2718 emphasizes "bringing down the cost of health care coverage." Enactment of the ACA offers a myriad of opportunities for the nursing profession to facilitate improvements to the health care system and the mechanisms by which care is delivered across various settings. Systemwide changes are needed that capture the full economic value of nurses and take into account the growing body of evidence that links nursing practice to improvements in the safety and quality of care. Advanced practice registered nurses (APRNs) should be called upon to fulfill and expand their potential as primary care providers across practice settings based on their

---

[1] For a list of nursing-related provisions included in the ACA, see http://championnursing.org/sites/default/files/nursingandhealthreformlawable.pdf.

education and competency. Nursing initiatives and programs should be scaled up to help bridge the gap between insurance coverage and access to care.

The nursing profession has the potential capacity to implement wide-reaching changes in the health care system. With more than 3 million members, the profession has nearly doubled since 1980 and represents the largest segment of the U.S. health care workforce (HRSA, 2010; U.S. Census Bureau, 2009). By virtue of their regular, close proximity to patients and their scientific understanding of care processes across the continuum of care, nurses have a considerable opportunity to act as full partners with other health professionals and to lead in the improvement and redesign of the health care system and its practice environment.

Nurses practice in many settings, including hospitals, schools, homes, retail health clinics, long-term care facilities, battlefields, and community and public health centers. They have varying levels of education and competencies—from licensed practical nurses, who greatly contribute to direct patient care in nursing homes, to nurse scientists, who research and evaluate more effective ways of caring for patients and promoting health. As described in Annex 1-1 at the end of this chapter, most nurses are registered nurses (RNs), who "complete a program of study at a community college, diploma school of nursing, or a four-year college or university and are required to pass a nationally standardized licensing exam in the state in which they begin practice" (AARP, 2010). Figure 1-1 shows that of the many settings where RNs practice, the majority practice in hospitals; Figure 1-2 shows the employment settings of nurses by highest nursing or nursing-related education. More than a quarter of a million nurses are APRNs (HRSA, 2010), who hold master's or doctoral degrees and pass national certification exams. APRNs deliver primary and other types of health care services. For example, they teach and counsel patients to understand their health problems and what they can do to get better, they coordinate care and advocate for patients in the complex health care system, and they refer patients to physicians and other health care providers. APRNs include nurse practitioners, clinical nurse specialists, certified registered nurse anesthetists, and certified nurse midwives (see Table 1-1). Annex 1-1 provides more detailed descriptions of the preparation and roles of nurses, pathways in nursing education, and numbers of nurses.

Nursing practice covers a broad continuum from health promotion, to disease prevention, to coordination of care, to cure—when possible—and to palliative care when cure is not possible. This continuum of practice is well matched to the current and future needs of the American population (see Chapter 2). Nurses have a direct effect on patient care. They provide the majority of patient assessments, evaluations, and care in hospitals, nursing homes, clinics, schools, workplaces, and ambulatory settings. They are at the front lines in ensuring that care is delivered safely, effectively, and compassionately. Additionally, nurses attend to patients and their families in a holistic way that often goes beyond physical health needs to recognize and respond to social, mental, and spiritual needs. Given their education, experience, and unique perspectives and the centrality of their role in

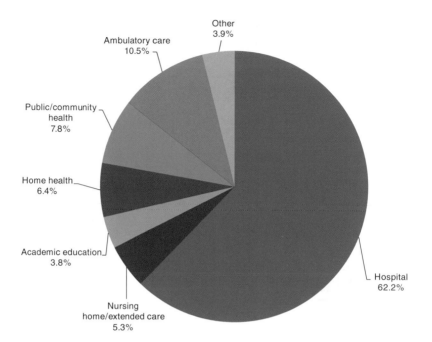
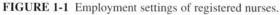

FIGURE 1-1 Employment settings of registered nurses.
NOTES: The totals may not add to 100 percent because of the effect of rounding. Only RNs for whom information on setting was available are included in the calculations used for this chart. Public/community health includes school and occupational health. Ambulatory care includes medical/physician practices, health centers and clinics, and other types of nonhospital clinical settings. Other includes insurance, benefits, and utilization review.
SOURCE: HRSA, 2010.

providing care, nurses will play a significant role in the transformation of the health care system. Likewise, while changes in the health care system will have profound effects on all providers, this will be undoubtedly true for nurses.

Traditional nursing competencies such as care management and coordination, patient education, public health intervention, and transitional care are likely to dominate in a reformed health care system as it inevitably moves toward an emphasis on prevention and management rather than acute care (O'Neil, 2009). Nurses have also begun developing new competencies for the future to help bridge the gap between coverage and access, to coordinate increasingly complex care for a wide range of patients, to fulfill their potential as primary care providers to the full extent of their education and training, to implement systemwide changes that take into account the growing body of evidence linking nursing practice to

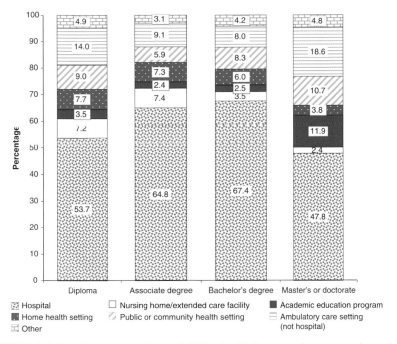

FIGURE 1-2 Employment settings of RNs, by highest nursing or nursing-related education.
NOTES: The total percent by setting may not equal the estimated total of all registered nurses due to incomplete information provided by respondents and the effect of rounding.
SOURCE: HRSA, 2010.

fundamental improvements in the safety and quality of care, and to capture the full economic value of their contributions across practice settings.

At the same time, the nursing profession has its challenges. While there are concerns regarding the number of nurses available to meet the demands of the health care system and the needs of patients, and there is reason to view as a priority replacing at least 900,000 nurses over the age of 50 (BLS, 2009), the composition of the workforce is turning out to be an even greater challenge for the future of the profession. The workforce is generally not as diverse as it needs to be—with respect to race and ethnicity (just 16.8 percent of the workforce is non-white), gender (approximately 7 percent of employed nurses are male), or age (the median age of nurses is 46, compared to 38 in 1988)—to provide culturally relevant care to all populations (HRSA, 2010). Many members of the profession lack the education and preparation necessary to adapt to new roles quickly in response to rapidly changing health care settings and an evolving health care sys-

TABLE 1-1 Types of Advanced Practice Registered Nurses (APRNs)

Who Are They?	How Many in United States?	What Do They Do?
Nurse Practitioners (NPs)	153,348	Take health histories and provide complete physical exams; diagnose and treat acute and chronic illnesses; provide immunizations; prescribe and manage medications and other therapies; order and interpret lab tests and x-rays; provide health teaching and supportive counseling.
Clinical Nurse Specialists (CNSs)	59,242*	Provide advanced nursing care in hospitals and other clinical sites; provide acute and chronic care management; develop quality improvement programs; serve as mentors, educators, researchers, and consultants.
Certified Registered Nurse Anesthetists (CRNAs)	34,821	Administer anesthesia and provide related care before and after surgical, therapeutic, diagnostic, and obstetrical procedures, as well as pain management. Settings include operating rooms, outpatient surgical centers, and dental offices. CRNAs deliver more than 65% of all anesthetics to patients in the United States.
Certified Nurse Midwives (CNMs)	18,492	Provide primary care to women, including gynecological exams, family planning advice, prenatal care, management of low-risk labor and delivery, and neonatal care. Practice settings include hospitals, birthing centers, community clinics, and patient homes.

*APRNs are identified by their responses to the National Sample Survey of Registered Nurses, and this number may not reflect the true population of CNSs.
SOURCE: AARP, 2010. Courtesy of AARP. All rights reserved.

tem. Restrictions on scope of practice and professional tensions have undermined the nursing profession's ability to provide and improve both general and advanced care. Producing a health care system that delivers the right care—quality care that is patient centered, accessible, evidence based, and sustainable—at the right time will require transforming the work environment, scope of practice, education, and numbers and composition of America's nurses. The remainder of this section examines the role of the nursing profession in health care reform according to the same three parameters by which all other health care reform initiatives are evaluated—quality, access, and value.

Nurses and Quality

Although it is difficult to prove causation, an emerging body of literature suggests that quality of care depends to a large degree on nurses (Kane et al., 2007; Lacey and Cox, 2009; Landon et al., 2006; Sales et al., 2008). The Joint Commission, the leading independent accrediting body for health care organizations, believes that "the future state of nursing is inextricably linked to the strides in patient care quality and safety that are critical to the success of America's health care system, today and tomorrow" (Joint Commission, 2010). While quality measures have historically focused on conditions or diseases, many of the quality measures used over the past few years address how well nurses are able to do their jobs (Kurtzman and Buerhaus, 2008).

In 2004, the National Quality Forum (NQF) endorsed the first set of nationally standardized performance measures, the National Voluntary Consensus Standards for Nursing-Sensitive Care, initially designed to assess the quality of care provided by nurses who work in hospitals (National Quality Forum, 2004). The NQF measures include prevalence of pressure ulcers and falls; nursing-centered interventions, such as smoking cessation counseling; and system-centered measures, such as voluntary turnover and nursing care hours per patient day. These measures have helped nurses and the organizations where they work identify targets for improvements in care delivery.

Another important vehicle for tracking and improving quality is the National Database of Nursing Quality Indicators, the nation's largest nursing registry. This database, which meets the new reporting requirement by the Centers for Medicare and Medicaid Services for nursing-sensitive care, is supported by the American Nurses Association.[2] More than 25 percent of hospitals participate in the database, which documents more than 21 measures of hospital performance linked to the availability and quality of nursing services in acute care settings. Participating facilities are able to obtain unit-level comparative data, including patient and staffing outcomes, to use for quality improvement purposes. Comparison data are publicly reported, which provides an incentive to improve the quality of care on a continuous basis. This database is now maintained at the University of Kansas School of Nursing and is available to researchers interested in improving health care quality.

Nurses and Access

Evidence suggests that access to quality care can be greatly expanded by increasing the use of RNs and APRNs in primary, chronic, and transitional care (Bodenheimer et al., 2005; Craven and Ober, 2009; Naylor et al., 2004; Rendell, 2007). For example, nurses serving in special roles created to increase access to care, such as care coordinators and primary care clinicians, have led to significant reductions in hospitalization and rehospitalization rates for elderly patients (Kane et al., 2003; Naylor et al., 2004). It stands to reason that one way to improve access to patient-centered care would be to allow nurses to make more care decisions at the point of care. Yet in many cases, outdated regulations, biases, and policies prevent nurses, particularly APRNs, from practicing to the full extent

---

[2] For more information, see http://www.nursingworld.org/MainMenuCategories/ThePracticeofProfessionalNursing/ PatientSafetyQuality/ Research-Measurement/The-National-Database.aspx.

of their education, skills, and competencies (Hansen-Turton et al., 2008; Ritter and Hansen-Turton, 2008; Safriet, 2010). Chapter 3 examines these barriers in greater depth.

Nurses also make significant contributions to access by delivering care where people live, work, and play. Examples include school nurses, occupational health nurses, public health nurses, and those working at so-called retail clinics in busy shopping centers. Nurses also work in migrant health clinics and nurse-managed health centers, organizations known for serving the most underserved populations. Additionally, nurses are often at the front lines serving as primary providers for individuals and families affected by natural or man-made disasters, delivering care in homes and designated community shelters.

Nurses and Value

"Value in health care is expressed as the physical health and sense of well-being achieved relative to the cost" (IOM Roundtable on Evidence-Based Medicine, 2008). Compared with support for the role of nurses in improving quality and access, there is somewhat less evidence that expanding the care provided by nurses will result in cost savings to society at large while also improving outcomes and ensuring quality. However, the evidence base in favor of such a conclusion is growing. Compared with other models of prenatal care, for example, pregnant women who receive care led by certified nurse midwives are less likely to experience antenatal hospitalization, and their babies are more likely to have a shorter hospital stay (Hatem et al., 2008) (see Chapter 2 for a case study of care provided by certified nurse midwives at the Family Health and Birth Center in Washington, DC). Another study examining the impact of nurse staffing on value suggests that increasing the proportion of nursing hours provided by RNs without increasing total nursing hours was associated with 1.5 million fewer hospital days, nearly 60,000 fewer inpatient complications, and a 0.5 percent net reduction in costs (Needleman et al., 2006). Chapter 2 includes a case study of the Nurse–Family Partnership Program, in which front-line RNs make home visits to high-risk young mothers over a 2.5-year period. This program has demonstrated significant value, resulting in a net savings of $34,148 per family served. The program has also reduced pregnancy-induced hypertension by 32 percent, child abuse and neglect by 50 percent, emergency room visits by 35 percent, and language-related delays by 50 percent (AAN, 2010).

THE NEED FOR A FUNDAMENTAL TRANSFORMATION OF THE NURSING PROFESSION

Given the crucial role of nurses with respect to the quality, accessibility, and value of care, the nursing profession itself must undergo a fundamental transformation if the committee's vision for health care is to be realized. As this report argues, the ways in which nurses were educated and practiced during the 20th century are no longer adequate for dealing with the realities of health care in the 21st century. Outdated regulations, attitudes, policies, and habits continue to restrict the innovations the nursing profession can bring to health care at a time of tremendous complexity and change.

In the course of its deliberations, the committee formulated four key messages that inform the discussion in Chapters 3–6 and structure its recommendations for transforming the nursing profession:

1. Nurses should practice to the full extent of their education and training.
2. Nurses should achieve higher levels of education and training through an improved education system that promotes seamless academic progression.
3. Nurses should be full partners, with physicians and other health professionals, in redesigning health care in the United States.
4. Effective workforce planning and policy making require better data collection and an improved information infrastructure.

These key messages speak to the need to transform the nursing profession in three crucial areas—practice, education, and leadership—as well as to collect better data on the health care workforce to inform planning for the necessary changes to the nursing profession and the overall health care system.

The Need to Transform Practice

Key Message #1: Nurses should practice to the full extent of their education and training.

To ensure that all Americans have access to needed health care services and that nurses' unique contributions to the health care team are maximized, federal and state actions are required to update and standardize scope-of-practice regulations to take advantage of the full capacity and education of APRNs. States and insurance companies must follow through with specific regulatory, policy, and financial changes that give patients the freedom to choose from a range of providers, including APRNs, to best meet their health needs. Removing regulatory, policy, and financial barriers to promote patient choice and patient-centered care should be foundational in the building of a reformed health care system.

Additionally, to the extent that the nursing profession envisions its future as confined to acute care settings, such as inpatient hospitals, its ability to help shape the future U.S. health care system will be greatly limited. As noted earlier, care in the future is likely to shift from the hospital to the community setting (O'Neil, 2009). Yet the majority of nurses still work in acute care settings; according to recent findings from the 2008 National Sample Survey of Registered Nurses, just over 62 percent of working RNs were employed in hospitals in 2008—up from approximately 57 percent in 2004 (HRSA, 2010). Nurses must create, serve in, and disseminate reconceptualized roles to bridge whatever gaps remain between coverage and access to care. More must become health coaches, care coordinators, informaticians, primary care providers, and health team leaders in a greater variety of settings, including primary care medical homes and accountable care organizations. In some respects, such a transformation would return the nursing profession to its roots in the public health movement of the early 20th century.

At the same time, new systems and technologies appear to be pushing nurses ever farther away from patients. This appears to be especially true in the acute care setting. Studies show that nurses on medical–surgical units spend only 31 to 44 percent of their time in direct patient activities (Tucker and Spear, 2006). A separate study of medical–surgical nurses found they walked nearly a mile longer while on than off duty in obtaining the supplies and equipment needed to perform their tasks. In general, less than 20 percent of nursing practice time was devoted specifically to patient care activities, the majority being consumed by documentation, medication administration, and communication regarding the patient (Hendrich et al., 2008). Several health care organizations, professional organizations, and consumer groups have endorsed a Proclamation for Change aimed at redressing inefficiencies in hospital design, organization, and technology infrastructure through a focus on patient-centered design; the implementation of systemwide, integrated technology; the creation of seamless workplace environments; and the promotion of vendor partnerships (Hendrich et al., 2009). Realizing the vision presented earlier in this chapter will require a practice environment that is fundamentally transformed so that nurses are efficiently employed—whether in the hospital or in the community—to the full extent of their education, skills, and competencies.

Chapter 3 examines these issues in greater depth.

The Need to Transform Education

Key Message #2: Nurses should achieve higher levels of education and training through an improved education system that promotes seamless academic progression.

Major changes in the U.S. health care system and practice environment will require equally profound changes in the education of nurses both before and after they receive their licenses. An improved education system is necessary to ensure that the current and future generations of nurses can deliver safe, quality, patient-centered care across all settings, especially in such areas as primary care and community and public health.

Interest in the nursing profession has grown rapidly in recent years, in part as a result of the economic downturn and the relative stability the health care sector offers. The number of applications to entry-level baccalaureate programs increased by more than 70 percent in just 5 years—from 122,000 applications in 2004 to 208,000 applications in 2009 (AACN, 2010). While nursing schools across the country have responded to this influx of interest, there are constraints, such as insufficient numbers of nurse faculty and clinical placements, that limit the capacity of nursing schools to accommodate all the qualified applicants. Thus, thousands of qualified students are turned away each year (Kovner and Djukic, 2009).

A variety of challenges limit the ability to ensure a well-educated nurse workforce. As noted, there is a shortage of faculty to teach nurses at all levels (Allan and Aldebron, 2008). Also, the ways in which nurses during the 20th century taught each other to care for people and learned to practice and make clinical decisions are no longer adequate for delivering care in the 21st century. Many nursing schools have dealt with the explosion of research and knowledge needed to provide health care in an increasingly complex system by adding layers of content that requires more instruction (Ironside, 2004). A fundamental rethinking of this approach is needed (Benner et al., 2009; Erickson, 2002; IOM, 2003, 2009; Lasater and Nielsen, 2009; Mitchell et al., 2006; Orsolini-Hain and Waters, 2009; Tanner et al., 2008). Additionally, nurses at all levels have few incentives to pursue further education, and face active disincentives to advanced education. Nurses and physicians—not to mention pharmacists and social workers—typically are not educated together, yet they are increasingly required to cooperate and collaborate more closely in the delivery of care.

The education system should provide nurses with the tools needed to evaluate and improve standards of patient care and the quality and safety of care while preserving fundamental elements of nursing education, such as ethics and integrity and holistic, compassionate approaches to care. The system should ensure nurses' ability to adapt and be flexible in response to changes in science, technology, and population demographics that shape the delivery of care. Nursing education at all levels needs to impart a better understanding of ways to work in the context of and lead change within health care delivery systems, methods for quality improvement and system redesign, methods for designing effective care delivery models and reducing patient risk, and care management and other roles involving expanded authority and responsibility. The nursing profession must adopt a framework of continuous, lifelong learning that includes basic education, residency programs, and continuing competence. More nurses must receive a solid education in how to manage complex conditions and coordinate care with multiple health professionals. They must demonstrate new competencies in systems thinking, quality improvement, and care management and a basic understanding of health policy and research. Graduate-level nurses must develop even greater competencies and deeper understanding in all of these areas. Innovative new programs to attract nurse faculty and provide a wider range of clinical education placements must clear long-standing bottlenecks in nursing education. Accrediting and certifying organizations must mandate demonstrated mastery of clinical skills, managerial competencies, and professional development at all levels to complement the completion of degree programs and written board examinations. Milestones for mandated skills, competencies, and professional development must be updated more frequently to keep pace with the rapidly changing demands of health care. And all health professionals should receive more of their education in concert with students from other disciplines. Interprofessional team training of nurses, physicians, and other health care providers should begin when they are students and proceed throughout their careers. Successful interprofessional education can be achieved only through committed partnerships across professions.

Nurses should move seamlessly through the education system to higher levels of education, including graduate degrees. Nurses with graduate degrees will be able to replenish the nurse faculty pool; advance nursing science and contribute to the knowledge base on how nurses can provide up-to-date, safe patient care; participate in health care decisions; and provide the leadership needed to establish nurses as full partners in health care redesign efforts (see the section on leadership below).

The Need to Transform Leadership

Key Message #3: Nurses should be full partners, with physicians and other health professionals, in redesigning health care in the United States.

Not all nurses begin their career with thoughts of becoming a leader. Yet strong leadership will be required to transform the U.S. health care system. A transformed system will need nurses with the adaptive capacity to take on reconceptualized roles in new settings, educating and reeducating themselves along the way—indispensable characteristics of effective leadership.

Whether on the front lines, in education, or in administrative positions and health policy roles, nurses have the well-grounded knowledge base, experience, and perspective needed to serve as full partners in health care redesign. Nurses' unique perspectives are derived from their experiences in providing direct, hands-on patient care; communicating with patients and their families about health status, medications, and care plans; and ensuring the linkage between a prescribed course of treatment and the desired outcome. In care environments, being a full partner involves taking responsibility for identifying problems and areas of waste, devising and implementing a plan for improvement, tracking improvement over time, and making necessary adjustments to realize established goals.

Being a full partner translates more broadly to the health policy arena. To be effective in reconceptualized roles, nurses must see policy as something they can shape rather than something that happens to them. Nurses should have a voice in health policy decision making, as well as being engaged in implementation efforts related to health care reform. Nurses also should serve actively on advisory committees, commissions, and boards where policy decisions are made to advance health systems to improve patient care. Yet a number of barriers prevent nurses from serving as full partners. Examples that are discussed later in the report include laws and regulations (Chapter 3), professional resistance and bias (Chapter 3), a lack of foundational competence (Chapter 5), and exclusion from decision-making bodies and boards (Chapter 5). If nurses are to serve as full partners, a culture change will be needed whereby health professionals hold each other accountable for improving care and setting health policy in a context of mutual respect and collaboration.

Finally, the health care system is widely understood to be a complex system, one in which responses to internal and external actions are sometimes predictable and sometimes not. Health care experts repeatedly encourage health professionals to understand the system's dynamics so they can be more effective in their individual jobs and help shape the larger system's ability to adapt successfully to changes and improve outcomes. In a field as intensively knowledge driven as health care, however, no one individual, group, or discipline can have all the answers. A growing body of research has begun to highlight the potential for collaboration among teams of diverse individuals to generate successful solutions in complex, knowledge-driven systems (Paulus and Nijstad, 2003; Pisano and Verganti, 2008; Singh and Fleming, 2010; Wuchty et al., 2007). Nurses must cultivate new allies in health care, government, and business and develop new partnerships with other clinicians, business owners, and philanthropists to help realize the vision of a transformed health care system. Many nurses have heard this call to develop new partnerships in a culture of collaboration and cooperation. However, the committee found no evidence that these initiatives have achieved the scale necessary to have an impact throughout the health care system. More intentional, large-scale initiatives of this sort are needed. These efforts must be supported by research that addresses such questions as what new models of leadership are needed for the increasingly knowledge-intensive health care environment and when collaboration is most appropriate (Singh and Fleming, 2010).

Chapter 5 further examines the need for expanded leadership opportunities in the nursing workforce.

The Need for Better Data on the Health Care Workforce

Key Message #4: Effective workforce planning and policy making require better data collection and an improved information infrastructure.

Key messages 1, 2, and 3 speak to the need to transform the nursing profession to achieve the vision of health care set forth at the beginning of this chapter.

At the same time, nurses do not function in a vacuum, but in the context of the skills and perspectives of physicians and other health professionals. Planning for the fundamental changes required to achieve a reformed health care system cannot be accomplished without a clear understanding of the necessary contributions of these various professionals and the numbers and composition of the health care workforce. That understanding in turn cannot be obtained without reliable, sufficiently granular data on the current workforce and projections of future workforce needs. Yet major gaps exist in the currently available workforce data. These gaps hamper the ability to identify and implement the necessary changes to the preparation and practice of nurses and to the overall health care system. Chapter 6 explores these issues in greater detail.

CONCLUSION

Most of the near-term challenges identified in the ACA speak to traditional and current strengths of the nursing profession in care coordination, health promotion, and quality improvement, among other things. Nurses are committed to improving the care they deliver by responding to health care challenges. If their full potential is to be realized, however, the nursing profession itself will have to undergo a fundamental transformation in the areas of practice, education, and leadership. During the course of this study, the committee formulated four key messages it believes must guide that transformation: (1) nurses should practice to the full extent of their education and training; (2) nurses should achieve higher levels of education and training through an improved education system that promotes seamless academic progression; (3) nurses should be full partners, with physicians and other health professionals, in redesigning health care in the United States; and (4) effective workforce planning and policy making require better data collection and an improved information infrastructure.

At the same time, the power to deliver better care—quality care that is accessible and sustainable—does not rest solely with nurses, regardless of how ably led or educated they are; it also lies with other health professionals, consumers, governments, businesses, health care institutions, professional organizations, and the insurance industry. The recommendations presented in Chapter 7 target individual policy makers; national, state, and local government leaders; payers; and health care researchers, executives, and professionals—including nurses and others—as well as larger groups such as licensing bodies, educational institutions, and philanthropic and advocacy and consumer organizations. Together, these groups have the power to transform the health care system to achieve the vision set forth at the beginning of this chapter.

REFERENCES

AACN (American Association of Colleges of Nursing). 2010. *Completed applications to entry-level baccalaureate nursing programs in the U.S.: 2004-2009.* http://www.aacn.nche.edu/Media/pdf/apps.pdf (accessed September 10, 2010).

AAN (American Academy of Nursing). 2010. *Edge Runner directory: Nurse-family partnership.* http://www.aannet.org/i4a/pages/index.cfm?pageid=3303 (accessed August 27, 2010).

AARP. 2010. *Preparation and roles of nursing care providers in America.* http://championnursing.org/resources/preparation-and-roles-nursing-care-providers-america (accessed August 17, 2010).

Allan, J. D., and J. Aldebron. 2008. A systematic assessment of strategies to address the nursing faculty shortage, U.S. *Nursing Outlook* 56(6):286-297.

Benner, P., M. Sutphen, V. Leonard, and L. Day. 2009. *Educating nurses: A call for radical transformation.* San Francisco, CA: Jossey-Bass.

BLS (Bureau of Labor Statistics). 2009. *Employment projections: Replacement needs.* http://www.bls.gov/emp/ep_table_110.htm (accessed September 10, 2010).

Bodenheimer, T., K. MacGregor, and N. Stothart. 2005. Nurses as leaders in chronic care. *BMJ* 330(7492):612-613.

Craven, G., and S. Ober. 2009. Massachusetts nurse practitioners step up as one solution to the primary care access problem: A political success story. *Policy, Politics, & Nursing Practice* 10(2):94-100.

Erickson, H. L. 2002. *Concept-based curriculum and instruction: Teaching beyond the facts.* Thousand Oaks, CA: Corwin Press.

Hansen-Turton, T., A. Ritter, and R. Torgan. 2008. Insurers' contracting policies on nurse practitioners as primary care providers: Two years later. *Policy, Politics, & Nursing Practice* 9(4):241-248.

Hatem, M., J. Sandall, D. Devane, H. Soltani, and S. Gates. 2008. Midwife-led versus other models of care for childbearing women. *Cochrane Database of Systematic Reviews* (4):CD004667.

Hendrich, A., M. P. Chow, B. A. Skierczynski, and Z. Lu. 2008. A time and motion study: How do medical-surgical nurses spend their time? *The Permanente Journal* 12(3):37-46.

Hendrich, A., M. P. Chow, and W. S. Goshert. 2009. A proclamation for change: Transforming the hospital patient care environment. *Journal of Nursing Administration* 39(6):266-275.

HRSA (Health Resources and Services Administration). 2010. *The registered nurse population: Findings from the 2008 National Sample Survey of Registered Nurses.* Rockville, MD: HRSA.

IOM (Institute of Medicine). 2003. *Health professions education: A bridge to quality.* Washington, DC: The National Academies Press.

IOM. 2009. *Redesigning continuing education in the health professions.* Washington, DC: The National Academies Press.

IOM Roundtable on Evidence-Based Medicine. 2008. *Learning healthcare system concepts, v. 2008.* Washington, DC: The National Academies Press.

Ironside, P. M. 2004. "Covering content" and teaching thinking: Deconstructing the additive curriculum. *Journal of Nursing Education* 43(1):5-12.

Joint Commission. 2010. Testimony submitted to inform the Forum on the Future of Nursing: Education. Houston, TX, February 22.

Kane, R. L., G. Keckhafer, S. Flood, B. Bershadsky, and M. S. Siadaty. 2003. The effect of Evercare on hospital use. *Journal of the American Geriatric Society* 51(10):1427-1434.

Kane, R. L., T. A. Shamliyan, C. Mueller, S. Duval, and T. J. Wilt. 2007. The association of registered nurse staffing levels and patient outcomes: Systematic review and meta-analysis. *Med Care* 45(12):1195-1204.

Kovner, C. T., and M. Djukic. 2009. The nursing career process from application through the first 2 years of employment. *Journal of Professional Nursing* 25(4):197-203.

Kurtzman, E. T., and P. I. Buerhaus. 2008. New Medicare payment rules: Danger or opportunity for nursing? *American Journal of Nursing* 108(6):30-35.

Lacey, S. R., and K. S. Cox. 2009. Nursing: Key to quality improvement. *Pediatric Clinics of North America* 56(4):975-985.

Landon, B. E., S. L. Normand, A. Lessler, A. J. O'Malley, S. Schmaltz, J. M. Loeb, and B. J. McNeil. 2006. Quality of care for the treatment of acute medical conditions in U.S. hospitals. *Archives of Internal Medicine* 166(22):2511-2517.

Lasater, K., and A. Nielsen. 2009. The influence of concept-based learning activities on students' clinical judgment development *Journal of Nursing Education* 48(8):441-446.

Mitchell, P. H., B. Belza, D. C. Schaad, L. S. Robins, F. J. Gianola, P. S. Odegard, D. Kartin, and R. A. Ballweg. 2006. Working across the boundaries of health professions disciplines in education, research, and service: The University of Washington experience. *Academic Medicine* 81(10):891-896.

National Quality Forum. 2004. *National voluntary consensus standards for nursing-sensitive care.* http://www.qualityforum.org/WorkArea/linkit.aspx?LinkIdentifier=id&ItemID=22094 (accessed September 2, 2010).

Naylor, M. D., D. A. Brooten, R. L. Campbell, G. Maislin, K. M. McCauley, and J. S. Schwartz. 2004. Transitional care of older adults hospitalized with heart failure: A randomized, controlled trial. *Journal of the American Geriatric Society* 52(5):675-684.

Needleman, J., P. I. Buerhaus, M. Stewart, K. Zelevinsky, and S. Mattke. 2006. Nurse staffing in hospitals: Is there a business case for quality? *Health Affairs* 25(1):204-211.

O'Neil, E. 2009. Four factors that guarantee health care change. *Journal of Professional Nursing* 25(6):317-321

Orsolini-Hain, L., and V. Waters. 2009. Education evolution: A historical perspective of associate degree nursing. *Journal of Nursing Education* 48(5):266-271.

Paulus, P. B., and B. A. Nijstad, eds. 2003. *Group creativity: Innovation through collaboration.* New York: Oxford University Press.

Pisano, G. P., and R. Verganti. 2008. Which kind of collaboration is right for you? *Harvard Business Review* 86(12):78-86.

Rendell, E. G. 2007. *Prescription for Pennsylvania: Right state, right plan, right now.* Harrisburg, PA: Office of the Governor.

Ritter, A., and T. Hansen-Turton. 2008. The primary care paradigm shift: An overview of the state-level legal framework governing nurse practitioner practice. *Health Lawyer* 20(4):21-28.

Safriet, B. J. 2010. *Federal options for maximizing the value of advanced practice nurses in providing quality, cost-effective health care.* Paper commissioned by the Committee on the RWJF Initiative on the Future of Nursing, at the IOM (see Appendix H on CD-ROM).

Sales, A., N. Sharp, Y. F. Li, E. Lowy, G. Greiner, C. F. Liu, A. Alt-White, C. Rick, J. Sochalski, P. H. Mitchell, G. Rosenthal, C. Stetler, P. Cournoyer, and J. Needleman. 2008. The association between nursing factors and patient mortality in the Veterans Health Administration: The view from the nursing unit level. *Medical Care* 46(9):938-945.

Singh, J., and L. Fleming. 2010. Lone inventors as sources of breakthroughs: Myth or reality? *Management Science* 56(1):41-56.

Stevens, R. 1999. *In sickness and wealth, American hospitals in the twentieth century.* Baltimore, MD: The Johns Hopkins University Press.

Tanner, C. A., P. Gubrud-Howe, and L. Shores. 2008. The Oregon Consortium for Nursing Education: A response to the nursing shortage. *Policy, Politics & Nursing Practice* 9(3):203-209.

Tucker, A. L., and S. J. Spear. 2006. Operational failures and interruptions in hospital nursing. *Health Services Research* 41(3 Pt 1):643-662.

U.S. Census Bureau. 2009. Table 603. Employed civilians by occupation, sex, race, and Hispanic origin: 2008. In *Statistical abstract of the United States: 2010.* 129th ed. Washington, DC: U.S. Census Bureau.

Wuchty, S., B. F. Jones, and B. Uzzi. 2007. The increasing dominance of teams in production of knowledge. *Science* 316(5827):1036-1039.

ANNEX 1-1
KEY TERMS AND FACTS ABOUT
THE NURSING WORKFORCE

DEFINITIONS FOR CORE TERMS

Throughout the report, the committee uses three terms—health, health care, and health care system—that are used routinely by policy makers, legislators, health care organizations, health professionals, the media, and the public. While these terms are commonly used, the definitions can vary and are often nuanced. In this section, the committee offers its definitions for these three core terms. In addition to the terms discussed below, other important terms are defined throughout the report in conjunction with relevant discussion. For example, value and primary care are defined and discussed in Chapter 2.

Health

In a previous Institute of Medicine (IOM) report, "health" is defined as "a state of well-being and the capability to function in the face of changing circumstances." It is "a positive concept emphasizing social and personal resources as well as physical capabilities" (IOM, 1997). Improving health is a shared responsibility of society, communities, health care providers, family, and individuals. Certain social determinants of health—such as income, education, family, and community—play a greater role than mere access to biomedical care in improving health outcomes for large populations (Commission on Social Determinants of Health, 2008; IOM, 1997). However, access to primary care, in contrast to specialty care, is associated with better population health outcomes (Starfield et al., 2005).

Health Care

"Health care" can be defined as the prevention, diagnosis, treatment, and management of disease and illness through a wide range of services provided by health professionals. These services are supplemented by the efforts of private individuals (patients), their families, and communities to achieve optimal mental and physical health and wellness throughout life. The committee considers the full range of services to be encompassed by the term "health care," including prevention and health promotion, mental and behavioral health, and primary care services; public health; acute care; chronic disease management; transitional care; long-term care; palliative care; end-of-life care; and other specialty health care services.

Health Care System

The term "health care system" refers to the organization, financing, payment, and delivery of health care. As described in greater detail in the IOM report *Crossing the Quality Chasm: A New Health System for the 21st Century* (IOM, 2001), the U.S. health care system is a complex, adaptive system (as opposed to a simple mechanical system). As a result, its many parts (including human beings and organizations) have the "freedom and ability to respond to stimuli in many different and fundamentally unpredictable ways." In addition, the system has many linkages so that changes in one part of the system often change the context for other parts (IOM, 2001). Throughout this report, the committee highlights what it believes to be one of the strongest linkages that has emerged within the U.S. health care system: that between health reform and the future of nursing. As the report emphasizes, the future of nursing—how it is shaped and the directions it takes—will have a major impact on the future of health care reform in the United States.

PREPARATION AND ROLES OF NURSING CARE PROVIDERS IN AMERICA[3]

The range of nursing care providers described below work in a variety of settings including ambulatory care, hospitals, community health centers, public health agencies, long-term care facilities, mental health facilities, war zones, prisons, and schools of nursing, as well as patients' homes, schools, places of worship, and workplaces. Basically anywhere there are health care needs, nurses can usually be found. Types of nursing care providers include

Nursing Assistants/Certified Nursing Assistants (NA/CNAs) provide basic patient care under the direction of licensed nurses: they feed, bathe, dress, groom, and move patients, change linens and may assume other delegated responsibilities. The greatest prevalence of these providers is in home care and in long-term care facilities. Training time varies from on-the-job training to 75 hours of state approved training for certification (CNA).

Licensed Practical/Licensed Vocational Nurses (LPN/LVNs) provide basic nursing care including monitoring vital signs, performing dressing changes and other ordered treatments, and dispense medications in most states. LPNs work under the supervision of a physician or registered nurse. While there is declining demand for LPNs in hospitals, demand is high in

---

[3] This section is reprinted from AARP, 2010b. Courtesy of AARP. All rights reserved. Original data provided by the American Academy of Nurse Practitioners, the American Association of Colleges of Nursing, the American Nurses Credentialing Center, the Bureau of Labor Statistics, the Health Resource and Service Administration, and the National League for Nursing.

long-term care facilities and to a lesser degree in out-patient settings, such as physicians' offices. They complete a 12–18 month education program at a vocational/technical school or community college and are required to pass a nationally standardized licensing exam in the state in which they begin practice. LPNs may become RNs by bridging into an Associate Degree or in some cases, Baccalaureate Nursing Program.

Registered Nurses (RNs) typically complete a program of study at a community college, diploma school of nursing or a four-year college or university and are required to pass a nationally standardized licensing exam in the state in which they begin practice. The essential core of their nursing practice is to deliver holistic, patient-centered care that includes assessment and monitoring, administering a variety of treatments and medications, patient and family education and serving as a member of an interdisciplinary team. Nurses care for individuals and families in all phases of the health and wellness continuum as well as provide leadership in health care delivery systems and in academic settings. There are over 57 RN specialty associations in nursing and others newly emerging. Many RNs practice in medical-surgical areas; some other common specialties among registered nurses, many of which offer specialty certification options, include:

Critical Care Nurses provide care to patients with serious, complex, and acute illnesses or injuries that require very close monitoring and extensive medication protocols and therapies. Critical care nurses most often work in intensive care units of hospitals; however, nurses also provide highly acute and complex care in emergency rooms.

Public Health Nurses work to promote and protect the health of populations based on knowledge from nursing, social, and public health sciences. Public Health Nurses most often work in municipal and State Health Departments.

Home Health/Hospice Nurses provide a variety of nursing services for both acute, but stable and chronically ill patients and their caregivers in the home, including end-of-life care.

Occupational/Employee Health Nurses provide health screening, wellness programs and other health teaching, minor treatments, and disease/medication management services to people in the workplace. The focus is on promotion and restoration of health, prevention of illness and injury, and protection from work related and environmental hazards.

Oncology Nurses care for patients with various types of cancer, administering chemotherapy, and providing follow-up care, teaching and monitoring. Oncology nurses work in hospitals, out-patient clinics and patients' homes.

Perioperative/Operating Room Nurses provide preoperative and postoperative care to patients undergoing anesthesia, or assist with surgical procedures by selecting and handling instruments, controlling bleeding, and suturing incisions. These nurses work in hospitals and out-patient surgical centers.

Rehabilitation Nurses care for patients with temporary and permanent disabilities within institutions and out-patient settings such as clinics and home health care.

Psychiatric/Mental Health Nurses specialize in the prevention of mental and behavioral health problems and the nursing care of persons with psychiatric disorders. Psychiatric nurses work in hospitals, out-patient clinics, and private offices.

School Nurses provide health assessment, intervention, and follow-up to maintain school compliance with healthcare policies and ensure the health and safety of staff and students. They refer students for additional services when hearing, vision, obesity, and other issues become inhibitors to successful learning.

Other common specialty areas are derived from a life span approach across healthcare settings and include maternal-child, neonatal, pediatric, and gerontological nursing.

There are several entry points as well as progression points for registered nurses:

Associate Degree in Nursing (ADN) or Diploma in Nursing prepared RNs provide direct patient care in various health care settings. The two to three years of education required is received primarily in community colleges and hospital-based nursing schools and graduates may bridge into a baccalaureate or higher degree program.

Baccalaureate Degree in Nursing (BSN) prepared RNs provide an additional focus on leadership, translating research for nursing practice, and population health; they practice across all healthcare settings. A BSN is often required for military nursing, case management, public health nursing, and school-based nursing services. Four-year BSN programs are offered primarily in a university setting. The BSN is the most common entry point into graduate education.

Master's Degrees in Nursing (MSN/Other) prepare RNs primarily for roles in nursing administration and clinical leadership, faculty, and for advanced practice in a nursing specialty area. The up to two years of education typically occurs in a university setting. Advanced Practice Registered Nurses (APRNs) receive advanced clinical preparation (generally a Master's degree and/or post Master's Certificate, although the Doctor of Nursing Practice degree is increasingly being granted). Specific titles and credentials vary by state approval processes, formal recognition and scope of practice as well as by board certification. APRNs fall into four broad categories: Nurse Practitioner, Clinical Nurse Specialist, Nurse Anesthetist, and Nurse Midwife:

> **Nurse Practitioners (NPs)** are Advanced Practice RNs who provide a wide range of healthcare services across healthcare settings. NPs take health histories and provide complete physical examinations; diagnose and treat many common acute and chronic problems; interpret laboratory results and X-rays; prescribe and manage medications and other therapies; provide health teaching and supportive counseling with an emphasis on prevention of illness and health maintenance; and refer patients to other health professionals as needed. Broad NP specialty areas include: Acute Care, Adult Health, Family Health, Geriatrics, Neonatal, Pediatric, Psychiatric/Mental Health, School Health, and Women's Health.

> **Clinical Nurse Specialists (CNS)** practice in a variety of health care environments and participate in mentoring other nurses, case management, research, designing and conducting quality improvement programs, and serving as educators and consultants. Specialty areas include but are not limited to: Adult Health, Community Health, Geriatrics, Home Health, Pediatrics, Psychiatric/Mental Health, School Health and Women's Health. There are also many sub-specialties.

> **Certified Registered Nurse Anesthetists (CRNAs)** administer anesthesia and related care before and after surgical, therapeutic, diagnostic and obstetrical procedures, as well as pain management and emergency services, such as airway management. Practice settings include operating rooms, dental offices and outpatient surgical centers. CRNAs deliver more than 65 percent of all anesthetics to patients in the United States.

> **Certified Nurse Midwives (CNMs)** provide primary care to women, including gynecological exams, family planning advice, prenatal care,

management of low risk labor and delivery, and neonatal care. Practice settings include hospitals, birthing centers, community clinics and patient homes.

Doctoral Degrees in Nursing include the Doctor of Philosophy in Nursing (PhD)[4] and the Doctor of Nursing Practice (DNP). PhD-prepared nurses typically teach in a university setting and conduct research, but are also employed increasingly in clinical settings. DNP programs prepare graduates for advanced practice and clinical leadership roles. A number of DNPs are employed in academic settings as well.

---

[4] There are also a very small number of Doctor of Nursing Science (DNS, DNSc) programs still in existence today. A significant number of doctorally-prepared RNs hold doctoral degrees in related fields.

TABLE 1-A1 Providers of Nursing Care: Numbers, Preparation/Training, and Roles

Type of Nursing Care Provider	Type of Degree	Preparation Time	Roles and Responsibilities	Salaries
Registered Nurses	Doctor of Philosophy (PhD) or Doctor of Nursing Practice (DNP) Degrees	4 to 6 years beyond baccalaureate degree	Serve as health system executives, educators, deans, clinical experts/ Advanced Practice Registered Nurses (APRNs), researchers, and senior policy analysts.	Mean faculty salaries range from $58,051.00 to $96,021.00 Administrators' and other non-faculty salaries not available but are generally higher
	Master's Degree (MSN/MS)	Typically up to 2 years beyond baccalaureate degree	Serve as educators, clinical leaders, administrators or APRNs certified as a Nurse Practitioner (NP), Clinical Nurse Specialist (CNS), Certified Nurse Midwife (CNM), or Certified Registered Nurse Anesthetist (CRNA).	Median salaries for APRNs range from $81,708.00 to $144,174.00 Mean Master's prepared instructor salary $54,426.00
	Baccalaureate Degree (BSN)	4 years	Provide direct patient care, nursing leadership, and translating research into nursing practice across all health care settings.	Mean salary $66,316
	Associate Degree (ADN) or a Diploma in Nursing	2 to 3 years	Provide direct patient care in various health care settings.	ADN mean salary $60,890 Diploma mean salary $65,349
Other Nursing Care Providers	Licensed Practical Nurse/Licensed Vocational Nurse (LPN/LVN)	12 to 18 months	Provide basic nursing care primarily in long-term-care or ambulatory settings under the supervision of the Registered Nurse or Physician.	Mean salary $40,110.00
	Nursing Assistant (NA)	Up to 75 hours training	Provide basic care to patients most commonly in nursing care facilities and patient homes.	Mean salary $26,110.00

SOURCE: Adapted from AARP, 2010c. Courtesy of AARP. All rights reserved. Original data provided by the American Association of Colleges of Nursing, the Bureau of Labor Statistics, the Health Resource and Service Administration, and the National League for Nursing.

TABLE 1-A2 Pathways in Nursing Education

Type of Degree	Description of Program
Doctor of Philosophy in Nursing (PhD) and Doctor of Nursing Practice (DNP)	PhD programs are research-focused, and graduates typically teach and conduct research, although roles are expanding. DNP programs are practice-focused and graduates typically serve in Advanced Practice Registered Nurse (APRN) roles and other advanced positions, including faculty positions. *Time to completion: 3–5 years. BSN or MSN to nursing doctorate options available.*
Masters Degree in Nursing (MSN/MS)	Prepares Advanced Practice Registered Nurses (APRNs), Nurse Practitioners, Clinical Nurse Specialists, Nurse-Midwives, and Nurse Anesthetists, as well as Clinical Nurse Leaders, nurse educators and administrators. *Time to completion: 18–24 months. Three years for ADN to MSN option.*
Accelerated BSN or Masters Degree in Nursing	Designed for students with baccalaureate degree in another field. *Time to completion: 12–18 months for BSN and three years for MSN depending on prerequisite requirements.*
Bachelor of Science in Nursing (BSN) Registered Nurse (RN)	Educates nurses to practice the full scope of professional nursing responsibilities across all health care settings. Curriculum provides additional content in physical and social sciences, leadership, research and public health. *Time to completion: Four years or up to two years for ADN/Diploma RNs and three years for LPNs depending on prerequisite requirements.*
Associate Degree (ADN) in Nursing (RN) and Diploma in Nursing (RN)	Prepares nurses to provide direct patient care and practice within the legal scope of professional nursing responsibilities in a variety of health care settings. Offered through community colleges and hospitals. *Time to completion: Two to three years for ADN (less in the case of LPN-entry) and three years for diploma (all hospital-based training programs) depending on prerequisite requirements.*
Licensed Practical Nurse (LPN)/Licensed Vocational Nurse (LVN)	Trains nurses to provide basic care, e.g. take vital signs, administer medications, monitor catheters and apply dressings. LPN/LVNs work under the supervision of physicians and registered nurses. Offered by technical/vocational schools and community colleges. *Time to completion: 12–18 months.*

REFERENCES

AARP. 2010a. *Pathways in nursing education.* http://championnursing.org/resources/pathways-nursing-education (accessed August 27, 2010).

AARP. 2010b. *Preparation and roles of nursing care providers in America.* http://championnursing.org/resources/preparation-and-roles-nursing-care-providers-america (accessed August 17, 2010).

AARP. 2010c. *Providers of nursing care: Numbers, preparation/training and roles: A fact sheet.* http://championnursing.org/resources/providers-nursing-fact-sheet (accessed August 26, 2010).

Commission on Social Determinants of Health. 2008. *Closing the gap in a generation: Health equity through action on the social determinants of health. Final report of the commission on social determinants of health.* Geneva, Switzerland: World Health Organization.

IOM (Institute of Medicine). 1997. *Improving health in the community: A role for performance monitoring.* Washington, DC: National Academy Press.

IOM. 2001. *Crossing the quality chasm: A new health system for the 21st century.* Washington, DC: National Academy Press.

Starfield, B., L. Shi, and J. Macinko. 2005. Contribution of primary care to health systems and health. *The Milbank Quarterly* 83(3):457-502.

2

Study Context

This chapter presents essential context for the remainder of the report, addressing in turn the evolving challenges faced by the health care system, which drive the need for a reformed system and the concomitant transformation of the nursing profession; the three primary concerns targeted by health care reform—quality, access, and value; and the principles the committee determined must guide any reform efforts. The final section summarizes the committee's conclusions about the implications of this discussion for the role of nurses in transforming the health care system.

EVOLVING HEALTH CARE CHALLENGES

For decades, the major focus of the U.S. health care system has been on treating acute illnesses and injuries, the predominant health challenges of the early 20th century. In the 21st century, the health challenges facing the nation have shifted dramatically:

- **Chronic conditions**—While acute injuries and illnesses will never disappear, most health care today relates to chronic conditions, such as diabetes, hypertension, arthritis, cardiovascular disease, and mental health conditions, which in 2005 affected nearly one of every two Americans (CDC, 2010). This shift can be traced in part to the increased capabilities of the health care system to treat these conditions and in part to the health challenges of an aging population, as the prevalence[1] of chronic conditions increases with age. Dramatic increases in the prevalence of many of these conditions since 1970 are expected to continue (DeVol et al., 2007). Increasing obesity levels in the United States have compounded the problem, as obesity is related to many chronic conditions.

- **An aging population**—According to the most recent census projections, the proportion of the U.S. population aged 65 or older is expected to rise from 12.7 percent in 2008 to 19.3 percent in 2030 (U.S. Census Bureau, 2008), in part as a result of increases in life expectancy and the aging of the Baby Boom generation. As the population continues to age, a dramatic growth in demand for health care services will be seen (IOM, 2008).

- **A more diverse population**—Minority groups, which currently make up about a third of the U.S. population, are projected to become the majority by 2042 and 54 percent of the total population by 2050 (U.S. Census Bureau, 2008). Diversity exists not only among but also within various ethnic and racial groups with respect to country of origin, primary language, immigrant status and generation, socioeconomic status, history, and other cultural features.

- **Health disparities**—Health disparities are inequities in the burden of disease, injury, or death experienced by socially disadvantaged groups relative to either whites or the general population. Such groups may be categorized by race, ethnicity, gender, sexual orientation, and/or income. Health disparities among these groups are driven in part by deleterious socioenvironmental conditions and behavioral risk factors, and in part by systematic biases that often result in unequal, inferior treatment (IOM, 2003b).

- **Limited English proficiency**—The number of people living in the United States with limited English proficiency is increasing (U.S. Census Bureau, 2003). To be effective, care and health information must be accessible and offered in a manner that is understandable, as well as culturally relevant (IOM, 2004a; Joint Commission, 2007). While there are national standards for linguistically and culturally relevant health care services, the rapid growth of diverse populations with limited English proficiency and varying cultural and health practices is emerging as an increasingly complex challenge that few health care providers and organizations are currently prepared to handle (HHS Office of Minority Health, 2007).

---

[1] Prevalence defines the total number of individuals with a condition, and incidence refers to the number of new cases reported in a given year.

PRIMARY CONCERNS IN HEALTH CARE
REFORM: QUALITY, ACCESS, AND VALUE

In the search for solutions to improve the health care system, experts target three primary concerns: quality, access, and cost or value (Goldman and Mc-Glynn, 2005). Substantial reforms designed to reshape and realign the major features of the entire health care system are needed to redress deficiencies in these three areas.

Quality

Despite unsustainable growth in health care spending in the United States (discussed below), the care received by individuals can often be too much, too little, too late, or too haphazard. Moreover, substantial geographic variations exist in the intensity of care provided across the nation, with attendant differences in quality, as well as cost (Fisher et al., 2009). The quality improvement movement in health care has grown significantly since the publication of two IOM reports: *To Err Is Human: Building a Safer Health System* and *Crossing the Quality Chasm: A New Health System for the 21st Century* (IOM, 2000, 2001). These reports helped shift discussions about quality away from assigning all responsibility and accountability to individual health professionals. They showed that improving quality requires an understanding of how such elements as systems and processes of care, equipment design, and organizational structure can fundamentally enhance or detract from the quality of care. Researchers also have emphasized the importance of building interprofessional teams and establishing collaborative cultures to identify and sustain continuous improvements in the quality of care (Kim et al., 2010; Knaus et al., 1986; Pronovost et al., 2008).

Access

Although the Affordable Care Act (ACA) provides insurance coverage for an additional 32 million Americans, millions of Americans will still lack coverage in 2019 (CBO, 2010). Even for those with insurance, out-of-pocket expenses, such as deductibles and copays, as well as limited coverage for necessary services and medications, create financial burdens that can limit access to care (Doty et al., 2005; Himmelstein et al., 2009). Other significant barriers to access include a lack of providers who are accepting new patients, especially those covered by Medicaid; a lack of providers who offer appointments outside of typical business hours; and for some a lack of transportation to and from appointments. Also hindering access is the above-discussed rapid growth of populations with limited English proficiency (U.S. Census Bureau, 2010), as well as limited health literacy among fluent English speakers.

Value

The term "value" has different meanings in different contexts. For the purposes of this report, the committee uses the following definition: "value in health care is expressed as the physical health and sense of well-being achieved relative to the cost" (IOM Roundtable on Evidence-Based Medicine, 2008). As one of the major components of value—quality—is discussed above, this section focuses on cost.

The United States spends more than any other nation—16.2 percent of gross domestic product in 2008—on health care (CMS, 2010a). Yet this investment is not matched by superlative health care outcomes (OECD, 2010), indicating deficiencies in the value of some aspects of the health care system. Moreover, while the United States spends too much on certain aspects of health care, such as hospital services and diagnostic tests, spending on other aspects is disproportionately low. For example, public health represents less than 3 percent of health care spending (CMS, 2010b).

Health care spending is responsible for large, and ultimately unsustainable, structural deficits in the federal budget (Dodaro, 2008), and many economists believe that rising health care costs are a principal reason why wages have increased so little in recent years (Emanuel and Fuchs, 2008). However, establishing and sustaining legislated cost controls and health care savings has proven elusive. Challenges with regard to costs and spending make achieving value within the health care system difficult.

Throughout its deliberations, the committee found it useful to focus on ensuring that the health care system delivers good value rather than focusing solely on cost. Accordingly, the committee paid particular attention to high-value innovations in nursing care that provide quality, patient-centered care at a lower price. Three specific examples are featured as case studies later in this chapter.

PRINCIPLES FOR CHANGE

The challenges faced by the U.S. health care system have been described and documented in recent years by many government agencies, researchers, policy analysts, and health professionals. From this work, a consensus has begun to emerge regarding some of the fundamental principles that should guide changes to meet these challenges. Broadly, the consensus is that care in the United States must become more patient centered; primary care and prevention must play a greater role relative to specialty care; care must be delivered more often within the community setting and even in people's homes; and care needs to be coordinated and provided seamlessly across health conditions, settings, and providers. It is also important that all providers practice to the fullest extent allowed by their education, training, and competencies and collaborate so that improvements can be achieved in both their own and each other's performance. This section provides an overview of these shifts in thinking and practice that a growing number of health care experts believe should be at the core of any proposed health care solutions.

The Need for Patient-Centered Care

Health care research is demonstrating the benefits of reorganizing the delivery of health care services around what makes the most sense for patients (Delbanco et al., 2001; Hibbard, 2004; Sepucha et al., 2004). As outlined in *Crossing the Quality Chasm*, patient-centered care is built on the principle that individuals should be the final arbiters in deciding what type of treatment and care they receive (IOM, 2001). Yet practice still is usually organized around what is most convenient for the provider, the payer, or the health care organization and not for the patient. Patients are repeatedly asked, for example, to change their expectations and schedules to fit the needs of the system. They are required to provide the same information to multiple caregivers or in sequential visits to the same provider. Primary care appointments typically are not available outside of work hours. The counseling, education, and coaching needed to help patients make informed decisions have historically been given insufficient attention (Hibbard, 2004). Additionally, patients' insurance policies often limit their choice of provider, especially if the provider is not a physician (Craven and Ober, 2009). Box 2-1 presents an example of how one health system, the University of Pittsburgh Medical Center, has implemented a truly patient-centered program.

How Patient-Centered Care Improves Quality, Access, and Value

A number of studies have linked patient-centered and quality care (Sepucha et al., 2004). For example, studies that compared surgery with watchful waiting for patients with benign prostatic hyperplasia showed how strong a role patient preference played in determining quality of life (Barry et al., 1988; Fowler et al., 1988; Wennberg et al., 1988). Likewise, involving patients more directly in the management of their own condition was found to result in significant improvements in health outcomes for individuals with insulin-dependent diabetes mellitus (Diabetes Control and Complications Trial Research Group, 1993). By 2001, so many different studies had found similar results that *Crossing the Quality Chasm* identified patient-centered care as one of six pillars on which a 21st-century health care system should be built (the others being safety, effectiveness, timeliness, efficiency, and equity) (IOM, 2001).

One of the hallmarks of patient-centered care is improving access to care, a key component of which is access to information. For example, a growing number of patients have greater access to their own laboratory results and diagnostic writeups about their procedures through such electronic forums as personal health records and patient portals. Many people participate in online communities to

BOX 2-1
Case Study: When Patients and Families Call a Code

The University of Pittsburgh Medical Center
Is Transforming Care at the Bedside

In 2001, 18-month-old Josie King was hospitalized at Johns Hopkins Children's Center with burns she had sustained in a bathtub accident. Josie responded well to treatment at first, but her condition quickly deteriorated. When her mother, Sorrel King, expressed concern, the staff nurses and physicians repeatedly dismissed them, and 2 days before her scheduled discharge Josie died. The cause was dehydration and a wrongly administered opioid—the result of a series of errors the hospital acknowledged.

Ms. King has since devoted herself to the elimination of medical errors, founding the Josie King Foundation (www.josieking.org) and addressing clinicians, policy makers, and consumers on the importance of creating a "culture of safety." And the need is pressing. According to a 2000 Institute of Medicine report, up to 98,000 people die from medical errors each year (IOM, 2000); nearly 10 years after that report's publication, despite improved patient-safety systems, a 2009 report gave a grade of C+ to efforts to empower patients to prevent errors (Wachter, 2009).

Tami Minnier, MSN, RN, FACHE, heard Ms. King speak in 2005, and the message was clear: if the staff had listened to her mother's concerns, Josie would have lived. "When I came back to work the following Monday," said Ms. Minnier, at the time chief nursing officer at the University of Pittsburgh Medical Center (UPMC) at Shadyside, "I told my chief medical officer, 'We're going to let patients and families call a rapid-response team'—a group of staff who are designated by the hospital to respond immediately to other staff's requests for help with critical or emergency patient situations. He thought I was insane."

As we've always known, when you give power and authority to patients, they treat it with great respect.

—Tami Minnier, MSN, RN, FACHE, chief quality officer, University of Pittsburgh Medical Center

---

Shadyside had been one of the first three hospitals to participate in Transforming Care at the Bedside (TCAB), an initiative of the Institute for Healthcare Improvement (IHI) and the Robert Wood Johnson Foundation, enabling front-line nurses to test their ideas for improving the safety and quality of care. Ms. Minnier called on Sorrel King to work with the nurses in Shadyside's TCAB unit in creating what they called Condition H (or Condition Help). They interviewed patients and families about when and why they might call for a rapid-response team, consisting of a nurse administrator, a physician, a staff nurse, and a patient advocate who would convene immediately in response to a patient's or visitor's call. They held drills with staff, and within

6 months, Condition H went live in the hospital's TCAB unit.

While some staff feared that patients would abuse the hotline, that concern was not borne out. Today, patients and families throughout UPMC's 13 acute care hospitals can use Condition H. They receive information on how to make the call (dial 3131 and say, "Condition H") during admission and through posters, a video, and stickers placed on patients' phones.

Ms. Minnier is now chief quality officer at UPMC and monitors the use of Condition H. At Shadyside, a 500-bed hospital, two or three calls are made each month, and only a few patients have called twice during the same admission. An analysis of the 45 calls made in the first 17 months showed that inadequately managed pain was the most frequent impetus

for calls, and more than 60 percent of the calls led to interventions that were deemed instrumental in preventing a patient-safety event.

Condition H is spreading and serves as one example of the changes hospitals have adopted using TCAB methods. Reports on TCAB have shown that it generates improved outcomes, greater patient and family satisfaction, and reduced turnover of nurses (Hassmiller and Bolton, 2009).

Sorrel King addressed medical and nursing students at an IHI-sponsored event in 2009 and spoke strongly in favor of Condition H. "Had I been able to push a button for a rapid-response team, that team would have come, they would have assessed Josie and . . . said one thing: the child is thirsty," Ms. King said. "They would have given her a drink, and she never would have died" (Matthews, 2009).

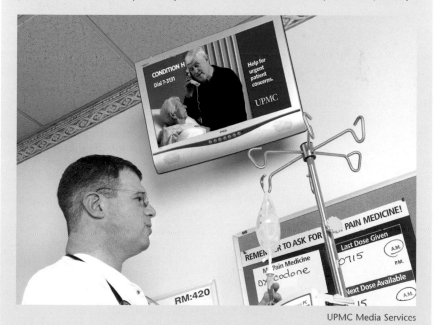

UPMC Media Services

Information about Condition H is clearly posted throughout UPMC at Shadyside, on patients' televisions, bulletin boards, and telephones.

learn more about or even how to manage their own conditions. Improving access also requires delivering care in a culturally relevant and appropriate manner so that patients can contribute positively to their own care.

Fewer studies have examined the economic value of patient-centered care. One such study found that offering a nurse advice phone number and a pediatric after-hours clinic resulted in a 17 percent decrease in emergency department visits (Wilson, 2005). Yet there is no reason to believe that enhancing patient-centered care will or even should always lead to lower costs. For example, truly patient-centered approaches to care may require new programs or additional services that go beyond current standards of practice.

Nurses and Patient-Centered Care

Nurses have long emphasized patient-centered care. The case study in Box 2-2 provides but one example—the patient-centered approach of midwifery care at the Family Health and Birth Center (FHBC) in Washington, DC. Through the FHBC, mothers-to-be who often have little control over their own lives develop a sense of control over one very important part of their lives. From such modest beginnings, many more hopeful futures have been launched.

The Need for Stronger Primary Care Services

Consensus is also strong on the need to make primary (rather than specialty) care a greater part of the health care system. Despite steps taken by the ACA to support the provision of primary care, however, the shortage of primary care providers is projected to worsen in the United States in the coming years (Boden-heimer and Pham, 2010; Doherty, 2010).

Primary care has been described in many ways. The IOM has defined it as "the provision of integrated, accessible health care services by clinicians who are accountable for addressing a large majority of personal health care needs, developing a sustained partnership with patients, and practicing in the context of family and community" (IOM, 1996). Starfield and colleagues identify the functions of primary care as "first-contact access for each new need; long-term person- (not disease) focused care; comprehensive care for most health needs; and coordinated care when it must be sought elsewhere" (Starfield et al., 2005). Similarly, the Government Accountability Office (GAO) has cited the following hallmarks of primary care: preventive care, care coordination for chronic illnesses, and continuity of care (Steinwald, 2008). Thus primary care is closely tied to two of the principles for change discussed below—the need to deliver more care in the community and the need for seamless, coordinated care.

How Primary Care Improves Quality, Access, and Value

Countries that build their health care systems on the cornerstone of primary care have better health outcomes and more equitable access to care than those that do not (Starfield et al., 2005). However, primary care plays a less central role in the U.S. health care system than many health policy experts believe it should (Bodenheimer, 2006; Cronenwett and Dzau, 2010; IOM, 1996; Starfield et al., 2005; Steinwald, 2008). Geographic variations nationwide illustrate the importance of primary care. Regions of the United States with a higher ratio of generalists to specialists provide more effective care at lower cost (Baicker and Chandra, 2004), and studies have shown that those states with a greater ratio of primary care providers to the general population experience lower mortality rates for all causes of death (Shi, 1992, 1994). The positive effect is more pronounced among African Americans who have access to primary care than among whites, thus indicating that this is a promising approach to decreasing health disparities (Starfield et al., 2005). Yet primary care services have been so difficult to access in parts of the United States that one in five adults has sought nonurgent care at an emergency department (IOM, 2009).

Nurses and Primary Care

Nurses with varying levels of education and preparation play important roles in primary care. Health promotion, education, and assessment are essential components of primary care that are also traditional strengths of the nursing profession; these services may be provided by either registered nurses (RNs) or advanced practice registered nurses (APRNs). RNs provide primary care services across the spectrum of health care settings—from acute care to home care to public health and community care. As visiting or home health nurses, RNs are positioned to identify new health problems or needs, such as medication education, prevention services, or nutrition counseling. In public health clinics, they may provide community assessments, developmental screenings, or disease surveillance. RNs in acute care settings may identify new health care problems and needs as they care for patients and their families. The range of possibilities for RNs providing primary care is significant, and their capacity for filling these roles is not always recognized.

APRNs, especially nurse practitioners (NPs), also provide primary care services across all levels of the health care system. In many situations, NPs provide care that is comparable in scope to that provided by primary care physicians. As discussed in Chapter 3, in many situations, APRNs are qualified to diagnose potential and actual health problems, develop treatment plans, in some case

BOX 2-2
Case Study: Nurse Midwives and Birth Centers

The Midwifery Model of Maternity Care Gives Mothers Control and Improves Outcomes

When Wendy Pugh delivered her first child at age 30 in a Washington, DC, hospital in 1999, her labor was induced—not out of medical necessity, she said, but because "there was a scheduling issue with the doctor." She didn't question the obstetrician's decision at the time, but when she got pregnant again, she polled her friends and discovered that many had had cesarean sections. When she asked why, few gave medical reasons. She decided she wanted "a more organic process."

Midwifery teaches you that the woman is the most important person in the relationship and that's why you should listen to her and try to give her what she wants and what she needs.

—Ruth Watson Lubic, EdD, CNM, FAAN, founder, Family Health and Birth Center

Seven months into her second pregnancy, Ms. Pugh arrived at the Family Health and Birth Center (FHBC) in northeast Washington, DC (www.yourfhbc.org), where certified nurse midwives provide pre- and postnatal care and assist with labor and delivery with little technological intervention. Delivery takes place at a homelike freestanding birth center or at a nearby hospital, depending on the woman's choice, her health, and such factors as whether she is homeless. The FHBC accepts Medicaid and private insurance and offers a sliding-scale fee for those ineligible for Medicaid. No one is turned away.

Ruth Watson Lubic, EdD, CNM, opened the FHBC in 2000 in response to the disproportionately high rates of infant and maternal death, cesarean section, and premature birth among poor and minority women in Washington, DC. In 2009 the infant mortality rate in the city was 12.22 per 1,000 live births, far exceeding that of any state in the nation (Heron et al., 2007). Nationwide, nearly four times as many black as white infants die as a result of premature birth or low birth weight (HRSA, 2006). Dr. Lubic had already founded the first freestanding birth center in the country (in 1975 in New York City) and has dedicated her career to reducing disparities in birth outcomes. "We're hoping to serve as a model for the whole country," Dr. Lubic said. There are now 195 such centers in the United States.

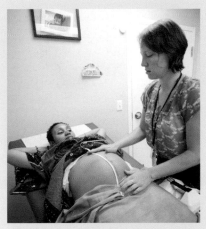

Sam Kittner/kittner.com
A pregnant woman receives prenatal care at the Family Health and Birth Center.

Ms. Pugh's case highlights the differences between the midwifery model of care, which promotes maternal and infant health, and the obstetrics model, which anticipates complications. During the hospital delivery of her first child, Ms. Pugh received pitocin to induce labor, saw her newborn for just a few moments before the child was taken away, and did not breastfeed until the second day. In contrast, during the delivery of her third child—her second delivery at the FHBC—she received assistance during labor from a doula, a trained volunteer who provided coaching and massage; her newborn was placed on her chest immediately after the birth; mother and child went home within hours of delivery; and when the infant showed difficulties with breastfeeding, a peer lactation counselor went to their home.

Two systematic reviews have found that women given midwifery care are more likely to have shorter labors, spontaneous vaginal births without hospitalization, less perineal trauma, higher breastfeeding rates, and greater satisfaction with their births (Hatem et al., 2008; Hodnett et al., 2007). Unpublished FHBC data show that, compared with all African American women giving birth in Washington, DC, women giving birth at the center have almost half the rate of cesarean sections, one-third the rate of births at less than 37 weeks' gestation, and half the rate of low-birth-weight newborns. The lower rates of complications added up to an estimated $1,231,000 in savings in 2005—more than the cost of operating the center that year. The FHBC reports a 100 percent breastfeeding rate among women giving birth at the center.

Obstacles to widespread use of the FHBC model include the fact that

continued

BOX 2-2 *continued*

Medicaid does not always pay mid-wives at birth centers at the rate paid to obstetricians for vaginal deliveries. Also, the high cost of malpractice insurance has forced some such centers to close, although nurse midwives have shown a lower risk of malpractice suits than that among obstetricians (Xu et al., 2008a, 2008b).

At age 83 Dr. Lubic has faced opposition to the midwifery model for decades. "There's this hangover from the days when midwives functioned on their own in communities," she

said. Even so, the enthusiasm of the FHBC's midwives is unflagging. Among the benefits of midwifery care, Lisa Betina Uncles, MSN, CNM, who attended Ms. Pugh's two births at the FHBC, highlighted one that cannot be easily measured. "A lot of our moms in the neighborhood don't have much control over their lives," she said. "This is something they have control over." Ms. Pugh agreed. "It was kind of a partnership," she said of her two FHBC births, "but they also let me guide the ship."

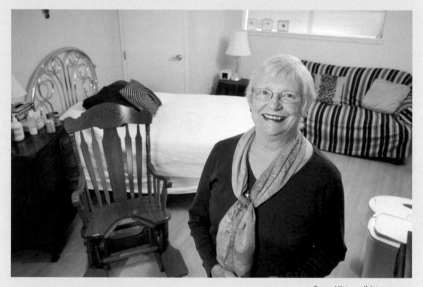

Sam Kittner/kittner.com

Family Health and Birth Center founder and nurse midwife Ruth Lubic is proud of the comfortable birthing rooms for new mothers.

prescribe medication, and create teams of providers to help manage the needs and care of patients and their families. APRNs are educated to refer patients to physicians or other providers when necessary.

Box 2-3 illustrates how one NP provides primary care both in a school, where she is required by the school district regulations to do less than she is trained to do, and in a low-cost clinic, where she may practice to the full extent of her training and licensure. Chapter 3 examines in detail why NPs, and more broadly APRNs, are often limited by regulations in the extent of the health services they may provide.

The Need to Deliver More Care in the Community

Care in the community—defined as those places where individuals live, work, play, and study—encompasses care that is provided in such settings as community and public health centers, long-term care and assisted-living facilities, retail clinics, homes, schools, and community centers. While acute care medical facilities will always be needed, the delivery of primary care and other health services in the community must grow significantly if the U.S. health care system is to be both widely accessible and sustainable (Dodaro, 2008; Steinwald, 2008).

Along with an emphasis on primary care, a key component of providing care in the community is a strong public health infrastructure to ensure the availability of a range of services that includes prevention, education, communication, and surveillance. The public health infrastructure and workforce are vulnerable and perpetually face fiscal and political barriers. As a 2002 IOM report notes, "public health infrastructure has suffered from political neglect and from the pressure of political agendas and public opinion that frequently override empirical evidence" (IOM, 2002). The public health workforce, including public health nurses, is aging rapidly. Between 20 and 50 percent of public health workers at the local, state, and national levels are eligible to retire in the next few years (ASPH, 2008; ASTHO, 2004; Perlino, 2006). Between 2008 and 2009, health departments at the local level lost 23,000 jobs—or approximately 15 percent of their total workforce—to recession-related layoffs and attrition in 2008 and 2009 (NACCHO, 2010). The number of nurses employed in public and community health settings underwent a marked decline from 18.3 percent of the RN workforce in 2000 to 15.2 percent in 2004 to 14.2 percent in 2008 (HRSA, 2010). The case study in Box 2-4 illustrates the value of nurses working in the public health sector, where many more nurses are needed.

Providing effective care in the community will require improvements in community infrastructures, resources, and the workforce. Health care providers, including nurses, will need to form new partnerships with community leaders and have strong community care–oriented competencies, such as the ability to develop, implement, and assess culturally relevant interventions.

BOX 2-3
Nurse Profile: Carolina Sandoval

A School Nurse Acts as Advocate for a
California Latino Community

"Did you eat breakfast?" This is often the first question school nurse Carolina Sandoval, MSN, PNP, RN, asks a student who comes to her office complaining of a stomachache. Usually, the child says no, and Ms. Sandoval takes the opportunity to discuss the value of a nutritious breakfast. "I give them a little speech," she said, "and then I give them a little snack."

What might sound like a simple interaction is anything but simplistic. Ms. Sandoval's work at a junior high school and an elementary school in Chino Hills, California, draws on her graduate education and incorporates many aspects of nursing: patient and community education, child advocacy, public health, infectious disease monitoring, trauma care, chronic illness management, nutritional counseling, reproductive health, and medication management, among others.

School nurses may be among the unsung heroes of health care, but occasionally they take the spotlight. "Hero," in fact, was how many described Mary Pappas, BSN, RN, the school nurse who first alerted infectious disease authorities to the outbreak of influenza A (H1N1)—swine flu—at her New York City high school in April 2009 (Jacobson, 2009). Not only did Ms. Pappas's decisive action

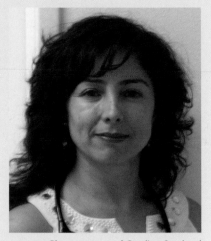

Photo courtesy of Carolina Sandoval
Carolina Sandoval, MSN, PNP, RN

protect the thousands of children in her charge, but within days she had prompted a worldwide alert for what would soon be declared a pandemic.

Yet even the smallest gesture, such as giving "a little snack," corresponds to the National Association of School Nurses (NASN) definition of school nursing: "nursing that advances the well-being, academic success and life-long achievement and health of students." At the same time, Ms. Sandoval does not sugar coat the fact that most school districts, including her own, fail to meet the NASN and

Healthy People 2010 recommendation of one nurse for every 750 healthy children. She is responsible for 2,000 children and works part time at each of the two schools.

Some of these kids—especially those without insurance in underserved areas—they have nobody. The school nurse is the only person they may see who can guide them and tell them where to go for resources for their health needs. So we are a good investment for the school district and community.

—Carolina Sandoval, MSN, PNP, RN, school nurse, Chino Hills, California

---

Indeed, California is 42nd on NASN's list of states ranked by student-to-registered nurse (RN) ratios, with 2,187 students for every school nurse (Vermont is first and Michigan is last, with 311 and 4,836 students per RN, respectively) (NASN, 2010). To fill the gap, some school districts hire non-nurse technicians, a move Ms. Sandoval said does not benefit students. She pointed out that nurses' skills in assessment and critical thinking come into play constantly in handling the conditions that affect students' ability to learn: obesity and chronic illness, vision deficits, behavioral problems, allergies, and asthma, to name the most common.

Having moved to Southern California at age 15 from Mexico, where, she said, a school nurse would have been an unthinkable luxury, Ms. Sandoval has a particular appreciation of the school nurse's role as child advocate. She now acts as a spokesperson for NASN's Voices of Meningitis Campaign (www.voicesof-meningitis.org), sponsored by Sanofi Pasteur, a vaccine manufacturer. Preteens and teens are at the greatest risk for meningococcal meningitis, a preventable infection that can rapidly be fatal and is spread through utensil sharing or kissing. Through radio, television, and other venues, Ms. Sandoval teaches parents and children, in Spanish, about prevention, symptoms, and treatment.

School district regulations do not permit Ms. Sandoval to use all of her skills as a nurse practitioner. She cannot diagnose or prescribe in the school, for example, even when children have symptoms of conjunctivitis or otitis media; she must refer them to other providers outside of the school. And because many of the children she sees come from uninsured families that may not have access to affordable care, she often refers families to a low-cost clinic where she works one evening a week as a nurse practitioner and can practice to the full extent of her training and licensure.

Ms. Sandoval tells the story of another routine intervention, involving a seventh-grader who was falling behind in his classes. She met with the boy and checked his vision; it was quite poor, and she gave his parents a certificate for a discounted eye exam and glasses. "We cannot change the whole world," she said. "But maybe we can change one student. And someday that student is going to go to college, and he'll remember the school nurse who took the time to look at his eyes."

BOX 2-4
Nurse Profile: Lisa Ayers

*A Public Health Nurse in Schenectady, New
York, Making Neighborhoods Healthier*

Lisa Ayers, BSN, RN, could tell from her initial inspection of the apartment, with its chipped paint, exposed electrical wires, and mice, that the situation was serious. As a public health nurse with Schenectady County Public Health Services near Albany, New York, she also quickly discerned that the deteriorating structure was not the only issue in need of her attention.

Ms. Ayers' patient, a pregnant woman whose toddlers had high blood lead levels, learned about the link between asthma and cigarette smoke, the dangers of a broken electrical plate, and the importance of testing her smoke detectors. Ms. Ayers also talked with the woman about prenatal care, scheduled a lead inspection of the home, reported the mice and electrical hazards to the city, and mailed a notice of the lead inspection to the landlord.

"It was a wonderful visit," Ms. Ayers said. "Very productive." A lifelong Schenectady native, she and her husband have reared three children there, and she has worked for 22 years as a public health nurse for the city and county health departments. She started out, as most nurses do, as a medical–surgical nurse, but after switching to home health care, she found it difficult to balance work and

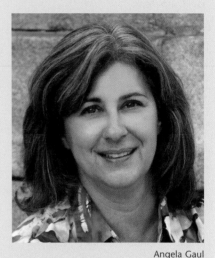

Angela Gaul

Lisa Ayers, BSN, RN

family demands and applied for a public health nursing position with the city. "It was the best decision I ever made," she said.

When she started in 1988, she and her 20 registered nurse (RN) co-workers cared for homebound older adults, pregnant women and infants, and patients with infectious diseases. In 1991 the health department expanded to cover the county, and her work in the years since has encompassed well-infant care, primary care pediatrics, and environmental health.

For 7 years, she investigated communicable diseases in the community.

Now, as one of the first nurses in the state to be certified as a lead risk inspector, she weaves environmental health into her practice. She assesses homes for sources of lead; works with landlords to fix problems; and supplies families with carbon monoxide detectors, cabinet locks, nightlights, buckets, mops—in short, anything they need to minimize hazards in their homes. At the same time, she is assessing the psychosocial aspects of families' health and helping them reduce tobacco use and prevent or control asthma. Ms. Ayers said, "Being a nurse, I can answer a lot more questions about asthma, medications, and inhalers than somebody who may not be a nurse." And she continues to take her turn as a home visitation nurse on weekends, seeing a child with leukemia, helping a new mother with breastfeeding, or checking on a newborn who is losing instead of gaining weight.

When I make home visits, I offer information on breastfeeding, nutrition, and lead poisoning, and I do environmental assessments. It's definitely public health and nursing combined.

—Lisa Ayers, BSN, RN, public health nurse, Schenectady County Public Health Services, Schenectady, New York

---

Usually, the health department will ask a landlord for permission to inspect a home only if a child has a blood lead level of at least 15 mcg/dL. But that requirement is waived for Healthy Neighborhoods, an initiative aimed at reducing environmental hazards in two zip codes—12307 and 12304—that have had high lead-poisoning rates. Anyone living in these zip codes can request a free home assessment of air quality, asthma triggers, fire safety, and other health issues, and the assessment can be done without the landlord's permission.

Ms. Ayers spends about 40 percent of her time on Healthy Neighborhoods and 60 percent on lead-poisoning prevention, and she finds ways to combine the work of the two programs. "When I'm out there doing prevention for air quality with Healthy Neighborhoods, I also do a visual lead inspection in the home," she said. And she teaches families measures such as handwashing; letting water run from lead-soldered pipes before drinking; and eating foods high in iron and calcium and low in fat, which prevents lead absorption.

The county has tracked cases of elevated blood lead levels in zip code 12307 for more than two decades. Since a peak of 34 cases in 1992, the number dropped to five or fewer annually from 2006 to 2009, according to unpublished data.

Nurses' contributions to these outcomes are not lost on Richard Daines, MD, New York State's health commissioner, who shadowed Ms. Ayers shortly after he took office. "He was very excited [by what he saw]," said Ms. Ayers. "I think they have recognized—all the way up to the commissioner level—what a nurse can bring to this position."

How Care in the Community Improves Quality, Access, and Value

In the 1990s, the state of New York pioneered quality assessment and im-provement in the management of HIV/AIDS in community health clinics, drug treatment centers, and hospitals (New York State Department of Health AIDS Institute, 2003). The program proved so successful that it soon became the model for a national effort at assessing and improving treatment and care for people with HIV (IOM, 2004b). Similarly, studies have found that improving nurse-to-student ratios in public schools results in higher immunization rates, increased vision screenings and more effective follow-up, and significant gains in identifying asthma and life-threatening conditions. As more care moves from the acute to the community setting, quality measurement must expand to ensure that quality care is maintained throughout the transition.

Investments in community care can improve access and value as well. In the 1990s, the Department of Veterans Affairs (VA) began shifting its programs from the acute care to the community setting, dramatically increasing the number of veterans who were able to access care (CBO, 2009; VA, 2003) while improving health outcomes and lowering costs per patient (Asch et al., 2004; CBO, 2009; Jha et al., 2003; Kerr et al., 2004). Likewise, community health centers and nurse-managed health centers have provided quality, high-value care in many socially disadvantaged neighborhoods.

Nurses and Care in the Community

Providing care for underserved populations in community settings has long been a major goal of the nursing profession. Box 2-4 illustrates how one public health nurse provides infant care, primary care, environmental health services, and care to individuals with infectious diseases in the community. In another ex-ample, Lilian Wald founded the Visiting Nurse Service of New York (VNSNY) in 1893 to help improve the health and social outcomes of those with lesser means. Today, VNSNY is the largest nonprofit home health care agency in the United States (IOM, 2010).

A growing number of nurses are embracing technology to expand care in the community. A study conducted in Florida showed that telehealth services brought directly to patients' communities and provided by nurses may increase access to care for children with special health care needs in rural, medically underserved parts of the state at no additional cost (Hooshmand, 2010). The alternative for these patients was to travel many miles, usually to an academic health center, to the site of a doctor's office.

The Need for Seamless, Coordinated Care

One of the major challenges facing the U.S. health care system is its high degree of fragmentation. Nowhere is this fragmentation more evident than in the transitions patients must undergo among multiple providers or different services for a single health problem. When care is seamless, these multiple aspects of care are coordinated to enhance the quality of care and the patient's experience of care. The ACA contains provisions that address coordination of care, but these initiatives are just the beginning of what is needed.

How Seamless, Coordinated Care Improves Quality, Access, and Value

In 2003, the IOM singled out coordination of care as indispensible to improving the quality of health care in the United States (IOM, 2003a). Likewise, the ACA highlights coordination of services as one of the required measures for reporting on the quality of care. The Medicare Payment Advisory Commission (MedPAC) also concluded that better coordination clearly improved the quality of beneficiaries' care. Proof that care coordination saves money was less apparent in part because measuring cost savings is so difficult. Investments in care coordination for a group of people with diabetes, for example, may take a long time to demonstrate cost savings because it can take years for poor glucose control to manifest itself as stroke, myocardial infarction, and other severe complications. However, the value of preventing these outcomes, from both a quality-of-life and financial perspective, is clear.

One particularly compelling example of the multiple benefits of seamless care is the On Lok program—an initiative that began in California in the 1970s (On Lok PACEpartners, 2006). Its successes inspired a new model of care—the Program of All-Inclusive Care for the Elderly (PACE), which now serves 19,000 frail older individuals in 31 states.[2] On Lok and the PACE programs that it inspired demonstrate that innovative programs that integrate care across the continuum can lead to synergistic improvements in quality, access, and value. The creativity and willingness to look beyond traditional solutions that animate these programs need to be adapted to other health care settings.

Nurses and Seamless, Coordinated Care

Coordinating care is one of the traditional strengths of the nursing profession, whether in the community or the acute care setting. For example, an interprofessional research team funded by the Robert Wood Johnson Foundation, called the Interdisciplinary Nursing Quality Research Initiative (INQRI), developed a Staff

---

[2] Personal communication, Shawn Bloom, President and CEO, National PACE Association, February 3, 2010.

Nurse Care Coordination model that features six nurse care coordination activities regularly performed by staff nurses in hospital settings as part of their daily activities—mobilizing, exchanging, checking, organizing, assisting, and backfilling (Lamb et al., 2008). Box 2-5 describes a program in the community setting called Living Independently for Life (LIFE), a PACE program in Pennsylvania that is led by nurse practitioners and provides interprofessional health services to low-income, frail, chronically ill older adults who are eligible for nursing home care (LIFE, 2010).

In acute care settings, care coordination is showing particular promise in efforts to reduce rehospitalizations. All 15 demonstration program sites under the Medicare Coordinated Care Demonstration program, for example, adopted interventions that relied on nurses as care coordinators (Peikes et al., 2009). Box 2-6 provides an in-depth look at the Transitional Care Model, developed by nursing researcher Mary Naylor. This model was designed to facilitate patients' transitions within and across settings and to break the cycle of acute flare-ups of chronic illness. The protocol goes beyond usual case management and home care by employing an APRN who is proficient in comprehensive in-hospital assessment, evaluation of medications, coordination of complex care, and in-home follow-up. By collaborating with the patient, family caregivers, specialists, primary care providers, and others, this nurse works to improve the management of multiple complex chronic conditions and thus reduce readmissions.

The Need for Reconceptualized Roles for Health Professionals

Many of the roles health professionals are being called upon to fill in the evolving U.S. health care system are not technically new. Nurses, physicians, and pharmacists, for example, have educated patients, helped coordinate care, and collaborated with other clinicians for decades. What is new is the extent and the centrality of these roles. Previous IOM studies have found that systemwide changes are necessary to meet higher standards for quality care, the growing requirements of an aging population, and the need to deliver more care in the community setting. *Crossing the Quality Chasm* introduced the idea of the advisability of expanding the scope of practice for many health workers (IOM, 2001). *Retooling for an Aging America* advised that meeting the needs of the growing geriatric population would require expanding the roles of health professionals "beyond the traditional scope of practice" (IOM, 2008).

In light of these considerations, the committee concludes that nurses, in concert with other health professionals, need to adopt reconceptualized roles as care coordinators, health coaches, and system innovators. This chapter has already provided examples of nurses working as care coordinators; the following subsections elaborate on what the committee means by health coaches and system innovators. Filling these roles, whether in entry-level nursing or advanced practice, will require that nurses receive greater education and preparation in leadership, care management, quality improvement processes, and systems thinking—a subject discussed in Chapter 4.

Nurses as Health Coaches

The committee envisions a health care system in which all individuals have a health coach who helps stay them healthy. The coach ensures that they understand why their primary care provider—whether a physician, physician assistant, or NP—has recommended a particular course of treatment. He/she coordinates patients' care with multiple providers so that, for example, an elderly grandfather with diabetes, arthritis, and heart disease can continue to live at home and avoid costly hospitalizations. The role of health coach has much in common with case management services, but it goes even further. The coach educates family, friends, and other informal caregivers about how they can help, addressing not just physical needs but also social, environmental, mental, and emotional factors that may promote or interfere with the maintenance of health. The coach helps overcome features in the health care system that may lead to inequities in care delivery. He/she also stays involved with patients if they enter the hospital and coordinates transitional services with APRNs and other care providers after discharge. Given all these job requirements, the health coach most often will be an RN. Box 2-7 presents a case study in which baccalaureate-trained RNs serve as health coaches for women who are first-time mothers and may be at risk of abusing or neglecting their children.

Nurses as System Innovators[3]

One of the fundamental insights of the quality improvement movement is that all health professionals should both perform their current work well and continuously look for ways to make their performance and that of the larger system better. Or as one nurse told a physician 20 years ago in a course on health care improvement, "I see. You're saying that I have two jobs: doing my job and making my job better" (Berwick, 2010).

The nursing profession is well positioned to produce system innovators. A few years ago, the Institute for Healthcare Improvement (IHI) launched a national project to reduce patient injuries, called the 100,000 Lives Campaign. The project translated the aims of safety and effectiveness into operational form as "bundles" of care procedures (Berwick et al., 2006; McCannon et al., 2006), such as the Central Line Bundle to prevent catheter-associated bloodstream infections. Hundreds of hospitals reported success in terms of improved patient outcomes.

---

[3] This section draws on a paper commissioned by the committee on "Preparing Nurses for Participation in and Leadership of Continual Improvement," by Donald M. Berwick, Institute for Healthcare Improvement (see Appendix I on CD-ROM).

BOX 2-5
Case Study: Living Independently for Elders (LIFE)

Nurses Supporting Older Adults to Stay in the Community

In 2002, when Lillie Mashore was in her late 50s, she was diagnosed with multiple sclerosis. Just a year later her diabetes was so severe she had to be placed in intensive care. Too ill in December 2003 to return to the West Philadelphia home she shared with her husband, who had cancer, she entered a nursing home. She was greeted there with the words, "You're going to leave here in a body bag."

But Ms. Mashore defied that prediction. In April 2005 she went home and spent the last year of her husband's life with him. With the support of the Living Independently for Elders (LIFE) program, she is still at home, receiving help twice a day from visiting nurses and aides and attending LIFE's adult day care center 3 days a week.

"I'm limited to certain things," Ms. Mashore, now age 66, said of her recovered independence. "But I can wash dishes. I didn't think I could do that. I was so proud when I washed those dishes."

Ms. Mashore is one of the nearly 700 elderly Philadelphians eligible for nursing home admission who have stayed in their homes with the help of LIFE—a program that provides all primary and specialty care services to low-income, frail, chronically ill older adults (age 55 or older). About 95 percent of members are African American. Nurse practitioner–led teams include nurses, physicians, social workers, physical and occupational therapists, dieticians, nurses' aides, and drivers.

Although home care is available for LIFE members like Ms. Mashore who need help managing household tasks or medications, it is not the primary focus. Many services are provided at the LIFE adult day care center, and groups take outings, such as to Phillies baseball games or a nearby Dave and Buster's restaurant. (Roughly 20 bed-bound members receive all LIFE services at home.) Also available are respite care for family caregivers, transportation to the center, and a "circle of care" for people with dementia. About 185 members are at the center each day.

The nurses are picking up subtle signs that could lead to deteriorating health—a slight fever or fluid retention—and because they're seeing the patient two or three times a week, they act on it quickly and prevent a further problem.

—Eileen M. Sullivan-Marx, PhD, FAAN, RN, associate dean for practice and community affairs,
University of Pennsylvania School of Nursing

As for outcomes, LIFE keeps nearly 90 percent of its members out of nursing homes, according to unpublished data. LIFE also reports reduced rates of falls, pressure

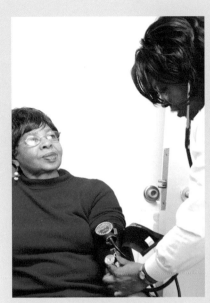

USEventPhotos.com

Among many services LIFE provides, routine preventive services such as measuring blood pressure enables older Philadelphia residents to stay healthy and remain in their own homes.

ulcers, preventable hospitalizations, and emergency room visits among members (LIFE, 2010).

LIFE is one of 72 programs in 31 states that are part of the Program for All-Inclusive Care for Elders (PACE)—a model of care begun in San Francisco in the 1970s that is now a national network offering services to elderly Medicare and Medicaid beneficiaries—and it is the only PACE program to be affiliated with a school of nursing, the University of Pennsylvania's. (See the websites of LIFE [www.lifeupenn.org] and PACE [www.npaonline.org] for more information.) And because

PACE programs receive capitated payments—per member, rather than per service provided—from government and private insurers, LIFE is both provider and payer for specific services, said Mary Austin, MSN, RN, NHA, LIFE's chief nursing officer and chief operating officer. "If members go to the hospital or a nursing home, we pay for all of that care as well," she said. The team makes all care decisions, including some that might seem unconventional, such as buying an air conditioner for a member with asthma.

Despite potential financial barriers—some might deem the $2 million required to start a PACE program prohibitive, and some private insurers do not cover PACE services—LIFE is fiscally sound. "We operate on a shoestring, to a degree. But we operate responsibly, and we get the money we need to run the program," said Eileen M. Sullivan-Marx, PhD, RN, FAAN, associate dean for practice and community affairs at the University of Pennsylvania School of Nursing. She also said that the state saves 15 cents on every dollar spent on LIFE members who would otherwise be in nursing homes. The program makes up about 41 percent of the nursing school's operating budget (Sullivan-Marx et al., 2009).

Ms. Mashore is quite clear that the program has strengthened her ability to care for herself. When a nurse suggested that she not use her electric wheelchair because using a manual one would strengthen her arms, Ms. Mashore was angry at first. "But I see what she's saying," Ms. Mashore said. "My arms are very strong. I pull my own self up in the bed. I can do things that I couldn't do when I was in the nursing home."

BOX 2-6
Case Study: The Transitional Care Model

Easing Transitions, Fostering Freedom: The Transitional Care Model "Speaks to What Nurses Really Do"

Mary Manley was accustomed to her independence. Having lived for many years on her own in North Philadelphia, worked until age 74, and cared for her infant great-granddaughter in her early 80s, she was undaunted by a diagnosis of diabetes in late 2007. "I didn't have to go to doctors too much," she said. "I was perfectly healthy, doing anything I wanted to do—"until 2009, that is, when 'the sickness' came."

"The sickness" was, in fact, many chronic conditions (among them hypertension, mild cognitive impairment, coronary artery disease, and chronic obstructive pulmonary disease) and two life-threatening acute conditions. The latter conditions—pneumonia and pancolitis, an intestinal inflammation caused by *Clostridium difficile*, a "superbug" that is often resistant to treatment—required hospitalization.

Ms. Manley received vancomycin intravenously for the *C. difficile* for two weeks as an inpatient. She was discharged on a Thursday afternoon with a prescription for oral vancomycin that her niece dropped off at a neighborhood pharmacy. But on Friday the pharmacy claimed not to have received the order and refused to dispense the drug.

While hospitalized, Ms. Manley had met a transitional care nurse, Ellen McPartland, MSN, APRN, BC, who made a home visit on Friday. When she heard about the potentially grave delay in antibiotic therapy, she called the pharmacy immediately, demanding to speak with a supervisor. The pharmacy dispensed enough medication to get Ms. Manley through the weekend at home until the full amount could be obtained on Monday—an outcome that prevented immediate rehospitalization and may have saved Ms. Manley's life.

We have not, as a health care system, figured out how best to respond to the needs of people with multiple chronic conditions. The Transitional Care Model is one approach to change the system to be more responsive to their needs.

—Mary D. Naylor, PhD, RN, FAAN, developer of the TCM

According to a recent study, 20 percent of hospitalized Medicare beneficiaries are readmitted within 30 days of discharge and 34 percent within 90 days, at an estimated cost in 2004 of "$17.4 billion of the $102.6 billion in hospital payments from Medicare" (Jencks et al., 2009). Among innovations aimed at reducing rehospitalization rates, the Transitional Care Model (TCM) relies on an advanced practice registered nurse (APRN), like Ms. McPartland, who meets with the patient and family caregivers during a hospitalization to devise a plan for managing chronic illnesses (see www.transitionalcare. info).

But the model involves more than discharge planning and home care, said TCM developer Mary D. Naylor, PhD, RN, FAAN, a professor of gerontology and director of the New-Courtland Center for Transitions and Health at the University of Pennsylvania. The first step is for the APRN to help the patient and family set goals during hospitalization. The nurse identifies the reasons for the patient's instability, designs a plan of care that addresses them, and coordinates various care providers and services.

The APRN then visits the home within 48 hours of discharge and provides telephone and in-person support as often as needed for up to 3 months. Assessing and counseling patients and accompanying them to medical appointments are aimed at helping patients and caregivers to learn the early signs of an acute problem that might require immediate help and to better manage patients' health care. Also essential is ensuring the presence of a primary care provider. "Patients might have six or seven specialists, but nobody who's taking care of the big picture," Dr. Naylor said.

In three randomized controlled trials of Medicare beneficiaries with multiple chronic illnesses, use of the TCM lengthened the period between hospital discharge and readmission or death and resulted in a reduction in the number of rehospitalizations (Naylor et al., 1994, 1999, 2004). The average annual savings was $5,000 per patient.

Until now, transitional care has not been covered by Medicare and private insurers. But the Affordable Care Act sets aside $500 million to fund pilot projects on transitional care services for "high-risk" Medicare beneficiaries (such as those with mul-tiple chronic conditions and hospital readmissions) at certain hospitals and community organizations over a 5-year period. The secretary of the Department of Health and Human Services is authorized to remove the pilot status of this program if it demonstrates cost savings.

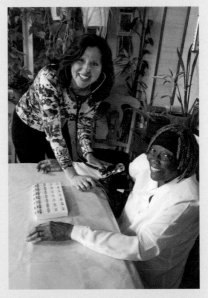

© 2010 Gregory Benson

Mary Manley relied heavily on her nurse, Ellen McPartland, during her transition from the hospital back to home.

Now age 85, Ms. Manley takes eight medications regularly, and with the help of Ms. McPartland and a new primary care team is spending more time with family and attending church again. Said Ms. McPartland, "Of all the roles I have had in nursing, this brings it all together. To see them going from so sick to back home and stable—the Transitional Care Model speaks to what nurses really do."

Recurrent patterns of success included actively engaged nurses supported in standardizing their own processes of care according to the IHI bundles and empowered and supported in monitoring and enforcing those standards across disciplines, including with their physician colleagues (Berwick et al., 2006). Encouraged to innovate locally to adapt changes to local contexts, nurses proved the ideal leaders for changing care systems and raising the bar on results.

One new role for nurses that taps their potential as innovators is the clinical nurse leader (CNL), an advanced generalist clinician role designed to improve clinical and cost outcomes for specific groups of patients. Responsible for coordinating care and in some cases actively providing direct care in complex situations, the CNL has the responsibility for translating and applying research findings to design, implement, and evaluate care plans for patients (AACN, 2007). This new role has been adopted by the VA system.

The Need for Interprofessional Collaboration

The need for greater interprofessional collaboration has been emphasized since the 1970s. Studies have documented, for example, the extent to which poor communication and lack of respect between physicians and nurses lead to harmful outcomes for patients (Rosenstein and O'Daniel, 2005; Zwarenstein et al., 2009). Conversely, a growing body of evidence links effective teams to better patient outcomes and more efficient use of resources (Bosch et al., 2009; Lemieux-Charles and McGuire, 2006; Zwarenstein et al., 2009), while good working relationships between physicians and nurses have been cited as a factor in improving the retention of nurses in hospitals (Kovner et al., 2007). As the delivery of care becomes more complex across a wide range of settings, and the need to coordinate care among multiple providers becomes ever more important, developing well-functioning teams becomes a crucial objective throughout the health care system.

Differing professional perspectives—with attendant differences in training and philosophy—can be beneficial. Nurses are taught to treat the patient not only from a disease management perspective but also from psychosocial, spiritual, and family and community perspectives. Physicians are experts in physiology, disease pathways, and treatment. Social workers are trained in family dynamics. Occupational and physical therapists focus on improving the patient's functional capacity. Licensed practical nurses provide a deeply ground-level perspective, given their routine of measuring vital signs and assisting patients in feeding, bathing, and movement. All these perspectives can enhance patients' well-being—provided the various professionals keep the patient and family at the center of their attention.

Finding the right balance of skills and professional expertise is important under the best of circumstances; in a time of increasing financial constraints, personnel shortages, and the growing need to provide care across multiple settings, it is crucial. Care teams need to make the best use of each member's education,

BOX 2-7
Case Study: The Nurse–Family Partnership

Nurses Visit the Homes of First-Time At-Risk Mothers, and the Results Are Wide-Ranging

In 2007 Crystalon Rodrigue, a recent high school graduate living in St. James, Louisiana, had an adverse reaction to an injectable contraceptive. She discontinued it and soon got pregnant. She was 19 years old and unemployed and living with her mother, and her relationship with her boyfriend was faltering. She turned to the state department of health; was referred to the Nurse–Family Partnership (NFP); and met "Miss Tina," a nurse who visited her at home.

"In the beginning of my pregnancy, and maybe all throughout, I was a little stressed out," the 21-year-old Ms. Rodrigue said recently. "I was depressed because I was having relationship problems with my child's father. Miss Tina helped me...." Ms. Rodrigue was interrupted by the chatter of her 19-month-old daughter, Nalayia, who was learning to read, her mother said with pride. Then she continued, "Miss Tina helped me to think about myself."

It was a quiet, almost offhand remark, but it represents the kind of shift in attitude that the NFP has helped foster among young women for more than 30 years. Now active in 375 counties in 29 states, the NFP sends registered nurses (RNs), usually with baccalaureate degrees, into the homes of at-risk, low-income, first-time mothers for 64 planned visits over the course of a pregnancy and the child's first 2 years.

When [the Nurse–Family Partnership nurse] came along, I was really down and out. I wouldn't get out of the house at all. She's helped me to be strong, to know that I can actually make it by myself and be a very good mom.

—Crystalon Rodrigue, 21-year-old Louisiana client of the Nurse–Family Partnership

---

Improving the lives of children is the chief aim of the NFP, yet the interventions target mothers. The

continued

BOX 2-7 *continued*

nurse discusses options for the mother's continued education and economic self-sufficiency; supports her in reducing or quitting smoking or drinking; teaches her about child development, nonviolent discipline, and breastfeeding; and helps her make decisions about family plan-

ning. The nurse does this by engaging the mother in a relationship that provides a model for interactions with others. The child's father and other family members are encouraged to participate.

"We don't look for the great big change," said Luwana Marts, BSN,

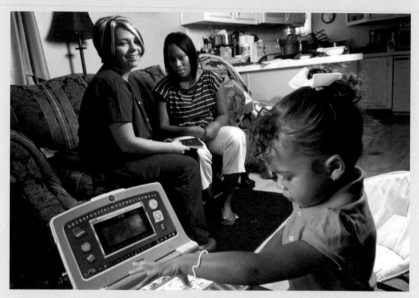

© 2010 Marc Pagani Photography, marcpagani.com

Tina Becnel, a nurse who provides home visits, helped Crystalon Rodrigue during her pregnancy and continued through her daughter Nalayia's second birthday.

RN, regional nurse consultant for the NFP in Louisiana. "A part of the model is that only a small change is necessary. So if a client never quits smoking but she doesn't smoke in the presence of her child, that's a plus."

In case-controlled, longitudinal trials conducted among racially and ethnically diverse populations—beginning in 1977 in Elmira, New York, and continuing in Memphis, Tennessee, and Denver, Colorado—the NFP has shown reductions in unintended second pregnancies and increases in mothers' employment. Children of mothers visited by nurses are less likely to be abused and by age 15 to be arrested. (For links to these and other studies of the NFP, visit www.nursefamilypartnership.org/proven-results/published-research.) The per-child cost is $9,118; for the highest-risk children, a return of $5.70 per dollar spent is realized (Karoly et al., 2005).

Several models of home visitation are in use, but the NFP relies on trained RNs for its interventions. A 2002 study compared home visits by untrained "paraprofessionals" and nurses. On almost all measures, the nurses produced far stronger outcomes (Olds et al., 2002). "People trust nurses," said Ruth A. O'Brien, PhD, RN, FAAN, professor of nursing at the University of Colorado in Denver and an author of the study.

"Low-income, minority people who have not had a lot of trust in the health care system might be willing to let a nurse in the door."

Barriers to implementation include the fact that states use various sources to fund the NFP, and in some the funding is limited. The Affordable Care Act mandates that $1.5 billion be spent over 5 years on home visitation programs for at-risk mothers and infants*—substantially less than the $8.5 billion over 10 years that President Obama requested in his 2010 budget (OMB, 2010). While the act establishes a federal agency to oversee such home visitation programs, it does not specify that nurses provide the care. Also, some municipalities increase the nurse's caseload beyond the recommended 25, diminishing the intensity and effectiveness of the interventions.

For her part, Ms. Rodrigue is looking ahead. She had completed a certified nursing assistant program while pregnant and will soon start nursing school, in which she had enrolled but quit shortly after high school. "I wasn't ready for it," she said. "But now I have a child and I know what to expect. I feel like I'm ready. I want to better myself."

Patient Protection and Affordable Care Act, HR 3590 § 2951, 111th Congress.

skill, and expertise, and all health professionals need to practice to the full extent of their license and education. Where the competency and skills of doctors and nurses safely overlap, it makes sense to rely on nurses to provide many of those services. Similarly, where the competency and skills of RNs and licensed practical or vocational nurses safely overlap, it makes sense to rely on the latter—or as the case may be, nurses' aides—to provide many of those services. In this way, more specialized skills and competencies are appropriately reserved for the most complex needs. This type of skill balancing should not, however, be used as a means of cutting costs by indiscriminately replacing more skilled with less skilled clinicians.

CONCLUSION

Nurses are well positioned to help meet the evolving needs of the health care system. They have vital roles to play in achieving patient-centered care; strengthening primary care services; delivering more care in the community; and providing seamless, coordinated care. They also can take on reconceptualized roles as health care coaches and system innovators. In all of these ways, nurses can contribute to a reformed health care system that provides safe, patient-centered, accessible, affordable care. Their ability to make these contributions, however, will depend on a transformation of nursing practice, education, and leadership, as discussed in Chapters 3, 4, and 5, respectively. Nurses must remodel the way they practice and make clinical decisions. They must rethink the ways in which they teach nurses how to care for people. They must rise to the challenge of providing leadership in rapidly changing care settings and in an evolving health care system. In short, nurses must expand their vision of what it means to be a nursing professional. At the same time, society must amend outdated regulations, attitudes, policies, and habits that unnecessarily restrict the innovative contributions the nursing profession can bring to health care.

REFERENCES

AACN (American Association of Colleges of Nursing). 2007. *White paper on the education and role of the clinical nurse leader.* Washington, DC: AACN.

Asch, S. M., E. A. McGlynn, M. M. Hogan, R. A. Hayward, P. Shekelle, L. Rubenstein, J. Keesey, J. Adams, and E. A. Kerr. 2004. Comparison of quality of care for patients in the Veterans Health Administration and patients in a national sample. *Annals of Internal Medicine* 141(12):938-945.

ASPH (Association of Schools of Public Health). 2008. *Confronting the public health workforce crisis.* Washington, DC: ASPH.

ASTHO (Association of State and Territorial Health Officials). 2004. *State public health employee worker shortage report: A civil service recruitment and retention crisis.* Washington, DC: ASTHO.

Baicker, K., and A. Chandra. 2004. Medicare spending, the physician workforce, and beneficiaries' quality of care. *Health Affairs* Suppl Web Exclusives:W184-197.

Barry, M. J., A. G. Mulley, Jr., F. J. Fowler, and J. W. Wennberg. 1988. Watchful waiting vs. immediate transurethral resection for symptomatic prostatism. The importance of patients' preferences. *JAMA* 259(20):3010-3017.

Berwick, D. M. 2010. *Preparing nurses for participation in and leadership of continual improvement.* Paper commissioned by the Committee on the RWJF Initiative on the Future of Nursing, at the IOM (see Appendix I on CD-ROM).

Berwick, D. M., D. R. Calkins, C. J. McCannon, and A. D. Hackbarth. 2006. The 100,000 lives campaign: Setting a goal and a deadline for improving health care quality. *JAMA* 295(3):324-327.

Bodenheimer, T. 2006. Primary care—will it survive? *New England Journal of Medicine* 355(9): 861-864.

Bodenheimer, T., and H. H. Pham. 2010. Primary care: Current problems and proposed solutions. *Health Affairs* 29(5):799-805.

Bosch, M., M. J. Faber, J. Cruijsberg, G. E. Voerman, S. Leatherman, R. P. Grol, M. Hulscher, and M. Wensing. 2009. Review article: Effectiveness of patient care teams and the role of clinical expertise and coordination: A literature review. *Medical Care Research and Review* 66(6 Suppl):5S-35S.

CBO (Congressional Budget Office). 2009. *Quality initiatives undertaken by the Veterans Health Administration.* Washington, DC: CBO.

CBO. 2010. *Cost estimates for the 111th Congress: H.R. 4872, Reconciliation Act of 2010 (final health care legislation).* http://www.cbo.gov/costestimates/CEBrowse.cfm (accessed June 28, 2010).

CDC (Centers for Disease Control and Prevention). 2010. *Chronic diseases and health promotion.* http://www.cdc.gov/chronicdisease/overview/index.htm (accessed July 23, 2010).

CMS (Centers for Medicare and Medicaid Services). 2010a. *National health expenditure data: Historical.* http://www.cms.gov/NationalHealthExpendData/02_NationalHealthAccountsHistorical.asp#TopOfPage (accessed May 17, 2010).

CMS. 2010b. *Table 2. National health expenditures aggregate amounts and average annual percent change, by type of expenditure: Selected calendar years 1960-2008.* Available from National Health Expenditure Data: Historical. https://www.cms.gov/NationalHealthExpendData/02_NationalHealthAccountsHistorical.asp#TopOfPage (accessed August 29, 2010).

Craven, G., and S. Ober. 2009. Massachusetts nurse practitioners step up as one solution to the primary care access problem: A political success story. *Policy, Politics, & Nursing Practice* 10(2):94-100.

Cronenwett, L., and V. J. Dzau. 2010. *Who will provide primary care and how will they be trained?, Proceedings of a conference sponsored by the Josiah Macy, Jr. Foundation.* Edited by B. Culliton and S. Russell. Durham, NC: Josiah Macy, Jr. Foundation.

Delbanco, T., D. M. Berwick, J. I. Boufford, S. Edgman-Levitan, G. Ollenschlager, D. Plamping, and R. G. Rockefeller. 2001. Healthcare in a land called peoplepower: Nothing about me without me. *Health Expectations* 4(3):144-150.

DeVol, R., A. Bedroussian, A. Charuworn, A. Chatterjee, I. Kim, S. Kim, and K. Klowden. 2007. *An unhealthy America: The economic burden of chronic disease.* Santa Monica, CA: The Milken Institute.

Diabetes Control and Complications Trial Research Group. 1993. The effect of intensive treatment of diabetes on the development and progression of long-term complications in insulin-dependent diabetes mellitus *New England Journal of Medicine* 329(14):977-986.

Dodaro, G. L. 2008. *Long-term fiscal outlook: Long-term federal fiscal challenge driven primarily by health care.* Washington, DC: GAO.

Doherty, R. B. 2010. The certitudes and uncertainties of health care reform. *Annals of Internal Medicine* 152(10):679-682.

Doty, M. M., J. N. Edwards, and A. L. Holmgren. 2005. *Seeing red: Americans driven into debt by medical bills: Results from a national survey.* New York: The Commonwealth Fund.

Emanuel, E. J., and V. R. Fuchs. 2008. Who really pays for health care? The myth of "Shared responsibility." *JAMA* 299(9):1057-1059.

Fisher, E., D. Goodman, J. Skinner, and K. Bronner. 2009. *Health care spending, quality, and outcomes: More isn't always better. A Dartmouth Atlas project topic brief.* Hanover, NH: The Dartmouth Atlas.

Fowler, F. J., Jr., J. E. Wennberg, R. P. Timothy, M. J. Barry, A. G. Mulley, Jr., and D. Hanley. 1988. Symptom status and quality of life following prostatectomy. *JAMA* 259(20):3018-3022.

Goldman, D. P., and E. A. McGlynn. 2005. *U.S. Health care: Facts about cost, access, and quality.* Santa Monica, CA: RAND.

Hassmiller, S. B., and L.B. Bolton (eds.). 2009. Transforming care at the bedside: Paving the way for change. *American Journal of Nursing* 109(11):3-80.

Hatem, M., J. Sandall, D. Devane, H. Soltani, and S. Gates. 2008. Midwife-led versus other models of care for childbearing women. *Cochrane Database of Systematic Reviews* (4):CD004667.

Heron, M., P. Sutton, J. Xu, S. Ventura, D. Strobino, and B. Guyer. 2007. Annual summary of vital statistics. *Pediatrics* 125(1):4-15.

HHS (Health and Human Services) Office of Minority Health. 2007. *National standards on culturally and linguistically appropriate services.* http://minorityhealth.hhs.gov/templates/browse. aspx?lvl=2&lvlID=15 (accessed June 30, 2010).

Hibbard, J. H. 2004. Moving toward a more patient-centered health care delivery system. *Health Affairs* Suppl Web Exclusives:VAR133-135.

Himmelstein, D. U., D. Thorne, E. Warren, and S. Woolhandler. 2009. Medical bankruptcy in the United States, 2007: Results of a national study. *American Journal of Medicine* 122(8):741-746.

Hodnett, E. D., S. Gates, G. Hofmeyr, and C. Sakala. 2007. Continuous support for women during childbirth. *Cochrane Database Systematic Reviews* 7(3).

Hooshmand, M. 2010. Comparison of telemedicine to traditional face-to-face care for children with special health care needs: Analysis of cost, caring, and family-centered care. School of Nursing and Health Studies, University of Miami, Coral Gables, FL.

HRSA (Health Resource and Services Administration). 2006. *Evidence of trends, risk factors, and intervention strategies: A report from the Healthy Start national evaluation 2006.* Rockville, MD: HRSA.

HRSA. 2010. *The registered nurse population: Findings from the 2008 National Sample Survey of Registered Nurses.* Rockville, MD: HRSA.

IOM (Institute of Medicine). 1996. *Primary care: America's health in a new era.* Washington, DC: National Academy Press.

IOM. 2000. *To err is human: Building a safer health system.* Washington, DC: National Academy Press.

IOM. 2001. *Crossing the quality chasm: A new health system for the 21st century.* Washington, DC: National Academy Press.

IOM. 2002. *The future of the public's health in the 21st century.* Washington, DC: The National Academies Press.

IOM. 2003a. *Priority areas for national action: Transforming health care quality.* Washington, DC: The National Academies Press.

IOM. 2003b. *Unequal treatment: Confronting racial and ethnic disparities in health care.* Washington, DC: The National Academies Press.

IOM. 2004a. *Health literacy: A prescription to end confusion.* Washington, DC: The National Academies Press.

IOM. 2004b. *Measuring what matters: Allocation, planning, and quality assessment for the Ryan White CARE Act.* Washington, DC: The National Academies Press.

IOM. 2008. *Retooling for an aging America: Building the health care workforce.* Washington, DC: The National Academies Press.

IOM. 2009. *The healthcare imperative: Lowering costs and improving outcomes: Brief summary of a workshop* Washington, DC: The National Academies Press.

IOM. 2010. *A summary of the December 2009 Forum on the Future of Nursing: Care in the community.* Washington, DC: The National Academies Press.

IOM Roundtable on Evidence-Based Medicine. 2008. *Learning healthcare system concepts, v. 2008.* Washington, DC: The National Academies Press.

Jacobson, J. 2009. School nurses nationwide respond to influenza A (H1N1) outbreaks. *American Journal of Nursing* 109(6):19.

Jencks, S. F., M. V. Williams, and E. A. Coleman. 2009. Rehospitalizations among patients in the Medicare fee-for-service program. *New England Journal of Medicine* 360(14):1418-1428.

Jha, A. K., J. B. Perlin, K. W. Kizer, and R. A. Dudley. 2003. Effect of the transformation of the Veterans Affairs health care system on the quality of care. *New England Journal of Medicine* 348(22):2218-2227.

Joint Commission. 2007. *What did the doctor say?: Improving health literacy to protect patient safety.* Oak Brook, IL: Joint Commission.

Karoly, L. A., M. R. Killburn, and J. S. Cannon. 2005. *Early childhood interventions: Proven results, future promise.* Arlington, VA: RAND Corporation.

Kerr, E. A., R. B. Gerzoff, S. L. Krein, J. V. Selby, J. D. Piette, J. D. Curb, W. H. Herman, D. G. Marrero, K. M. Narayan, M. M. Safford, T. Thompson, and C. M. Mangione. 2004. Diabetes care quality in the Veterans Affairs health care system and commercial managed care: The triad study. *Annals of Internal Medicine* 141(4):272-281.

Kim, M. M., A. E. Barnato, D. C. Angus, L. A. Fleisher, and J. M. Kahn. 2010. The effect of multidisciplinary care teams on intensive care unit mortality. *Archives of Internal Medicine* 170(4):369-376.

Knaus, W. A., E. A. Draper, D. P. Wagner, and J. E. Zimmerman. 1986. An evaluation of outcome from intensive care in major medical centers. *Annals of Internal Medicine* 104(3):410-418.

Kovner, C. T., C. S. Brewer, S. Fairchild, S. Poornima, H. Kim, and M. Djukic. 2007. Newly licensed RNs' characteristics, work attitudes, and intentions to work. *American Journal of Nursing* 107(9).58-70; quiz 70-51.

Lamb, G., M. Schmitt, P. Edwards, F. Sainfort, I. Duva, and M. Higgins. 2008 October 2-4. Measuring staff nurse care coordination in the hospital. Paper presented at National State of the Science Congress on Nursing Research, Washington, DC.

Lemieux-Charles, L., and W. L. McGuire. 2006. What do we know about health care team effectiveness? A review of the literature. *Medical Care Research and Review* 63(3):263-300.

LIFE (Living Independently for Elders). 2010. *LIFE receives innovative care model award.* http://www.lifeupenn.org/innovative%20care%20models%20award.pdf (accessed March 28, 2010).

Matthews, S. 2009. Channeling grief into action: Creating a culture of safety conference call, February 25, 2009, Hosted by Institute for Healthcare Improvement.

McCannon, C. J., M. W. Schall, D. R. Calkins, and A. G. Nazem. 2006. Saving 100,000 lives in US hospitals. *BMJ* 332(7553):1328-1330.

NACCHO (National Association of County and City Health Officials). 2010. *LHD budget cuts and job losses.* http://www.naccho.org//topics/infrastructure/lhdbudget/index.cfm (accessed July 2, 2010).

NASN (National Association of School Nurses). 2010. *Healthy children learn better! School nurses make a difference.* Silver Spring, MD: NASN. Available from http://www.nasn.org/Portals/0/about/2009_press_room_faq.pdf.

Naylor, M. D., D. Brooten, R. Jones, R. Lavizzo-Mourey, M. Mezey, and M. Pauly. 1994. Comprehensive discharge planning for the hospitalized elderly. A randomized clinical trial. *Annals of Internal Medicine* 120(12):999-1006.

Naylor, M. D., D. Brooten, R. Campbell, B. S. Jacobsen, M. D. Mezey, M. V. Pauly, and J. S. Schwartz. 1999. Comprehensive discharge planning and home follow-up of hospitalized elders: A randomized clinical trial. *JAMA* 281(7):613-620.

Naylor, M. D., D. A. Brooten, R. L. Campbell, G. Maislin, K. M. McCauley, and J. S. Schwartz. 2004. Transitional care of older adults hospitalized with heart failure: A randomized, controlled trial. *Journal of the American Geriatrics Society* 52(5):675-684.

New York State Department of Health AIDS Institute. 2003. *Clinical management of HIV infection: Quality of care performance in New York State 1999-2001.* Albany, NY: New York State Department of Health.

OECD (Organisation for Economic Co-operation and Development). 2010. *OECD health data 2010—frequently requested data.* http://www.oecd.org/document/16/0,3343,en_2649_34631_2085200_1_1_1_1,00.html (accessed July 21, 2010).

Olds, D. L., J. Robinson, R. O'Brien, D. W. Luckey, L. M. Pettitt, C. R. Henderson, Jr., R. K. Ng, K. L. Sheff, J. Korfmacher, S. Hiatt, and A. Talmi. 2002. Home visiting by paraprofessionals and by nurses: A randomized, controlled trial. *Pediatrics* 110(3):486-496.

OMB (Office of Management and Budget). 2010. *President Obama's fiscal 2010 budget.* http://www.whitehouse.gov/omb/fy2010_key_education (accessed March 27, 2010).

On Lok PACEpartners. 2006. *History.* http://www.pacepartners.net/history.php (accessed August 20, 2010).

Peikes, D., A. Chen, J. Schore, and R. Brown. 2009. Effects of care coordination on hospitalization, quality of care, and health care expenditures among Medicare beneficiaries: 15 randomized trials. *JAMA* 301(6):603-618.

Perlino, C. M. 2006. *The public health workforce shortage: Left unchecked, will it be protected?* Washington, DC: APHA.

Pronovost, P. J., S. M. Berenholtz, C. Goeschel, I. Thom, S. R. Watson, C. G. Holzmueller, J. S. Lyon, L. H. Lubomski, D. A. Thompson, D. Needham, R. Hyzy, R. Welsh, G. Roth, J. Bander, L. Morlock, and J. B. Sexton. 2008. Improving patient safety in intensive care units in Michigan. *Journal of Critical Care* 23(2):207-221.

Rosenstein, A. H., and M. O'Daniel. 2005. Disruptive behavior and clinical outcomes: Perceptions of nurses and physicians. *American Journal of Nursing* 105(1):54-64; quiz 64-65.

Sepucha, K. R., F. J. Fowler, Jr., and A. G. Mulley, Jr. 2004. Policy support for patient-centered care: The need for measurable improvements in decision quality. *Health Affairs* Suppl Web Exclusives:VAR54-62.

Shi, L. 1992. The relationship between primary care and life chances. *Journal of Health Care for the Poor and Underserved* 3(2):321-335.

Shi, L. 1994. Primary care, specialty care, and life chances. *International Journal of Health Services* 24(3):431-458.

Starfield, B., L. Shi, and J. Macinko. 2005. Contribution of primary care to health systems and health. *The Milbank Quarterly* 83(3):457-502.

Steinwald, A. B. 2008. *Primary care professionals: Recent supply trends, projections, and valuation of services.* Washington, DC: GAO.

Sullivan-Marx, E., C. Bradway, and J. Barnsteiner. 2009. Innovative collaborations: A case study for academic owned nursing practice. *Journal of Nursing Scholarship* 42(1):50-57.

U.S. Census Bureau. 2003. *Language use and English-speaking ability: 2000.* Washington, DC: U.S. Census Bureau.

U.S. Census Bureau. 2008. *An older and more diverse nation by midcentury.* http://www.census.gov/newsroom/releases/archives/population/cb08-123.html (accessed July 9, 2010).

U.S. Census Bureau. 2010. *New Census Bureau report analyzes nation's linguistic diversity: Population speaking a language other than English at home increases by 140 percent in past three decades.* http://www.census.gov/newsroom/releases/archives/american_community_survey_acs/cb10-cn58.html (accessed June 30, 2010).

VA (Department of Veterans Affairs). 2003. *VHA vision 2020*. Washington, DC: VA.

Wachter, R. M. 2009. Patient safety at ten: Unmistakable progress, troubling gaps. *Health Affairs* 29(1):165-173.

Wennberg, J. E., A. G. Mulley, Jr., D. Hanley, R. P. Timothy, F. J. Fowler, Jr., N. P. Roos, M. J. Barry, K. McPherson, E. R. Greenberg, D. Soule, T. Bubolz, E. Fisher, and D. Malenka. 1988. An assessment of prostatectomy for benign urinary tract obstruction. Geographic variations and the evaluation of medical care outcomes. *JAMA* 259(20):3027-3030.

Wilson, C. F. 2005. Community care of North Carolina: Saving state money and improving patient care. *North Carolina Medical Journal* 66(3):229-233.

Xu, X., J. R. Lori, K. A. Siefert, P. D. Jacobson, and S. B. Ransom. 2008a. Malpractice liability burden in midwifery: A survey of Michigan certified nurse-midwives. *Journal of Midwifery & Women's Health* 53(1):19-27.

Xu, X., K. A. Siefert, P. D. Jacobson, J. R. Lori, and S. B. Ransom. 2008b. The effects of medical liability on obstetric care supply in Michigan. *American Journal of Obstetrics and Gynecology* 198(2):205, e201-e209.

Zwarenstein, M., J. Goldman, and S. Reeves. 2009. Interprofessional collaboration: Effects of practice-based interventions on professional practice and healthcare outcomes. *Cochrane Database of Systematic Reviews* (3):CD000072.

Part II

A Fundamental Transformation of the Nursing Profession

3

Transforming Practice

Key Message #1: Nurses should practice to the full extent of their education and training.

Patients, in all settings, deserve care that is centered on their unique needs and not what is most convenient for the health professionals involved in their care. A transformed health care system is required to achieve this goal. Transforming the health care system will in turn require a fundamental rethinking of the roles of many health professionals, including nurses. The Affordable Care Act of 2010 outlines some new health care structures, and with these structures will come new opportunities for new roles. A number of programs and initiatives have already been developed to target necessary improvements in quality, access, and value, and many more are yet to be conceived. Nurses have the opportunity to play a central role in transforming the health care system to create a more accessible, high-quality, and value-driven environment for patients. If the system is to capitalize on this opportunity, however, the constraints of outdated policies, regulations, and cultural barriers, including those related to scope of practice, will have to be lifted, most notably for advanced practice registered nurses.

The Affordable Care Act of 2010 (ACA) will place many demands on health professionals and offer them many opportunities to create a system that is more patient centered. The legislation has begun the long process of shifting the focus of the U.S. health care system away from acute and specialty care. The need for this shift in focus has become particularly urgent with respect to chronic conditions; primary care, including care coordination and transitional care; prevention and wellness; and the prevention of adverse events, such as hospital-acquired infections. Given the aging population, moreover, the need for long-term and palliative care will continue to grow in the coming years (see Chapter 2). The increase in the insured population and the rapid increase in racial and ethnic minority groups who have traditionally faced obstacles in accessing health care will also demand that care be designed for a more socioeconomically and culturally diverse population.

This chapter examines how enabling nurses to practice to the full extent of their education and training (key message #1 in Chapter 1) can be a major step forward in meeting these challenges. The first section explains why transforming nursing practice to improve care is so important, offering three examples of how utilizing the full potential of nurses has increased the quality of care while achieving greater value. The chapter then examines in detail the barriers that constrain this transformation, including regulatory barriers to expanding nurses' scope of practice, professional resistance to expanded roles for nurses, fragmentation of the health care system, outdated insurance policies, high turnover rates among nurses, difficulties encountered in the transition from education to practice, and demographic challenges. The third section describes the new structures and opportunities made possible by the ACA, as well as through technology. The final section summarizes the committee's conclusions regarding the vital contributions of the nursing profession to the success of these initiatives as well as the overall transformation of the health care system, and what needs to be done to transform practice to ensure that this contribution is realized. Particular emphasis is placed on advanced practice registered nurses (APRNs), including their roles in chronic disease management and increased access to primary care, and the regulatory barriers preventing them from taking on these roles. This is not to say that general registered nurses (RNs) should not have the opportunity to improve their practice and take on new roles; the chapter also provides such examples.

THE IMPORTANCE OF TRANSFORMING
NURSING PRACTICE TO IMPROVE CARE

As discussed in Chapter 2, the changing landscape of the health care system and the changing profile of the population require that the system undergo a fundamental shift to provide patient-centered care; deliver more primary as opposed to specialty care; deliver more care in the community rather than the acute care setting; provide seamless care; enable all health professionals to practice to the full extent of their education, training, and competencies; and foster interprofessional collaboration. Achieving such a shift will enable the health care system to provide higher-quality care, reduce errors, and increase safety. Providing care in this way and in these areas taps traditional strengths of the nursing profession. This chapter argues that nurses are so well poised to address these needs by virtue of their numbers, scientific knowledge, and adaptive capacity that the health care system should take advantage of the contributions they can make by assuming enhanced and reconceptualized roles.

Nursing is one of the most versatile occupations within the health care workforce.[1] In the 150 years since Florence Nightingale developed and promoted the concept of an educated workforce of caregivers for the sick, modern nursing has reinvented itself a number of times as health care has advanced and changed (Lynaugh, 2008). As a result of the nursing profession's versatility and adaptive capacity, new career pathways for nurses have evolved, attracting a larger and more broadly talented applicant pool and leading to expanded scopes of practice and responsibilities for nurses. Nurses have been an enabling force for change in health care along many dimensions (Aiken et al., 2009). Among the many innovations that a versatile, adaptive, and well-educated nursing profession have helped make possible are

- the evolution of the high-technology hospital;
- the possibility for physicians to combine office and hospital practice;
- lengths of hospital stay that are among the shortest in the world;
- reductions in the work hours of resident physicians to improve patient safety;
- expansion of national primary care capacity;
- improved access to care for the poor and for rural residents;
- respite and palliative care, including hospice;
- care coordination for chronically ill and elderly people; and
- greater access to specialty care and focused consultation (e.g., incontinence consultation, home parenteral nutrition services, and sleep apnea evaluations) that complement the care of physicians and other providers.

With every passing decade, nursing has become an increasingly integral part of health care services, so that a future without large numbers of nurses is impossible to envision.

---

[1] This discussion draws on a paper commissioned by the committee on "Nursing Education Policy Priorities," prepared by Linda H. Aiken, University of Pennsylvania (see Appendix I on CD-ROM).

Nurses and Access to Primary Care

Given current concerns about a shortage of primary care health professionals, the committee paid particular attention to the role of nurses, especially APRNs,[2] in this area. Today, nurse practitioners (NPs), together with physicians and physician assistants, provide most of the primary care in the United States. Physicians account for 287,000 primary care providers, NPs for 83,000, and physician assistants for 23,000 (HRSA, 2008; Steinwald, 2008). While the numbers of NPs and physician assistants are steadily increasing, the numbers of medical students and residents entering primary care have declined in recent years (Naylor and Kurtzman, 2010). The demand to build the primary care workforce, including APRNs, will grow as access to coverage, service settings, and services increases under the ACA. While NPs make up slightly less than a quarter of the country's primary care professionals (Bodenheimer and Pham, 2010), it is a group that has grown in recent years and has the potential to grow further at a relatively rapid pace.

The Robert Wood Johnson Foundation (RWJF) Nursing Research Network commissioned Kevin Stange, University of Michigan, and Deborah Sampson, Boston College, to provide information on the variation in numbers of NPs across the United States. Figures 3-1 and 3-2, respectively, plot the provider-to-primary care doctor of medicine (MD) ratio for NPs and physician assistants by county for 2009.[3] The total is calculated as the population-weighted average for states with available data. Between 1995 and 2009, the number of NPs per primary care MD more than doubled, from 0.23 to 0.48, as did the number of physician assistants per primary care MD (0.12 to 0.28) (RWJF, 2010c). These figures suggest that it is possible to increase the supply of both NPs and physician assistants in a relatively short amount of time, helping to meet the increased demand for care.

In addition to the numbers of primary care providers available across the United States and where specifically they practice, it is worth noting the kind of care being provided by each of the primary care provider groups. According to the complexity-of-care data shown in Table 3-1, the degree of variation among primary care providers is relatively small. Much of the practice of primary care—whether provided by physicians, NPs, physician assistants, or certified nurse midwives (CNMs)—is of low to moderate complexity.

---

[2] APRNs include nurse practitioners (NPs), certified nurse midwives (CNMs), clinical nurse specialists (CNSs), and certified registered nurse anesthetists (CRNAs). When the committee refers to NPs, the term denotes only NPs.

[3] To get a sense of the size and proportion of the NP workforce across the country, Stange and Sampson computed the ratio of the total number of licensed NPs to the total number of primary care MDs, physician assistants, and NPs in a given area. The physician assistant share was computed similarly. These computations are for proportion and growth analysis purposes only; they are not to suggest that all NPs or physician assistants are providing primary care.

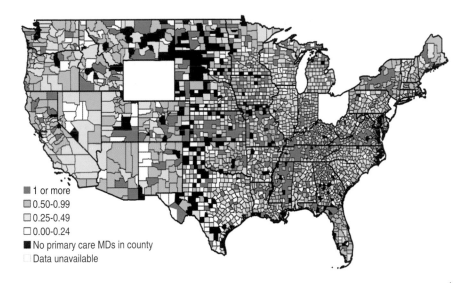

FIGURE 3-1 Map of the number of NPs per primary care MD by county, 2009.
SOURCE: RWJF, 2010a. Reprinted with permission from Lori Melichar, RWJF.

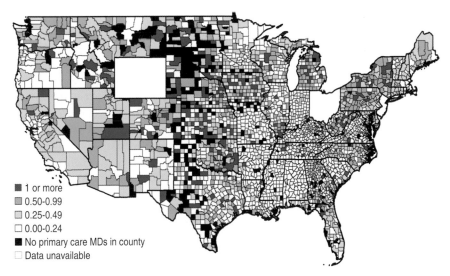

FIGURE 3-2 Map of the number of physician assistants per primary care MD by county, 2009.
SOURCE: RWJF, 2010b. Reprinted with permission from Lori Melichar, RWJF.

TABLE 3-1 Complexity of Evaluation and Management Services Provided Under Medicare Claims Data for 2000, by Practitioner Type

Practitioner Type	Low Complexity (%)	Moderate Complexity (%)	High Complexity (%)
Primary care physician	55	34	11
Nurse practitioner	57	35	9
Physician assistant	59	34	7
Certified nurse midwife	77	19	4

NOTES: For evaluation and management services, low-complexity services are defined as those requiring straightforward or low-complexity decision making; moderate-complexity services are those defined as requiring a moderate level of decision making; and high-complexity services are defined as those requiring a high level of decision making.
SOURCE: Chapman et al., 2010. Copyright © 2010 by the authors. Reprinted by permission of SAGE Publications.

Nurses and Quality of Care

Beyond the issue of pure numbers of practitioners, a promising field of evidence links nursing care to a higher quality of care for patients, including protecting their safety. According to Mary Naylor, director of the Robert Wood Johnson Foundation's Interdisciplinary Nursing Quality Research Initiative (INQRI), several INQRI-funded research teams have provided examples of this link. "[Nurses] are crucial in preventing medication errors, reducing rates of infection and even facilitating patients' transition from hospital to home."[4]

INQRI researchers at The Johns Hopkins University have found that substantial reductions in central line–associated blood stream infections can be achieved with nurses leading the infection control effort. Hospitals that adopted INQRI's intensive care unit safety program, as well as an environment that supported nurses' involvement in quality improvement efforts, reduced or eliminated bloodstream infections (INQRI, 2010b; Marsteller et al., 2010).

Other INQRI researchers linked a core cluster of nurse safety processes to fewer medication errors. These safety processes include asking physicians to clarify or rewrite unclear orders, independently reconciling patient medications, and providing patient education. A positive work environment was also important. This included having more RNs per patient, a supportive management structure, and collaborative relationships between nurses and physicians (Flynn et al., 2010; INQRI, 2010a).

---

[4] Personal communication, Mary Naylor, Marian S. Ware Professor in Gerontology, Director of New Courtland Center for Transitions and Health, University of Pennsylvania School of Nursing, June 16, 2010.

Examples of Redesigned Roles for Nurses

Many examples exist in which organizations have been redesigned to better utilize nurses, but their scale is small. As Marilyn Chow, vice president of the Patient Services Program Office at Kaiser Permanente, declared at a public forum hosted by the committee, "The future is here, it is just not everywhere" (IOM, 2010b). For example, over the past 20 years, the U.S. Department of Veterans Affairs (VA) has expanded and reconceived the roles played by its nurses as part of a major restructuring of its health care system. The results with respect to quality, access, and value have been impressive. In addition, President Obama has lauded the Geisinger Health System of Pennsylvania, which provides comprehensive care to 2.6 million people at a greater value than is achieved by most other organizations (White House, 2009). Part of the reason Geisinger is so effective is that it has aligned the roles played by nurses to accord more closely with patients' needs, starting with its primary care sites and ambulatory areas. The following subsections summarize the experience of the VA and Geisinger, as well as Kaiser Permanente, in expanding and reconceptualizing the roles of nurses. Because these institutions also measured outcomes as part of their initiatives, they provide real-world evidence that such an approach is both possible and necessary. Of note in these examples is not only how nurses are collaborating with physicians, but also how nurses are collaborating with other nurses.

Department of Veterans Affairs[5]

In 1996, Congress greatly expanded the number of veterans eligible to receive VA services, which created a need for the system to operate more efficiently and effectively (VHA, 2003). Caring for the wounded from the wars in Afghanistan and Iraq has further increased demand on the VA system, particularly with respect to brain injuries and posttraumatic stress disorder. Moreover, the large cohort of World War II veterans means that almost 40 percent of veterans are aged 65 or older, compared with 13 percent of the general population (U.S. Census Bureau, 2010; VA, 2010).

Anticipating the challenges it would face, the VA began transforming itself in the 1990s from a hospital-based system into a health care system that is focused on primary care, and it also placed emphasis on providing more services, as appropriate, closer to the veteran's home or community (VHA, 2003, 2009). This strategy required better coordination of care and chronic disease management—a role that was filled by experienced front-line RNs. More NPs were hired as primary care providers, and the VA actively promoted a more collaborative professional culture by organizing primary care providers into health teams. It

---

[5] See http://www1.va.gov/health/.

also developed a well-integrated information technology system to link its health professionals and its services.

The VA uses NPs as primary care providers to care for patients across all settings, including inpatient and outpatient settings. In addition to their role as primary care providers, NPs serve as health care researchers who apply their findings to the variety of settings in which they practice. They also serve as educators, some as university faculty, providing clinical experiences for 25 percent of all nursing students in the country. As health care leaders, VA NPs shape policy, facilitate access to VA health care, and impact resource management (VA, 2007).

The results of the VA's initiatives using both front-line RNs and APRNs are impressive. Quality and outcome data consistently demonstrate superior results for the VA's approach (Asch et al., 2004; Jha et al., 2003; Kerr et al., 2004). One study found that VA patients received significantly better health care—based on various quality-of-care indicators[6]—than patients enrolled in Medicare's fee-for-service program. In some cases, the study showed, between 93 and 98 percent of VA patients received appropriate care in 2000; the highest score for comparable Medicare patients was 84 percent (Jha et al., 2003). In addition, the VA's spending per enrollee rose much more slowly than Medicare's, despite the 1996 expansion of the number of veterans who could access VA services. After adjusting for different mixes of population and demographics, the Congressional Budget Office determined that the VA's spending per enrollee grew by 30 percent from 1999 to 2007, compared with 80 percent for Medicare over the same period.

Geisinger Health System[7]

The Geisinger Health System employs 800 physicians; 1,900 nurses; and more than 1,000 NPs, physician assistants, and pharmacists. Over the past 18 years, Geisinger has transformed itself from a high-cost medical facility to one that provides high value—all while improving quality. It has borrowed several restructuring concepts from the manufacturing world with an eye to redesigning care by focusing on what it sees as the most critical determinant of quality and cost—actual caregiving. "What we're trying to do is to have [our staff] work up to the limit of their license and . . . see if redistributing caregiving work can increase quality and decrease cost," Glenn Steele, Geisinger's president and CEO, said in a June 2010 interview (Dentzer, 2010).

Numerous improvements in the quality of care, as well as effective innovations proposed by employees, have resulted. For example, the nurses who

---

[6] Quality-of-care indicators included those in preventive care (mammography, influenza vaccination, pneumococcal vaccination, colorectal cancer screening, cervical cancer screening), outpatient care (care for diabetes [e.g., lipid screening], hypertension [e.g., blood pressure goal <140/90 mm Hg], depression [annual screening]), and inpatient care (acute myocardial infarction [e.g., aspirin within 24 hr of myocardial infarction], congestive heart failure [e.g., ejection fraction checked]).

[7] See http://www.geisinger.org/about/index.html.

used to coordinate care and provide advice through the telephone center under Geisinger's health plan suspected that they would be more effective if they could build relationships with patients and meet them at least a few times face to face. Accordingly, some highly experienced general-practice nurses moved from the call centers to primary care sites to meet with patients and their families. The nurses used a predictive model to identify who might need to go to the hospital and worked with patients and their families on creating a care plan. Later, when patients or families received a call from a nurse, they knew who that person was. The program has worked so well that nurse coordinators are now being used in both Geisinger's Medicare plan and its commercial plan.[8] Some of the nation's largest for-profit insurance companies, including WellPoint and Cigna, are now trying out the approach of employing more nurses to better coordinate their patients' care (Abelson, 2010). As a result, an innovation that emerged when a few nurses at Geisinger took the initiative and changed an already well-established program to deliver more truly patient-centered care may now spread well beyond Pennsylvania. Geisinger was also one of the very first health systems in the country to create its own NP-staffed convenient care clinics[9]—another innovation that reflects the organization's commitment to providing integrated, patient-centered care throughout its community.

Kaiser Permanente[10,11]

As one of the largest not-for-profit health plans, Kaiser Permanente provides health care services for more than 8.6 million members, with an employee base of approximately 165,000. Kaiser Permanente has facilities in nine states and the District of Columbia, and has 35 medical centers and 454 medical offices. The system provides prepaid health plans that emphasize prevention and consolidated services designed to keep as many services as possible in one location (KP, 2010). Kaiser is also at the forefront of experimenting with reconceptualized roles for nurses that are improving quality, satisfying patients, and making a difference to the organization's bottom line.

Nurses in San Diego have taken the lead in overseeing the process for patient discharge, making it more streamlined and efficient and much more effective. Discharge nurses now have full authority over the entire discharge process until home health nurses, including those in hospice and palliative care, step in to take over the patient's care. They have created efficiencies relative to previous

---

[8] Personal communication, Bruce H. Hamory, Executive Vice President and Chief Medical Officer Emeritus, Geisinger Health System, April 27, 2010.

[9] Personal communication, Tine Hansen-Turton, CEO, National Nursing Centers Consortium, and Vice President, Public Health Management Corporation, August 11, 2010.

[10] See https://members.kaiserpermanente.org/kpweb/aboutus.do.

[11] Personal communication, Marilyn Chow, Vice President, Patient Care Services, Program Office, Kaiser Permanente, August 23, 2010.

processes by using time-sensitive, prioritized lists of only those patients who are being discharged over the next 48 hours (instead of patients who are being discharged weeks into the future). Home health care nurses and discharge planners stay in close contact with one another on a daily basis to make quick decisions about patient needs, including the need for home health care visitation. In just 3 months, the number of patients who saw a home health care provider within 24 hours increased from 44 to 77 percent (Labor Management Partnership, 2010).

In 2003, Riverside Medical Center implemented the Riverside Proactive Health Management Program (RiPHM)™, an integrated, systematic approach to health care management that promotes prevention and wellness and coordinates interventions for patients with chronic conditions. The model strengthens the patient-centered medical home concept and identifies members of the health care team (HCT)—a multidisciplinary group whose staff is centrally directed and physically located in small units within the medical office building. The team serves panel management and comprehensive outreach and inreach functions to support primary care physicians and proactively manage the care of members with chronic conditions such as diabetes, hypertension, cardiovascular disease, asthma, osteoporosis, and depression. The expanded role of nurses as key members of the HCT is a major factor in RiPHM's success. Primary care management nurse clinic RNs and licensed practical nurses (LPNs) provide health care coaching and education for patients to promote self-management of their chronic conditions through face-to-face education visits and telephone follow-up. Using evidence-based clinical guidelines, such as diabetes and hypertension treat-to-target algorithms, nurses play important roles in the promotion of changes in chronic conditions and lifestyles, coaching and counseling, self-monitoring and goal setting, depression screening, and the use of advanced technology such as interactive voice recognition for patient outreach.

Through this model of care, nurses and pharmacists have become skilled users of health information technology to strengthen the primary care–based, patient-centered medical home. Nurses use disease management registries to work with assigned primary care physicians, and review clinical information that addresses care gaps and evaluate treatment plans. RiPHM has provided a strong foundation for the patient-centered medical home. By implementing this program and expanding the role of nurses, Riverside has sustained continuous improvement in key quality indicators for patient care.

Guided care is a new model for chronic care that was recently introduced within the Kaiser system. Guided care is intended to provide, within a primary care setting, quality care to patients with complex needs and multiple chronic conditions. An RN, who assists three to four physicians, receives training in such areas as the use of an electronic health record (EHR), interviewing, and the particulars of health insurance coverage. RNs are also provided skills in managing chronic conditions, providing transitional care, and working with families and community organizations (Boult et al., 2008).

The nurse providing guided care offers eight services: assessment; planning care; monitoring; coaching; chronic disease self-management; educating and supporting caregivers; coordinating transitions between providers and sites of care; and facilitating access to community services, such as Meals-on-Wheels, transportation services, and senior centers. Results of a pilot study comparing surveys of patients who received guided care and those who received usual care revealed improved quality of care and lower health care costs (according to insurance claims) for guided care patients (Boult et al., 2008).

Summary

The VA, Geisinger, and Kaiser Permanente are large integrated care systems that may be better positioned than others to invest in the coordination, education, and assessment provided by their nurses, but their results speak for themselves. If the United States is to achieve the necessary transformation of its health care system, the evidence points to the importance of relying on nurses in enhanced and reconceptualized roles. This does not necessarily mean that large regional corporations or vertically integrated care systems are the answer. It does mean that innovative, high-value solutions must be developed that are sustainable, easily adopted in other locations, and rapidly adaptable to different circumstances. A website on "Innovative Care Models" illustrates that many other solutions have been identified in other types of systems.[12] As patients, employers, insurers, and governments become more aware of the benefits offered by nurses, they may also begin demanding that health care providers restructure their services around the contributions that a transformed nursing workforce can make. As discussed later in the chapter, the committee believes there will be numerous opportunities for nurses to help develop and implement care innovations and assume leadership roles in accountable care organizations and medical homes as a way of providing access to care for more Americans. As the next section describes, however, it will first be necessary to acknowledge the barriers that prevent nurses from practicing to the full extent of their education and training, as well as to generate the political will on the part of policy makers to remove these barriers.

BARRIERS TO TRANSFORMING PRACTICE

Nurses have great potential to lead innovative strategies to improve the health care system. As discussed in this section, however, a variety of historical, regulatory, and policy barriers have limited nurses' ability to contribute to widespread transformation (Kimball and O'Neil, 2002). This is true of all RNs, including those practicing in acute care and public and community health settings, but is most notable for APRNs in primary care. Other barriers include

---

[12] See http://www.innovativecaremodels.com/ and http://www.rwjf.org/reports/grr/057241.htm.

professional resistance to expanded roles for nurses, fragmentation of the health care system, outdated insurance policies, high rates of nurse turnover, difficulties for nurses transitioning from school into practice, and an aging workforce and other demographic challenges. Many of these barriers have developed as a result of structural flaws in the U.S. health care system; others reflect limitations of the present work environment or the capacity and demographic makeup of the nursing workforce itself.

Regulatory Barriers

As the committee considered how the additional 32 million people covered by health insurance under the ACA would receive care in the coming years, it identified as a serious barrier overly restrictive scope-of-practice regulations for APRNs that vary by state. Scope-of-practice issues are of concern for CNMs, certified registered nurse anesthetists (CRNAs), NPs, and clinical nurse specialists (CNSs). The committee understands that physicians are highly trained and skilled providers and believes strongly that there clearly are services that should be provided by these health professionals, who have received more extensive and specialized education and training than APRNs. However, regulations in many states result in APRNs not being able to give care they were trained to provide. The committee believes all health professionals should practice to the full extent of their education and training so that more patients may benefit.

History of the Regulation of the Health Professions

A paper commissioned by the committee[13] points out that the United States was one of the first countries to regulate health care providers and that this regulation occurred at the state—not the federal—level. Legislatively, physician practice was recognized before that of any other health profession (Rostant and Cady, 1999). For example, legislators in Washington defined the practice of medicine broadly as any action to "diagnose, cure, advise or prescribe for any human disease, ailment, injury, infirmity, deformity, pain or other condition, physical or mental, real or imaginary, by any means or instrumentality" or to administer or prescribe "drugs or medicinal preparations to be used by any other person" or to "[sever or penetrate] the tissues of human beings."[14] Even more important were corresponding provisions making it illegal for anyone not licensed as a physician to undertake any of the acts included in this definition. These provisions

---

[13] This and the following paragraph draw on a paper commissioned by the committee on "Federal Options for Maximizing the Value of Advanced Practice Registered Nurses in Providing Quality, Cost-Effective Health Care," prepared by Barbara J. Safreit, Lewis & Clark Law School (see Appendix H on CD-ROM).

[14] *Washington Rev. Code* §18.71.011 (1)-(3) (1993).

rendered the practice of medicine not only comprehensive but also (in medicine's own view) exclusive,[15] a preemption of the field that was reinforced when physicians obtained statutory authority to control the activities of other health care providers.

Most APRNs are in the opposite situation. Because virtually all states still base their licensure frameworks on the persistent underlying principle that the practice of medicine encompasses both the ability and the legal authority to treat all possible human conditions, the scopes of practice for APRNs (and other health professionals) are exercises in legislative exception making, a "carving out" of small, politically achievable spheres of practice authority from the universal domain of medicine. As a result, APRNs' scopes of practice are so circumscribed that their competence extends far beyond their authority. At any point in their career, APRNs can do much more than they may legally do. As APRNs acquire new skills, they must seek administrative or statutory revision of their defined scopes of practice (a costly and often difficult enterprise).

As the health care system has grown over the past 40 years, the education and roles of APRNs have continually evolved so that nurses now enter the workplace willing and qualified to provide more services than they previously did. As the services supported by evolving education programs expanded, so did the overlap of practice boundaries of APRNs and physicians. APRNs are more than physician extenders or substitutes. They cover the care continuum from health promotion and disease prevention to early diagnosis to prevent or limit disability. These services are grounded in and shaped by their nursing education, with its particular ideology and professional identity. NPs also learn how to work with teams of providers, which is perhaps one of the most important factors in the successful care of chronically ill patients. Although they use skills traditionally residing in the realm of medicine, APRNs integrate a range of skills from several disciplines, including social work, nutrition, and physical therapy.

Almost 25 years ago, an analysis by the Office of Technology Assessment (OTA) indicated that NPs could safely and effectively provide more than 90 percent of pediatric primary care services and 75 percent of general primary care services, while CRNAs could provide 65 percent of anesthesia services. OTA concluded further that CNMs could be 98 percent as productive as obstetricians in providing maternity services (Office of Technology Assessment, 1986). APRNs also have competencies that include the knowledge to refer patients with complex problems to physicians, just as physicians refer patients who need services they are not trained to provide, such as medication counseling, developmental screening, or case management, to APRNs. As discussed in Chapter 1 and reviewed in Annex 1-1, APRNs provide services, in addition to primary care, in a wide range of areas, including neonatal care, acute care, geriatrics, community health, and

---

[15] Sociologist Eliot Freidson has aptly characterized this statutory preemption as "the exclusive right to practice" (Freidson, 1970).

psychiatric/mental health. Most NPs train in primary care; however, increasing numbers are being trained in acute care medicine and other specialty disciplines (Cooper, 1998).

The growing use of APRNs and physician assistants has helped ease access bottlenecks, reduce waiting times, increase patient satisfaction, and free physicians to handle more complex cases (Canadian Pediatric Society, 2000; Cunningham, 2010). This is true of APRNs in both primary and specialty care. In orthopedics, the use of APRNs and physician assistants is a long-standing practice. NPs and physician assistants in gastroenterology help meet the growing demand for colon cancer screenings in either outpatient suites or hospital endoscopy centers. Because APRNs and physician assistants in specialty practice typically collaborate closely with physicians, legal scope-of-practice issues pose limited obstacles in these settings.

Variation in Nurse Practitioner Scope-of-Practice Regulations

Regulations that define scope-of-practice limitations vary widely by state. In some states, they are very detailed, while in others, they contain vague provisions that are open to interpretation (Cunningham, 2010). Some states have kept pace with the evolution of the health care system by changing their scope-of-practice regulations to allow NPs to see patients and prescribe medications without a physician's supervision or collaboration. However, the majority of state laws lag behind in this regard. As a result, what NPs are able to do once they graduate varies widely across the country for reasons that are related not to their ability, their education or training, or safety concerns (Lugo et al., 2007) but to the political decisions of the state in which they work. For example, one group of researchers found that 16 states plus the District of Columbia have regulations that allow NPs to see primary care patients without supervision by or required collaboration with a physician (see Figure 3-3). As with any other primary care providers, these NPs refer patients to a specialty provider if the care required extends beyond the scope of their education, training, and skills.

Other legal practice barriers include on-site physician oversight requirements, chart review requirements, and maximum collaboration ratios for physicians who collaborate with more than a single NP. See Safriet (2010, Appendix H on the CD-ROM in the back of this book) for further discussion of inconsistencies in the regulation of NP practice at the state level.

There are fundamental contradictions in this situation. Educational standards—which the states recognize—support broader practice by all types of APRNs. National certification standards—which most states also recognize—likewise support broader practice by APRNs. Moreover, the contention that APRNs are less able than physicians to deliver care that is safe, effective, and efficient is not supported by the decades of research that has examined this question (Brown and Grimes, 1995; Fairman, 2008; Groth et al., 2010; Hatem et al.,

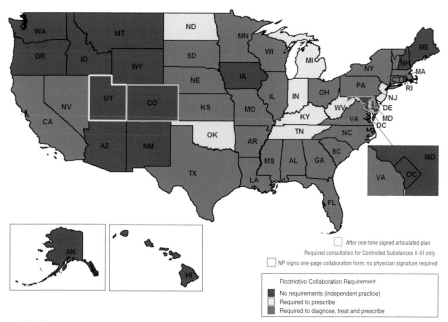

FIGURE 3-3 Requirements for physician–nurse collaboration, by state, as a barrier to access to primary care.

NOTE: Collaboration refers to a mutually agreed upon relationship between nurse and physician.

SOURCE: AARP, 2010b. Courtesy of AARP. All rights reserved. This figure combines Map 1, Overview of Diagnosing and Treating Aspects of NP Practice and Map 2, Overview of Prescribing Aspects of NP Practice, both developed by Linda Pearson (2010).

2008; Hogan et al., 2010; Horrocks et al., 2002; Hughes et al., 2010; Laurant et al., 2004; Mundinger et al., 2000; Office of Technology Assessment, 1986). No studies suggest that care is better in states that have more restrictive scope-of-practice regulations for APRNs than in those that do not. Yet most states continue to restrict the practice of APRNs beyond what is warranted by either their education or their training.

Depending on the state, restrictions on an APRN's scope of practice may limit or prohibit the authority to prescribe medications, admit patients to hospitals, assess patient conditions, and order and evaluate tests. Box 3-1 provides an example of the variation in state licensure regulations, detailing examples of the services an APRN would not be permitted to provide if she practiced in a more restrictive state (Safriet, 2010). In addition to variations among states, the scope of practice for APRNs in some cases varies within a state by geographic location of the practice within the state or nature of the practice setting.

BOX 3-1*
Variation in State Licensure Regulations

Several states permit APRNs to provide a broad list of services, such as independently examining patients, ordering and interpreting laboratory and other tests, diagnosing and treating illness and injury, prescribing indicated drugs, ordering or referring for additional services, admitting and attending patients in a hospital or other facility, and directly receiving payment for services. In other states, however, those same APRNs would be prohibited from providing many of these services. The following list provides examples of restrictions that APRNs face in states that have adopted more restrictive scope-of-practice regulations. These restrictions could greatly limit the ability of APRNs to fully utilize their education and training.

Examination and Certification

A nurse may not examine and certify for:

- worker's compensation;
- department of motor vehicles (DMV) disability placards and license plates and other DMV testing;
- excusal from jury service;
- mass transit accommodation (reduced fares, access to special features);
- sports physicals (she may perform them, but cannot sign the forms);
- declaration of death;
- school physicals and forms, including the need for home-bound schooling;
- clinician order for life-sustaining treatment (COLST), cardiopulmonary resuscitation (CPR), or do not resuscitate (DNR) directives;
- disability benefits;
- birth certificates;
- marriage health rules;
- treatment in long-term-care facilities;
- involuntary commitment for alcohol and drug treatment;
- psychiatric emergency commitment;
- hospice care; or
- home-bound care (including signing the plan of care).

Referrals and Orders

A nurse may not refer for and order:

- diagnostic and laboratory tests (unless the task has been specifically delegated by protocol with a supervising physician),
- occupational therapy,
- physical therapy,
- respiratory therapy, or
- durable medical equipment or devices.

---

*This box draws on Safriet (2010).

Examination and Treatment

A nurse may not:

- treat chronic pain (even at the direction of a supervising physician);
- examine a new patient, or a current patient with a major change in diagnosis or treatment plan, unless the patient is seen and examined by a supervising physician within a specified period of time;
- set a simple fracture or suture a laceration;
- perform:
  - cosmetic laser treatments or Botox injections,
  - first-term aspiration abortions,
  - sigmoidoscopies, or
  - admitting examinations for patients entering skilled nursing facilities; or
- provide anesthesia services unless supervised by a physician, even if she has been trained as a certified registered nurse anesthetist.

Prescriptive Authority

A nurse may not:

- have her name on the label of a medication as prescriber;
- accept and dispense drug samples;
- prescribe:
  - some (or, in a few jurisdictions, any) scheduled drugs, and
  - some legend drugs;
- prescribe even those drugs that she is permitted to prescribe except as follows:
  - as included in patient-specific protocols,
  - with the cosignature of a collaborating or supervising physician,
  - if the drugs are included in a specific formulary or written protocol or practice agreement,
  - if a specified number or percentage of charts are reviewed by a collaborating or supervising physician within a specified time period,
  - if the physician is on site with the APRN for a specified percentage of time or number of hours per week or month,
  - if the APRN is practicing in a limited number of satellite offices of the supervising physician,
  - if the prescription is only for a sufficient supply for 1 or 2 weeks or provides no refills until the patient sees a physician,
  - if a prescribing/practice agreement is filed with the state board of nursing and/or board of medicine and/or board of pharmacy both annually and when the agreement is modified in any way,
  - pursuant to rules jointly promulgated by the boards named above, and
  - if the collaborating or supervising physician's name and Drug Enforcement Administration (DEA) number are also on the script; or
- admit or attend patients in hospitals
  - if precluded from obtaining clinical privileges or inclusion in the medical staff,

continued

BOX 3-1 *continued*

> - if state rules require physician supervision of NPs in hospitals,
> - if medical staff bylaws interpret "clinical privileges" to exclude "admitting privileges," or
> - if hospital policies require a physician to have overall responsibility for each patient.

Compensation

A nurse may not be:

- empaneled as a primary care provider for Medicaid or Medicare Advantage managed care enrollees;
- included as a provider for covered services for Workers Compensation;

Current laws are hampering the ability of APRNs to contribute to innovative health care delivery solutions. Some NPs, for example, have left primary care to work as specialists in hospital settings (Cooper, 2007), although demand in those settings has also played a role in their movement. Others have left NP practice altogether to work as staff RNs. For example, restrictive state scope-of-practice regulations concerning NPs have limited expansion of retail clinics, where NPs provide a limited set of primary care services directly to patients (Rudavsky et al., 2009). Similarly, the roles of NPs in nurse-managed health centers and patient-centered medical homes can be hindered by dated state practice acts.

Credentialing and payment policies often are linked to state practice laws. A 2007 survey of the credentialing and reimbursement policies of 222 managed care organizations revealed that 53 percent credentialed NPs as primary care providers; of these, 56 percent reimbursed primary care NPs at the same rate as primary care providers, and 38 percent reimbursed NPs at a lower rate (Hansen-Turton et al., 2008). Rationales stated by managed care staff for not credentialing NPs as primary care providers included the fact that NPs have to bill under a physician's provider number, NPs do not practice in physician shortage areas, NPs do not meet company criteria for primary care providers, state law does not require them to credential NPs, and the National Committee for Quality Assurance (NCQA) accreditation process prevents them from recognizing NPs as primary care provider leads in medical homes. As discussed above, some states require NPs to be supervised by physicians in order to prescribe medications, while others do not. In this survey, 71 percent of responding insurers credentialed NPs as primary care providers in states where there was no requirement for physicians to supervise NPs in prescribing medications. In states that required more physician involvement in NP prescribing, insurers were less likely to credential

- paid other than at differential rates (65, 75, or 85 percent of physician scale) by Medicaid, Medicare, or other payers and insurers;
- paid directly by Medicaid;
- certified as leading a patient-centered medical home or primary care home; or
- paid for services unless supervised by a physician.

A nurse may:

- indirectly affect the eligibility of other providers for payment because
  - pharmacies cannot obtain payment from some private insurers unless the supervising or collaborating physician's name is on the script, and
  - hospitals cannot bill for APRNs' teaching or supervising of medical students and residents and advanced practice nursing students (as they can for physicians who provide those same services).

NPs. Of interest, this was the case even though the actual level of involvement by the physician may be the same in states where supervision is required as in states where it is not. Also of note is that Medicaid plans were more likely than any other category of insurer to credential NPs.

Although there is a movement away from a fee-for-service system, Table 3-2 shows the current payment structure for those providing primary care.

The Federal Government and Regulatory Reform[16]

Precisely because many of the problems described in this report are the result of a patchwork of state regulatory regimes, the federal government is especially well situated to promote effective reforms by collecting and disseminating best practices from across the country and incentivizing their adoption. The federal government has a compelling interest in the regulatory environment for health care professions because of its responsibility to patients covered by federal programs such as Medicare, Medicaid, the VA, and the Bureau of Indian Affairs. Equally important, however, is the federal government's responsibility to all American taxpayers who fund the care provided under these and other programs to ensure that their tax dollars are spent efficiently and effectively. Federal actors already play a central role in a number of areas that would be essential to effective reform of nursing practice, especially that of APRNs. They pay for the majority of health care services delivered today, they pay for research on the safety and effectiveness of existing and innovative practice models and encourage

---

[16] This section is based on a September 10, 2010, personal communication with Barbara J. Safriet, Lewis & Clark Law School.

TABLE 3-2 Medicare Claims Payment Structure by Provider Type

Provider	Office Services	Hospital Services	Incident to a Physician's Services[a]	Surgery Services	Medicare Provider ID	Direct Reimbursement
Physician	100% of physician fee	100% of physician fee	N/A	Usually receives a global fee	Own provider ID required	Physician or employer may be reimbursed directly
Nurse practitioner (NP)	85% of physician fee, 100% if billed "incident to"[a] in a physician's office or clinic using MD's provider ID	Usually salaried; nursing costs are part of hospital payment	100% of physician fee (must bill under the MD's provider ID)	Usually accounted for in surgeon's global fee	Own ID possible, but not required	NP or employer may be reimbursed directly
Certified nurse midwife (CNM)	65% of physician fee[b]		100% if billed "incident to" in a physician office or clinic using MD's provider ID	Usually accounted for in surgeon's global fee	Own ID possible, but not required	CNM or employer may be reimbursed directly
Physician assistant (PA)	Lesser of the actual charge or 85% of physician fee	Lesser of the actual charge or 75% of physician fee	100% if billed "incident to" in a physician office or clinic using MD's provider ID	Use assistant surgeon modifier	Own ID required	Only employer can be reimbursed directly

[a]"Incident to" is used by Medicare to denote cases in which work is performed under the direction and supervision of a physician. Criteria for "incident to" billing require that the physician be on site (in the suite of offices) at the time the service is performed, that the physician treat the patient on the patient's first visit to the office, and that the service be within the NP scope of practice in the state.

[b]CNM payment will increase to 100 percent of physician fee as of January 1, 2011.

SOURCE: Chapman et al., 2010. Copyright © 2010 by the authors. Reprinted by permission of SAGE Publications.

their adoption, and they have a compelling interest in achieving more efficient and value-driven health care services. The federal government also appropriates substantial funds for the education and training of health care providers, and it has an understandable interest in ensuring that the ever-expanding skills and abilities acquired by graduates of these programs are fully utilized for the benefit of the American public.

In particular, the Federal Trade Commission (FTC) has a long history of targeting anticompetitive conduct in health care markets, including restrictions on the business practices of health care providers, as well as policies that could act as a barrier to entry for new competitors in the market. The FTC has responded specifically to potential policies that might be viewed predominantly as guild protection rather than consumer protection, for example, taking antitrust actions against the American Medical Association (AMA) for policies restricting access to clinical psychologists to cases referred by a physician and for ethical prohibitions on collaborating with chiropractors, podiatrists, and osteopathic physicians. In 2008, the FTC evaluated proposed laws in Massachusetts, Illinois, and Kentucky, finding that several provisions could be considered anticompetitive, including limits on advertising, differential cost sharing, more stringent physician supervision requirements, restrictions on clinic locations and physical configurations or proximity to other commercial ventures, and limits on the scope of professional services that can be provided that are not applicable to professionals with similar credentials who practice in similar "limited care settings" (for example, urgent care centers) (DeSanti et al., 2010; Ohlhausen et al., 2007, 2008). Likewise, the FTC initiated an administrative complaint against the North Carolina Board of Dental Examiners in June 2010 (FTC, 2010). The Board had prohibited nondentists from providing teeth-whitening services. The FTC alleged that by doing this the Board had hindered competition and made it more difficult and costly for consumers in the state to obtain this service.

As a payer and administrator of health insurance coverage for federal employees, the Office of Personnel Management (OPM) and the Federal Employees Health Benefits program have a responsibility to promote and ensure employee/subscriber access to the widest choice of competent, cost-effective health care providers. Principles of equity would suggest that this subscriber choice would be promoted by policies ensuring that full, evidence-based practice is permitted for all providers regardless of geographic location.

Finally, the Centers for Medicare and Medicaid Services (CMS) has the responsibility to promulgate rules and policies that promote access of Medicare and Medicaid beneficiaries to appropriate care. CMS therefore should ensure that its rules and polices reflect the evolving practice abilities of licensed providers, rather than relying on dated definitions drafted at a time when physicians were the only authorized providers of a wide array of health care services.

Expanding Scopes of Practice for Nurses

For several decades, the trend in the United States has been toward expansion of scope-of-practice regulations for APRNs, but this shift has been incremental and variable. Most recently, the move to expand the legal authority of all APRNs to provide health care that accords with their education, training, and competencies appears to be gathering momentum. In 2008, after 5 years of study, debate, and negotiation, a group of nursing accreditation, certification, and licensing organizations, along with several APRN groups, developed a consensus model for the education, training, and regulation of APRNs (see Appendix D). The stated goals of the APRN consensus process are to:

- "strive for harmony and common understanding in the APRN regulatory community that would continue to promote quality APRN education and practice;
- develop a vision for APRN regulation, including education, accreditation, certification, and licensure;
- establish a set of standards that protect the public, improve mobility, and improve access to safe, quality APRN care; and
- produce a written statement that reflects consensus on APRN regulatory issues" (see Appendix D).

The consensus document will help schools and programs across the United States standardize the education and preparation of APRNs. It will also help state regulators establish consistent practice acts because of education and certification standardization. And of importance, this document reflects the consensus of nursing organizations and leaders and accreditation and certification boards regarding the need to eliminate variations in scope-of-practice regulations across states and to adopt regulations that more fully recognize the competence of APRNs.

In March 2010, the board of directors of AARP concluded that statutory and regulatory barriers at the state and federal levels "are short-changing consumers." Acknowledging that nurses, particularly APRNs, can provide much of the care that Americans need and that barriers to their doing so must be lifted, the organization updated its policy on scope of practice. AARP states that "the policy change allows us to work together to ensure that our members and all health care consumers, especially in underserved settings such as urban and rural communities, have increased access to high quality care." The amended policy reads as follows:

> Current state nurse practice acts and accompanying rules should be interpreted and/or amended where necessary to allow APRNs to fully and independently practice as defined by their education and certification. (AARP, 2010a)

Meanwhile, after passage of the ACA, 28 states began considering expanding their scope-of-practice regulations for NPs (Johnson, 2010). Expanding the scope of practice for NPs is particularly important for the rural and frontier areas of the country. Twenty-five percent of the U.S. population lives in these areas; however, only 10 percent of physicians practice in these areas (NRHA, 2010). People who live in rural areas are generally poorer and have higher morbidity and mortality rates than their counterparts in suburban and urban settings, and they are in need of a reliable source of primary care providers (NRHA, 2010). The case study in Box 3-2, describing an NP in rural Iowa, demonstrates the benefits of a broad scope of practice with respect to the quality of and access to care.

Scope of Practice for Non-APRN Nurses

Generalist nurses are expanding their practices across all settings to meet the needs of patients. Expansions include procedure-based skills (involving, for example, IVs and cardiac outputs), as well as clinical judgment skills (e.g., taking health histories and performing physical examinations to develop a plan of nursing care). According to Djukic and Kovner (2010), there has been "no formal examination of the impact of RN role expansion on care cost or on physician and RN workload." The authors describe the expansion as a shifting of skills and activities, which in the long run, given the physician shortage, could free up physician resources, especially in long-term care, community health, and school-based health. On the other hand, given the projected nursing shortage, task shifting to overworked nurses could create unsafe patient care environments, especially in acute care hospitals. To avert this situation, nurses need to delegate to others, such as LPNs, nursing assistants, and community health workers, among others. A transformed nursing education system that is able to respond to changes in science and contextual factors, such as population demographics, will be able to incorporate needed new skills and support full scopes of practice for non-APRNs to meet the needs of patients (see Chapter 4).

Professional Resistance

Increasing access to care by expanding state scope-of-practice regulations so they accord with the education and competency of APRNs is a critical and controversial topic. Practice boundaries are constantly changing with the emergence of new technologies, evolving patient expectations, and workforce issues. Yet the movement to expand scopes of practice is not supported by some professional medical organizations. Professional tensions surrounding practice boundaries are not limited to nurses and physicians, but show a certain continuity across many disciplines. Psychiatrists and psychologists have been disagreeing about prescriptive privileges for more than two decades (Daly, 2007). In the dental field, one new role, the advanced dental hygiene practitioner, functions under a broadened scope similar to that of an APRN. The American Dental Association does not

BOX 3-2
Case Study: Advanced Practice Registered Nurses

Promoting Access to Care in Rural Iowa

The passage of the Affordable Care Act will give millions of Americans better access to primary care—if there are enough providers. The United States has a shortage of primary care physicians, especially in rural areas, but Alison Mitchell, president of Texas Nurse Practitioners, told the *Dallas Morning News* in April 2010 that nurse practitioners (NPs) are ready to step in: "We would be happy to help in the trenches and be primary care providers." Many states are considering ways to permit NPs to function in this capacity with fewer restrictions (AP, 2010).

In 2001, 23 percent of NPs in the United States worked in rural areas and almost 41 percent in urban communities, where most provided primary care services to underserved populations (Hooker and Berlin, 2002). The NP's scope of practice is governed by state laws and regulations that differ in their requirements for physician supervision and prescriptive authority—the ability to prescribe medications. In rural communities, NPs may be the only available primary care providers, and it is important that they be able to practice independently, if need be, although they value collaboration with physicians and other providers regardless of state authorization.

Iowa is one of 22 states where advanced practice registered nurse (APRNs)—NPs, certified nurse midwives, certified registered nurse anesthetists (CRNAs), and clinical nurse specialists—practice without physi-

cian oversight and one of 12 states that permit them to prescribe without restriction (Phillips, 2010). Iowa's APRNs must be nationally certified in their specialty; meet state requirements for continuing education; provide evidence of their education; and collaborate with a physician on "medically delegated tasks," such as circumcision and hospital admission. Several studies have shown that APRNs produce outcomes comparable to those of physicians and that the care they provide encompasses 80 to 90 percent of the services provided by physicians (Lenz et al., 2004; Mundinger et al., 2000; Office of Technology Assessment, 1986).

A qualified health care professional is a terrible thing to waste.

—*Cheryll Jones, BSN, ARNP, BC, CPNP, pediatric NP, Ottumwa, Iowa*

One pediatric NP in Ottumwa, Iowa, has worked to remove barriers faced by APRNs for more than three decades. Cheryll Jones, BSN, ARNP, BC, CPNP, said that permitting all nurses to practice to the fullest extent of their education has been essential to improving access to care for rural Iowans. Iowa's gains have been realized largely through regulations rather than through incremental changes to the state's nurse practice act, as has been the case in other states. Ms. Jones attributes those successes to the diligence of Iowa nurses and others interested in promoting access to care, who:

- emphasized the issue of access to care for rural and disadvantaged populations;
- ensured that policy makers knew what APRNs do (Ms. Jones invited legislators to her clinic);
- promoted unity among Iowa nursing groups and with organizations such as the Iowa Hospital Association; and
- partnered with leaders, such as former Iowa governor Tom Vilsack (now U.S. secretary of agriculture), the first governor to opt out of Medicare's requirement that the state's CRNAs be supervised by physicians.

Evidence that it is safe to remove restrictions on APRNs comes from an annual review of state laws and regulations governing APRNs that now includes malpractice claims in its analysis. The 2010 *Pearson Report* documents no increase in claims registered in the Healthcare Integrity and Protection Data Bank in states where APRNs have full authority to practice and prescribe independently. The report also notes that the overall ratio of claims against NPs is 1 for every 166 NPs in the nation, compared with 1 for every 4 physicians (Pearson, 2010).

In June 2010 President Barack Obama addressed the House of Delegates of the American Nurses Association to announce "a number of investments to expand the primary care workforce." These included increased funding for NP students and for nurse- and NP-run clinics— two important steps, the President said, in "a larger effort to make our system work better for nurses and for doctors, and to improve the quality of care for patients" (White House, 2010).

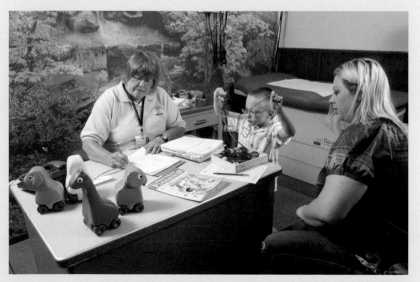

Susan McClellen, University of Iowa

A mother brings her son for an appointment with nurse practitioner Cheryll Jones, who provides high-quality care in the rural community of Ottumwa, IA.

recognize this new type of practitioner as an independent clinician, but mandates that all dental teams be headed by a professional dentist (Fox, 2010). Likewise, physical therapists are challenging traditional scope-of-practice boundaries established by chiropractors (Huijbregts, 2007).

Physician Challenges to Expanded Scope of Practice

The AMA has consistently issued resolutions, petitions, and position papers supporting opposition to state efforts to expand the scope of practice for professional groups other than physicians.[17] The AMA's Citizens Petition, submitted to the Health Care Financing Administration in June 2000, and the AMA-sponsored Scope of Practice Partnership (SOPP), announced in January 2006, both focused on opposing scope-of-practice expansion. The SOPP in particular, an alliance of the AMA and six medical specialty organizations, was an effort on the part of organized medicine to oppose boundary expansion and to defeat proposed legislation in several states to expand scope of practice for allied health care providers, including nurses (Croasdale, 2006; Cys, 2000).

The SOPP, with the assistance of a special full-time legislative attorney hired for the purpose, spearheaded several projects designed to obstruct expansion of scopes of practice for nurses and others. These projects included comparisons between the medical profession and specific allied health professions on education standards, certification programs, and disciplinary processes; development of evidence to discredit access-to-care arguments made by various allied health professionals, particularly in rural areas of a state; and identification of the locations of physicians by specialty to counter claims of a lack of physicians in certain areas (Cady, 2006). One of the policies pursued by the SOPP is the AMA's 2006 resolution H-35.988,[18] Independent Practice of Medicine by "Nurse Practitioners." This resolution opposes any legislation allowing the independent practice of medicine by individuals who have not completed state requirements to practice medicine.

The AMA has released a set of 10 documents for members of state medical associations to help them explain "to regulators and legislators the limitations in the education and training of non-physician providers" (AMA, 2009). One of these, the *AMA Scope of Practice Data Series: Nurse Practitioners*, uses the term "limited licensure health care providers." The document argues that these providers—NPs—seek scope-of practice expansions that may be harmful to the public (AMA, 2009). Other organizations, such as the American Society of Anesthesiologists and the American Association of Family Physicians (AAFP), have also issued statements that do not support nurses practicing to their fullest

[17] See for example, AMA. 2000. Res. H-360.988. "Nurse Practitioner Reimbursement Under Medicare"; AMA. 2000. H.D. Res. H-160.947, Physician Assistants and Nurse Practitioners."

[18] AMA. 2006. Res. H-35.988, "Independent Practice of Medicine by 'Nurse Practitioners'."

ability (ASA, 2004), although the AAFP supports nurses and physicians working together in collaborative teams (Phillips et al., 2001). The AAFP recently released a press packet—a "nurse practitioner information kit."[19] The kit includes a set of five papers and a new piece of legislation "clarifying" why NPs cannot substitute for physicians in primary care, although as Medicare and Medicaid data show, they already are doing so. There are also new guidelines on how to supervise CNMs, NPs, and physician assistants. The AAFP notes that its new proposed legislation, the Health Care Truth and Transparency Act of 2010, "ensures that patients receive accurate health care information by prohibiting misleading and deceptive advertising or representation of health care professionals' credentials and training." The legislation is also endorsed by 13 other physician groups.

Action has been taken at the state level as well. For example, in 2010, the California Medical Association (CMA) and the California Society of Anesthesiologists (CSA) sued the state of California after Governor Schwarzenegger decided to opt out of a Medicare provision requiring physician supervision of CRNAs (Sorbel, 2010). At the time of release of this report, the case had not yet been heard.

Reasons for Physician Resistance

The CMA and CSA both cited patient safety as the reason for protesting the governor's decision—although evidence shows that CRNAs provide high-quality care to California citizens, there is no evidence of patient harm from their practice, and 14 other states have taken similar opt out actions (Sorbel, 2010). A study by Dulisse and Cromwell (2010) found no increase in inpatient mortality or complications in states that opted out of the CMS requirement that an anesthesiologist or surgeon oversee the administration of anesthesia by a CRNA. As noted earlier in this chapter, the contention that APRNs are less able than physicians to deliver care that is safe, effective, and efficient is not supported by research that has examined this question (Brown and Grimes, 1995; Fairman, 2008; Groth et al., 2010; Hatem et al., 2008; Hogan et al., 2010; Horrocks et al., 2002; Hughes et al., 2010; Laurant et al., 2004; Mundinger et al., 2000; Office of Technology Assessment, 1986).

Some physician organizations argue that nurses should not be allowed to expand their scope of practice, citing medicine's unique education, clinical knowledge, and cognitive and technical skills. Opposition to this expansion is particularly strong with regard to prescriptive practice. However, evidence does not support an association between a physician's type and length of preparation and the ability to prescribe correctly and accurately or the quality of care (Fairman, 2008). Similar questions have been raised about the content of nursing education (see the discussion of nursing curricula in Chapter 4).

---

[19] See http://www.aafp.org/online/en/home/media/kits/fp-np.html.

Support for Expanded Scope of Practice for Nurse Practitioners

Some individual physicians support expanded scope of practice for NPs. The Robert Wood Johnson Foundation Nursing Research Network (described in Appendix A) conducted a survey of 100 physician members of the online physician site Sermo.com[20] and found that more than 50 percent of respondents agreed either somewhat or strongly that "allowing NPs to practice independently would increase access to primary care in the U.S." (RWJF, 2010e). As Figure 3-4 shows, however, physicians were more skeptical that expanding NPs' scope of practice in this way would decrease costs, and they feared a decrease in average quality of care provided to patients.

In addition to support for expanded scope of practice for NPs among some physicians, public support for NP practice is indicated by satisfaction ratings for retail-based health clinics. Approximately 95 percent of providers in these clinics are NPs, with the remaining 5 percent comprising physician assistants and some physicians.[21] According to a survey of U.S. adults by the Wall Street Journal.com/ Harris Interactive (Harris Interactive, 2008), almost all respondents who had used a retail-based health clinic (313 total) were very or somewhat satisfied with the quality of care, cost, and staff qualifications (see Figure 3-5). Such public support can be backed up with high-quality clinical outcomes (Mehrotra et al., 2008).

Despite opposition by some physicians and specialty societies, the strong trend over the past 20 years has been a growing receptivity on the part of state legislatures to expanded scopes of practice for nurses. There simply are not enough primary care physicians to care for an aging population now, and their patient load will dramatically increase as more people gain access to care. For example, in 2007 Pennsylvania Governor Edward Rendell announced a blueprint for reform, known as Prescription for Pennsylvania (Rx for PA), to promote access to care for the state's residents and reduce health care expenses (see the case study in Chapter 5). One initiative under Rx for PA was expanding the legal scope of practice for physician assistants, APRNs, CNSs, CNMs, and dental hygienists. This initiative has had an important impact on access to care. Outcome data after the first year of Rx for PA show an increase in the number of people with diabetes receiving eye and foot examinations and a doubling of the number of children with asthma who have a plan in place for controlling exacerbations (Pennsylvania Governor's Office, 2009).

The experience of states that have led these changes offers important reas-

---

[20] Sermo.com respondents are all members of the online community sermo.com. Sermo.com members are distributed across age, gender, geography, and specialty groups in patterns that mimic those of the U.S. population. For this study, respondents were randomly recruited to participate in the IOM survey activity via e-mail; others were allowed to join the survey by volunteering when they visited the site. The majority of respondents have specialties in cardiology (6 percent), family medicine (35 percent), internal medicine (26 percent), and oncology (4 percent). The remaining physicians surveyed are distributed across a wide range of specialties.

[21] Personal communication, Tine Hansen-Turton, CEO, National Nursing Centers Consortium, and Vice President, Public Health Management Corporation, August 6, 2010.

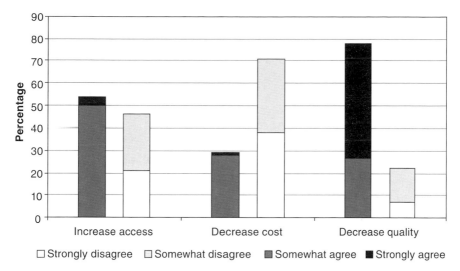

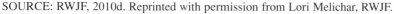

FIGURE 3-4 Physician opinions about the impact of allowing nurse practitioners to practice independently.
SOURCE: RWJF, 2010d. Reprinted with permission from Lori Melichar, RWJF.

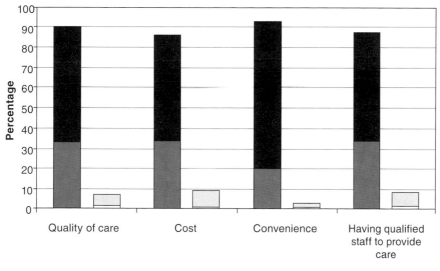

FIGURE 3-5 Patient satisfaction with retail-based health clinics.
NOTES: Question asked: Overall, how satisfied were you with your or your family member's experience using an onsite health clinic in a pharmacy or retail chain on the following items?
Percentages may not add up to 100 because of the small percentage not included here that chose "not sure."
SOURCE: Harris Interactive, 2008.

surance to physicians who continue to believe that patient care may be adversely affected, or that expanded nursing practice autonomy threatens the professional and economic roles of physicians. States with broader nursing scopes of practice have experienced no deterioration of patient care. In fact, patient satisfaction with the role of APRNs is very high. Nor has expansion of nursing scopes of practice diminished the critical role of physicians in patient care or physician income (Darves, 2007). With regard to the quality of care and the role of physicians, it is difficult to distinguish states with restrictive and more expanded scopes of practice. Finally, the committee believes that the new medical home concept, based on professional collaboration, represents a perfect opportunity for nurses and physicians to work together for the good of patient care in their community.

Fragmentation of the Health Care System

The U.S. health care system is characterized by a high degree of fragmentation across many sectors, which raises substantial barriers to building value. A fragmented health care system is characterized by weak connections among multiple component parts. Fragmentation makes simple tasks—such as assigning responsibility for payment—much more difficult than they need to be, while more complex tasks—such as coordination of home health care, family support, transportation, and social services after a hospital stay—become more difficult because they require following many separate sets of often contradictory rules. As a result, people may simply give up trying rather than take advantage of the services to which they are entitled. An examination of fragmentation in hospital services explores its origins in American pluralism, historical accident, and the hybridization of business and charity (Stevens, 1999). A review by Cebul and colleagues identifies three broad areas of fragmentation: (1) the U.S. health insurance system; (2) the provision of care; and (3) the inability of health information systems to allow a "seamless flow of information between hospitals, providers and insurers" (Cebul et al., 2008).

In the United States, there is a disconnect between public and private services, between providers and patients, between what patients need and how providers are trained, between the health needs of the nation and the services that are offered, and between those with insurance and those without (Stevens, 1999). Communication between providers is difficult, and care is redundant because there is no means of sharing results. For example, a patient with diabetes covered by Medicaid may have difficulty finding a physician to help him control his blood sugar. If he is able to find a physician, that individual may not have admitting privileges at the hospital to which the patient is transported after a hypoglycemic reaction. After the patient has been admitted to the emergency room, a new cadre of physicians is responsible for him but has no information about previous blood sugar determinations, other medications he is taking, or other health problems. The patient is stabilized and a discharge is arranged, but he is ineligible under his insurance plan for reimbursement for the further education in diet and glucose control, materials (such as a glucometer), and referral to an ophthalmologist that are indicated. Home follow-up is needed, but the visiting nurse agency is certified to provide only two visits when the patient could use five. No one calls the initial primary care physician to share discharge planning or information, and no one gives the patient a summary of the visit to take to that physician. The ophthalmologist will not accept the patient because of his status as a Medicaid recipient. A major challenge to repairing this fragmentation lies in the fee-for-service structure of the payment system, which indiscriminately rewards increasing volume of services regardless of whether it improves health outcomes or provides greater value (MedPAC, 2006).

Effect of Fragmentation on Realizing the Value of Nurses

Within this system, the contributions of nursing are doubly hidden. Accounting systems of most hospitals and health care organizations are not designed to capture or differentiate the economic value provided by nurses. Thus, all nursing care is treated equally in its effect on revenue. A 2007 review of 100 demonstration projects that provided incentives for high-value care to hospitals and physicians found no examples that specifically delineated or rewarded nurses' contributions (Kurtzman et al., 2008). Yet nurses' work is estimated to vary by 15 to 40 percent for any given diagnosis-related group (Laport et al., 2008). The effect on the provision of health care is difficult to document, but a closer look at staffing ratios suggests some of the consequences. Generally speaking, as an analysis by the Lewin Group concludes, because health care facilities cannot capture the full economic value of the services nurses provide, they have an economic incentive—whether they decide to heed it or not—to staff their organizations "at levels below where the benefit to society equals the cost to employ an additional nurse" (Dall et al., 2009).

Barriers to measuring and realizing the economic value generated by nurses exist outside the hospital setting as well. In many states, APRNs are not paid directly but must be reimbursed through the physician with whom they have a collaboration agreement. Payments are funneled through the physician provider number, and the nurse is salaried.

For years, professional nursing organizations have sought to counter the inequitable aspects of the fee-for-service payment system by lobbying to increase the types of services for which NPs can independently bill Medicare, Medicaid, and other providers. They have had some success in that regard in the past (Sullivan-Marx, 2008). However, according to Mark McClellan and Gail Wilensky, both former directors of CMS, this approach has become a losing proposition. As McClellan and Wilensky testified to the committee in September 2009, while fee-for-service is not going to disappear any time soon, its future is severely limited in any sustainable health care system.

Proposals to Address Fragmentation

Alternative proposals for financing the health care system have coalesced around the idea of providing "global payments" that are shared among a predetermined group of providers, such as hospitals, physicians, nurses, social workers, nutritionists, and other professionals, and "bundled payments" that are linked to a single episode of care, such as treatment of and recovery from a heart attack. A full exploration of all the benefits and caveats of such alternative payment proposals is beyond the scope of this report. However, as the Medicare Payment Advisory Commission (MedPAC) noted in its June 2008 report to Congress, "[b]undling payment raises a range of implementation issues because under bundled payment the entity accepting the payment—rather than Medicare—has discretion in the amount it pays providers for care provided, whether to pay for services not now covered by Medicare, and how it rewards providers for reducing costs and improving quality" (MedPAC, 2008). It will be up to the entity accepting payment to determine how and indeed whether to valuate nurses' contributions. Yet the tendency of human nature is to follow the practices and behaviors with which one is most familiar. Without the presence of nurses in decision-making positions in these new entities, the legacy of undervaluing nurses, characteristic of the fee-for-service system, will carry over into whatever new payment schemes are adopted. The services of nurses must be properly and transparently valued so that their contributions can fully benefit the entire system.

Outdated Policies of Insurance Companies

As noted in Chapter 2, many NPs and CNMs have cared for underserved populations that are either uninsured or rely on Medicaid. Expanding their services to the private insurance market is another matter altogether. The health care reform experience of Massachusetts shows the extent to which corporate policy can negate government regulation. An estimated 5,600 NPs work in Massachusetts (Pearson, 2010), falling under the authority of the Commonwealth's Board of Nursing as well as its Board of Medicine. NPs are required to collaborate with a physician and may prescribe drugs only under a written collaborative agreement with a physician (Christian et al., 2007). The law allows them to act as primary care providers (PCPs), and the Massachusetts Medicaid program formally named NPs as PCPs.

Despite the shortage of PCPs that occurred after the Massachusetts legislature enacted health care reform in 2006, no private insurance companies listed NPs as PCPs in Massachusetts. As a matter of policy, one major New England carrier stated that it would not list NPs as PCPs unless required to do so by the legislature. This same carrier, however, listed NPs as PCPs in its service directories for the neighboring states of New Hampshire and Maine. Eventually, Massachusetts passed a second health care reform law in 2008 that amended the state's insurance regulations to recognize NPs as PCPs in the private as well as the public market. Massachusetts was thereby able to expand the supply of its PCPs without changing its scope-of-practice laws (Craven and Ober, 2009). The policy differences among states may have to do with different scope-of-practice regulations or differences in the states' insurance industries. There is some evidence that insurers are more likely to recognize NPs as PCPs in states where NPs have independent practice authority (Hansen-Turton et al., 2008).

The actions of private insurance companies toward APRNs are having an effect on government-funded programs as well. Nurse-managed health centers (NMHCs) have long provided care for populations served by Medicare, Medicaid, and children's health insurance programs. However, federal and state governments are increasingly turning to the private sector to manage these programs (Hansen-Turton et al., 2006). The insurance companies' continued policy of not credentialing and/or recognizing NPs as PCPs—and the federal government's refusal to mandate that they do so—creates a barrier for NMHCs as they seek to continue serving these populations (Hansen-Turton et al., 2006).

One specific model of the medical/health home—the Patient-Centered Medical Home™ (PCMH)—does not permit management by nurses. In other words, a nurse may manage an organization that in every way adheres to the principles of PCMHs, but the practice will not be recognized as a PCMH by NCQA, a "not-for-profit organization dedicated to improving health care quality" (NCQA, 2010). Without public recognition, nurse-led medical/health homes cannot qualify for insurance reimbursement, which in turn leaves substantial populations underserved. NCQA, which administers the recognition for the medical homes, is a physician-dominated organization receiving its member dues from physicians. Its board, although currently reconsidering its stance on whether NPs can lead medical homes, has decided that physicians are more able to serve in PCMH leadership positions. The original concept for the medical home came from physicians, and NCQA adopted their principles of operation.[22] Several state agencies have contacted NCQA to request that it recognize NPs' ability to lead PCMHs. NCQA has appointed an advisory committee to review the policy that medical homes must be physician led. Meanwhile, the Joint Commission is developing a competitive certification program that will allow for leadership by NPs.[23]

High Turnover Rates

As the health care system undergoes transformation, it will be imperative that patients have highly competent nurses who are adept at caring for them across all settings. It will be just as important that the system have enough nurses at any

---

[22] Personal communication, Greg Pawlson, Executive Vice President, NCQA, January 5, 2010.

[23] Personal communication, Greg Pawlson, Executive Vice President, NCQA, January 5, 2010.

given time. Both having enough nurses and having the right kind of highly skilled nurses will contribute to the overall safety and quality of a transformed system. Although the committee did not focus solely on the upcoming shortage of nurses, it did devote time to considering how to retain experienced nurses and faculty.

Some solutions have been researched, proposed, and reproposed for so long that it is difficult to understand why they have not yet been implemented more widely. High turnover rates continue to destabilize the nurse workforce in the United States and other countries (Hayes et al., 2006). Figure 3-6 indicates some of the reasons that have been cited for not working in the nursing profession. For nurses under 50, personal or family reasons were most frequently cited.

The costs associated with high turnover rates are significant, particularly in hospitals and nursing homes (Aiken and Cheung, 2008). The literature shows that the workplace environment plays a major role in nurse turnover rates (Hayes et al., 2006; Tai et al., 1998; Yin and Yang, 2002). Staff shortages, increasing work-

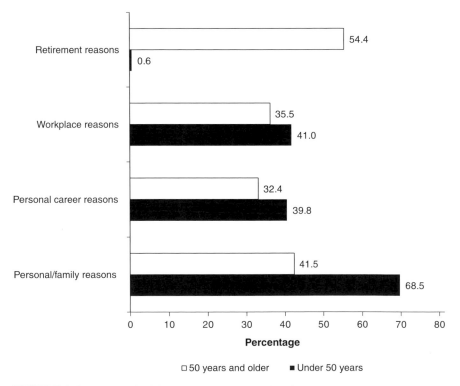

FIGURE 3-6 Reasons cited for not working in nursing, by age group.
NOTES: Percents do not add to 100 because registered nurses may have provided more than one reason. Includes only RNs who are not working in nursing.
SOURCE: HRSA, 2010.

loads, inefficient work and technology processes, and the absence of effective pathways for nurses to propose and implement improvements all have a negative impact on job satisfaction and contribute to the decision to leave. Tables 3-3 and 3-4, respectively, show the intentions of nurses with regard to their employment situation (e.g., plan to leave current job) and the percentage of nurses who left their job in 2007–2008, by setting. New research has also highlighted the contribution to the problem of disruptive behavior—ranging from verbal abuse to physical assault or sexual harassment of nurses, often by physicians but also by other nurses (Rosenstein and O'Daniel, 2005, 2008). For more than a quarter century, blue ribbon commissions and policy experts have concluded that widereaching changes in nurses' practice environments would significantly reduce their high turnover rates and improve productivity (Aiken and Cheung, 2008).

Many individual facilities and programs have adopted those recommenda-

TABLE 3-3 Plans Regarding Nursing Employment, by Graduation Cohort, 2008

Plans	Graduated before 2001 (%)	Graduated 2001–2008 (%)
Plans regarding current position		
No plans to leave job	57.8	42.8
Undecided about plans	15.1	17.8
Have left job or plan to leave in 12 months	14.5	23.2
Plan to leave in 1 to 3 years	12.6	16.2
Total that plan to leave within 3 years	27.1	39.3
For those who plan to leave their job		
Plan to remain in nursing work	77.9	96.7
Plan to leave nursing	22.1	3.3

SOURCE: HRSA, 2010.

TABLE 3-4 Changes in Position Setting, by 2007 Setting, for Registered Nurses Who Graduated in 2001–2008

Setting in 2007	Percent Who Left Setting Between 2007 and 2008
Hospital	11.1
Nursing home/extended care	25.8
Home health	21.2
Public/community health	23.2
Ambulatory care	20.8
Other	18.9

NOTES: Public/community health includes school health and occupational health. Other settings include academic education and insurance/benefits/utilization review.
SOURCE: HRSA, 2010.

tions. Much of the data showing the impact of reducing turnover by focusing on workplace environment comes from the acute care setting. Nonetheless, these data are instructive in their demonstration of a triple win: improving the workplace environment reduces nurse turnover, lowers costs, and improves health outcomes of patients. For example, the Transforming Care at the Bedside (TCAB) initiative is a national program that engages nurses to lead process improvement efforts so as to improve health outcomes for patients, reduce costs, and improve nurse retention (Bolton and Aronow, 2009). TCAB relies on nurses developing small tests of change that are continuously planned, assessed, and rapidly adopted or dropped, with each round building on previous successes. According to Bolton and Aronow (2009), as the TCAB principles and locally proposed and tested interventions spread throughout Cedars-Sinai Hospital, administrators noted the emergence of "a culture that emphasizes performance improvement and value-adding activities on nursing units." Physician–nurse rounding, physician–nurse education teams, recognition programs, and collaborative efforts of nursing staff with other, non-nursing departments were the major reason, the authors believe, behind a decrease in nurse turnover rates from 7 percent in 2004 to 3 percent in 2008.

Some employers have also discovered that making it easier for nurses to obtain advanced degrees while continuing to work has increased retention rates. Chapter 4 includes an example of this phenomenon from the Carondelet Health Network in Tucson, Arizona. Based on workforce data Carondelet regularly collects for use in its strategic planning, the network has concluded that its educational efforts have had a positive effect on recruiting and retention. Its percentage of staff (as opposed to contract) nurses has increased from 81.7 to 89.2 percent. Because so many newly graduated nurses have begun seeking work at Carondelet, the average age of its staff nurses fell from 50 years in 2004 to 45.2 years in 2007 (The Lewin Group, 2009).

Difficulties of Transition to Practice

High turnover rates among newly graduated nurses highlight the need for a greater focus on managing the transition from school to practice (Kovner et al., 2007). Some turnover is to be expected—and is even appropriate if new nurses discover they are not really suited to the care setting or employer they have chosen. However, some entry-level nurses who leave first-time hospital jobs leave the profession entirely, a situation that needs to be avoided when possible. In a 2007 survey of entry-level nurses, those who had already left their first job cited reasons such as poor management, stress, and a desire for experience in a different clinical area (Kovner et al., 2007).

In 2002, the Joint Commission recommended the development of nurse residency programs—planned, comprehensive periods of time during which nursing graduates can acquire the knowledge and skills to deliver safe, quality care that meets defined (organization or professional society) standards of practice. This recommendation was most recently endorsed by the 2009 Carnegie study on the nursing profession (Benner et al., 2009). Versant[24] and other organizations have launched successful transition-to-practice residency programs for nurses in recent years, while the University HealthSystem Consortium (UHC) and the American Association of Colleges of Nursing (AACN) have developed a model for postbaccalaureate nurse residencies (Goode and Williams, 2004; Krugman et al., 2006; Williams et al., 2007). The residency model developed by the UHC/AACN addresses needs identified by new nursing graduates and organizations that employ them. These needs included developing skills in ways to organize work and establish priorities; communicate with physicians, other professionals as well as patients and their families. In addition, nurses and employers indicated the need for nurses to develop leadership and technical skills in order to provide quality care (Beecroft et al., 2001, 2004; Halfer and Graf, 2006). As an example, in one hospital, the total cost for a residency program is $93,100, with a cost per resident of $2,023.91. Given that the average cost of replacing just one new graduate RN is $45,000, a return on investment can be significantly dependent on a reduction in RN turnover (AAN, 2010a).

The AACN has also adopted accreditation standards for these programs (AACN, 2008). Meanwhile, the National Council of State Boards of Nursing, after reviewing the evidence in favor of nursing residencies, has developed a regulatory model for transition-to-practice programs, recommending that state boards of nursing enforce a transition program through licensure (NCSBN, 2008).

Residencies Outside of Acute Care

Residency programs are supported predominantly in hospitals and larger health systems, with a focus on acute care. This has been the area of greatest need since most new graduates gain employment in acute care settings, and the proportion of new hires (and nursing staff) that are new graduates is rapidly increasing (Kovner et al., 2007). It is essential, however, that residency programs outside of acute care settings be developed and evaluated. Chapter 2 documents the demographic changes on the horizon; the shift of care from hospital to community-based settings; and the need for nursing expertise in chronic illness management, care of older adults in home settings, and transitional services. In this context, nurses need to be prepared for new roles outside of the acute care setting.

---

[24] Versant is a nonprofit organization that provides, supervises, and evaluates nurse transition-to-practice residency programs for children's and general acute care hospitals. See http://www.versant.org/item.asp?id=35.

It follows that new types of residency programs appropriate for these types of roles need to be developed.[25]

Several community care organizations are already acting on their own perceived need for a residency-type program lasting 3 months or longer for new employees. At the Visiting Nurse Services of New York, nurses receive a great deal of education and training on the job. New nurses with a bachelor's degree participate in an internship that provides hands-on experience and mentoring from experienced staff that prepares them for home-based nursing. "We really have to do a lot of our own education and training to compensate for the fact that most of the nurses don't come with the experience, the competencies, or the comfort and confidence with technology that we think they need," said Carol Raphael, the organization's president and CEO (IOM, 2010a).

There are a few successful transition-to-practice initiatives in the field of public health, although they are commonly called internships, orientations, or mentoring programs. For example, the North Carolina State Health Department has begun a pilot effort with four public health departments in an effort to educate new nurses about population-based health. The 6-month mentoring program is being used as a recruitment and retention tool and has very explicit objectives, including an increase in retention and understanding of population health and a willingness to serve as a mentor as the program goes forward.[26] Another successful community-based transition-to-practice program, called LEAP (Linking Education and Practice for Excellence in Public Health Nursing), was recently demonstrated in Milwaukee Wisconsin. Two public health departments and three community health centers not only collaborated to diversify the nurses entering public and community health settings, but also offered them paid traineeships to transition into their settings. The public health departments partnered with the Wisconsin Center for Nursing and a collaborative of five baccalaureate schools of nursing to first boost the community health curriculum in those schools and then help with the development of the internship upon graduation for 17 nurses. The program has been successful in recruiting more minorities into community and public health settings with the knowledge they need to practice successfully outside of the acute care setting. Financial support was secured from a variety of sources, including foundations, corporations, and partnership members themselves. The program is new and is currently undergoing an evaluation to deter-

---

[25] This paragraph draws on a paper commissioned by the committee on "Transforming Pre-licensure Nursing Education: Preparing the New Nurse to Meet Emerging Health Care Needs," prepared by Christine A. Tanner, Oregon Health & Science University School of Nursing (see Appendix I on CD-ROM).

[26] Personal communication, Joy Reed, Head, Public Health Nursing for the NC Division of Public Health, August 24, 2010.

mine its financial sustainability.[27] Such programs are not widespread, however, and need to be.

Evidence in Support of Residencies

Much of the evidence supporting the success of residencies has been produced through self-evaluations by the residency programs themselves. For example, Versant has demonstrated a profound reduction in turnover rates for new graduate RNs—from 35 to 6 percent at 12 months and from 55 to 11 percent at 24 months—compared with new graduate RN control groups hired at a facility prior to implementation of the residency program (Versant, 2010). Other research suggests residencies may be useful to help new graduates transition into practice settings (Goode et al., 2009; Krozek, 2008).

The UHC/AACN nurse residency program described above also reports reduced rates of turnover and cites cost savings to its participants. According to the UHC (2009) and AACN,[28] since 2002 the program:

- saved participating organizations over $6 million per year on the costs of turnover for a first-year nurse (the cost to recruit and retain a replacement nurse was estimated at $88,000);
- increased its retention rate from 87 percent in 2004 to 94 percent in 2009;
- increased stability in staffing levels, thereby reducing stress, improving morale, increasing efficiency, and promoting safety;
- achieved a return on investment of up to 14:1; and
- helped first-year nurses in the program achieve the following:
  - develop their ability in clinical decision making,
  - develop clinical autonomy in providing patient care,
  - incorporate research-based evidence into their practices, and
  - increase commitment to nursing as a career.

The committee focused its attention on residencies for newly licensed RNs because these residencies have been most studied. Looking forward, however, the committee acknowledges the need for RNs with more experience to take part in residency programs as well. Such programs may be necessary to help nurses transition from, for example, the acute care to the community setting. As a growing number of nurses pursue advanced practice degrees immediately after receiving a bachelor's degree—with no break between for employment in

---

[27] See http://pindev.forumone.com/faye-mcbeath-foundation-with-greater-milwaukee-foundation-northwestern-mutual-foundation-wisconsin-2/.

[28] This section also draws on a June 2010 personal communication with Geraldine Bednash, CEO, AACN.

a clinical setting—the benefit to APRNs of completing a residency is likely to grow as well. The committee believes that regardless of where the residency takes place—whether in the acute care setting or the community—nurses should be paid a salary, although the committee does not take a position on whether this should be a full or reduced salary. Loan repayment and educational debt should be postponed during residency, especially if a reduced salary is offered.

At the committee's December 2009 Forum on the Future of Nursing: Care in the Community, Margaret Flinter, vice president and clinical director, Community Health Center, Inc., spoke about her organization's decision to develop nurse residency programs for APRNs. The intensity and demands of providing service in the complex setting of a federally qualified health center (FQHC), Flinter testified, often discourage newly graduated NPs from joining an FQHC and the clinics from hiring newly graduated NPs. In 2006, she continued, her organization started the country's first formal NP residency training program. The goal was to ensure that new NPs would find the training and transition support they needed to be successful as PCPs. The program is a 12-month, full-time, intensive residency that provides extensive precepting, specialty rotations, and additional didactic education in the high-risk/high-burden problems commonly seen in FQHCs. The NP residents are trained in a chronic care/planned care approach that features both prevention and chronic disease management, advance access to eliminate waits and delays, integrated behavioral health and primary care, and expert use of the electronic health record. In Flinter's view and that of her organization, the initial year of residency training is essential to transitioning a new NP into a fully accountable PCP (Flinter, 2009). And indeed, the ACA allocates $200 million from 2012 to 2015 as part of a demonstration project that will pay hospitals for the costs of clinical training to prepare APRNs with the skills necessary to provide primary and preventive care, transitional care, chronic care management, and other nursing services appropriate for the Medicare population.

Residency provides a continuing opportunity to apply important knowledge for the purpose of remaining a safe and competent provider in a continuous learning environment. Paying for residencies is a challenge, but the committee believes that funds received from Medicare can be used to help with these costs. In 2006, about half of all Medicare nursing funding went to five states that have the most hospital-based diploma nursing programs (Aiken et al., 2009). The diploma programs in these states directly benefit from receiving these funds. Most states, however, and most hospitals do not receive Medicare funding for nursing education. The committee believes it would be more equitable to spread these funds more widely and use it for residency programs that would be valuable for all nurses across the country.

Demographic Challenges

As discussed in Chapter 2, the population of the United States is growing older and is becoming increasingly diverse in terms of race, ethnicity, and language. To achieve the goal of increasing access to high-quality, culturally relevant care among the diverse populations in the United States, the nursing profession must increase its appeal to young people, men, and nonwhite racial/ ethnic groups.

An Aging Workforce

Like the U.S. population, the nurse workforce continues to grow older. Over the past three decades, there has been a profound shift in the age composition of nurses. In 1983, approximately 50 percent (596,000 full-time equivalents [FTEs]) of the workforce was between the ages of 20 and 34, while only 17 percent (202,000 FTEs) was over the age of 50. Since the 1980s, the number of FTEs in the nursing workforce has doubled, and there has been a dramatic increase in the number of middle-aged and older RNs. From 1983 to 2009, the number of nurses over age 50 more than quadrupled, and the number of middle-aged nurses (aged 35–49) doubled to approximately 39 percent (977,000). These older and middle-aged nurses now represent almost three-quarters of the nursing workforce, while nurses younger than 34 now make up only 26 percent (Buerhaus et al., 2009a). Figure 3-7 shows the age shift in the nursing workforce that has occurred over the past two decades.

The figure shows that since 1980, the nursing workforce has grown older, as reflected by more RNs reporting that they fall within the older age categories with each successive survey. At the same time, the figure indicates that in both 2004 and especially 2008, the number of young RNs in the workforce was growing relative to earlier years. This increase may reflect, in part, the impact of the John-son & Johnson Campaign for Nursing's Future, which launched a large national media initiative in 2002 aimed at attracting people into nursing. As other similar recruitment initiatives followed, more, younger people chose to become nurses, reversing a 20-year trend of declining entry into nursing by young people.

The shift in the age composition of the nursing workforce can be attributed in part to the large number of baby boomers who became RNs in the 1970s and 1980s, followed by much smaller cohorts in the later decades (Buerhaus et al., 2009a). These smaller cohorts were a result of not only the decrease in births, but also a decrease in interest in the profession during the 1980s and 1990s when women began entering other professions that had typically been dominated by men (Staiger et al., 2000). The physician workforce has also been aging, but in much smaller numbers. Figure 3-8 compares the average age of nurses with vary-ing levels of education with that of physicians and physician faculty. Between 2001 and 2009, the number of physicians aged 50–64 grew by 77,000 FTEs, while the number of RNs in that same age group grew by almost five times as many (368,000 FTEs) (Staiger et al., 2009). Compared with the size of the nurs-ing workforce, however, the size of the physician workforce is less dependent on interest in profession. The supply of physicians is influenced more by institutional factors that govern the number of available slots in medical schools and residency

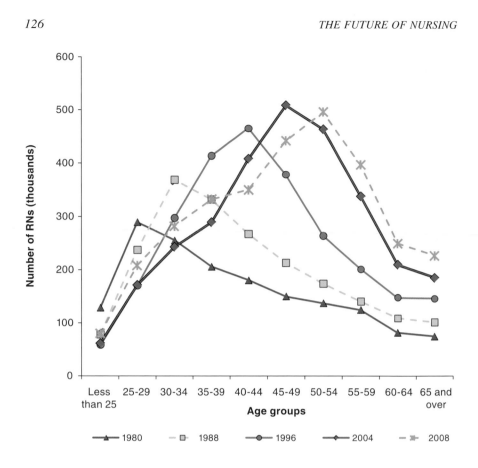

FIGURE 3-7 Age distribution of registered nurses, 1980–2008.
SOURCE: HRSA, 2010.

programs. For example, the supply of physicians was deliberately expanded in the 1960s with the introduction of the Medicare and Medicaid programs but has remained fairly constant since then. This pattern has resulted in large successive cohorts of physicians who are replacing smaller groups of retiring physicians (Staiger et al., 2009).

As the coming decades unfold, nurses and physicians will continue to age. Many of the large numbers of older RNs will retire, and increasing numbers of middle-aged RNs will enter their 50s. Although the number of younger RNs has recently begun to grow, the increase is not expected to be large enough to offset the number of RNs anticipated to retire over the next 15 years (Buerhaus et al., 2009b). To fill gaps created by retirement and the increasing demand for nursing services, resulting in part from an aging population and increased rates of insurance coverage, the nursing workforce will need to expand by attracting younger

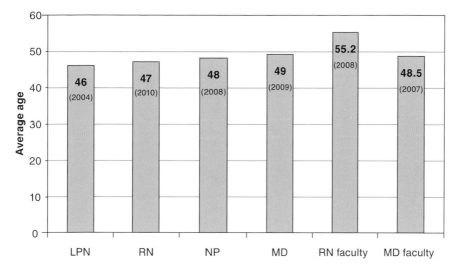

FIGURE 3-8 Average age of nurses at various levels of education and of MDs.
NOTE: LPN = licensed practical nurse; MD = doctor of medicine; NP = nurse practitioner; RN = registered nurse.
SOURCE: Based on data for LPNs (HRSA, 2004); for RNs (HRSA, 2010); for NPs (AANP, 2010); for MDs (Sermo.com, 2009); for RN faculty (AACN, 2010b); for MD faculty (AAMC, 2009).

individuals into the profession—a challenge that has been more difficult for the nursing profession than it has been for medicine (Kimball and O'Neil, 2002).

Gender Diversity

Throughout much of the 20th century, the nursing profession was composed mainly of women. While the absolute number of men who become nurses has grown dramatically in the last two decades, from 45,060 in 1980 to 168,181 in 2004 (HRSA, 2006), men still make up just over 7 percent of all RNs (HRSA, 2010). Overall, male RNs tend to be younger than female RNs, with an average age of 44.6 years. Men are also more likely to begin their careers with slightly more advanced nursing degrees (HRSA, 2006).

Efforts to recruit more men into the civilian nursing profession have had minimal success, and a body of research indicates gender-based reasons for entering the nursing profession. The evidence is generally thin, but men tend to list factors associated with security and professional growth that led them to the nursing profession: salary, ease of obtaining work, job security, and opportunities for leadership. By contrast, women tend to list factors that represent social encouragement from family or friends (Zysberg and Berry, 2005). While more men are being drawn to nursing, especially as a second career, the profession needs to continue efforts to recruit men; their unique perspectives and skills are important to the profession and will help contribute additional diversity to the workforce.

Racial and Ethnic Diversity

To better meet the current and future health needs of the public and to provide more culturally relevant care, the current nursing workforce will need to grow more diverse. Previous IOM reports have found that greater racial and ethnic diversity among providers leads to stronger relationships with patients in nonwhite communities. These reports argue that the benefits of such diversity are likely to be felt across health professions and to grow as the U.S. population becomes increasingly diverse (IOM, 2004, 2006). The IOM's report *Unequal Treatment: Addressing Racial and Ethnic Disparities in Health Care* identifies the diversification of the health care workforce as an important step toward responding to racial and ethnic disparities in the health care system (IOM, 2003). Because nurses make up the largest proportion of the health care workforce and work across virtually every health care and community-based setting, changing the demographic composition of nurses has the potential to effect changes in the face of health care in America.

Although nurses need to develop the ability to communicate and interact with people from differing backgrounds, the demographic characteristics of the nursing workforce should be closer to those of the population at large to foster better interaction and communication (AACN, 2010a). The 2008 National Sample Survey of Registered Nurses (NSSRN) documented the lack of diversity in the nursing workforce, with 5.4 percent of nurses describing themselves as Black/African American, 3.6 percent as Hispanic/Latino, 5.8 percent as Asian or Native Hawaiian/Pacific Islander, 0.3 percent as American Indian/Alaska Native, and 1.7 percent as multiracial (HRSA, 2010). Figure 3-9 compares the racial/ethnic diversity of RNs with that of the U.S. population.

Numerous programs nationwide are aimed at increasing the number of health professionals from underrepresented ethnic and racial groups. One program that seeks to increase diversity while also responding to the health needs of underserved populations is the Harambee Nursing Center (HNC) in Louisville, Kentucky (AAN, 2010c). The name refers to an African tribal word that means "let's pull together." HNC was founded in 2003 by the University of Louisville School of Nursing, in partnership with the University of Louisville hospital and several religious groups, "to improve the health of the approximately 11,000 low-income, primarily African-American, urban, underserved Smoketown-Shelby Park-Phoenix Hill neighborhood" (Roberts and Hayes, 2005). It is managed by nurses with the help of a volunteer family practice physician. Since its inception, a goal of the program has included attracting greater numbers of minority persons into nursing and other health professions and providing opportunities to enhance

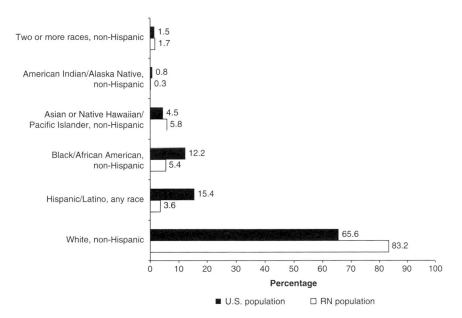

FIGURE 3-9 Distribution of registered nurses and the U.S. population by racial/ethnic background.
SOURCE: HRSA, 2010.

the cultural competence of nursing students and faculty.[29] Strategies to increase diversity in nursing include

- providing supervised clinical experiences for nursing and other health professional students at HNC;
- offering group educational programs to community members and persons working in community agencies and one-to-one mentoring of community residents who are interested in a nursing career (which includes providing clinical experiences, taking participants to planning meetings, having them talk directly to student advisers at the School of Nursing, arranging experiences at the hospital or nursing home, and holding conversations with interested persons);
- creating structured opportunities for nursing students and faculty to be engaged in service to the community so they can begin to comprehend the life experiences of the residents and be more sensitive to their needs when advising and creating recruitment programs;

[29] This section draws on a September 8, 2010, personal communication with Kay T. Roberts, Executive Director, Harambee Nursing Center.

- distributing literature and pictures related to the history of African Americans in nursing; and
- collaborating with other community agencies to include nursing education and career options in their educational and jobs programs.

Outcomes cited by Dr. Roberts include the following:

- Nursing careers and educational pathways are now formally included in job-related programs implemented by the Presbyterian Community Center (PCC). For example, over the past 2 years, PCC has selected 50 community residents into the Changemaker program, which targets 19- to 25-year-olds to engage them in self-discovery, goal setting, and progress toward career goals, with the condition of giving back to the community. Each year about four to six Changemakers examine health careers in depth. HNC included nursing and health careers in the proposal that funded this pathway and provides supervised clinical experiences, mentoring, part-time job opportunities where possible, and education about nursing.
- Arrangements have been made to connect interested residents with entry into a medical assistant program that provides articulation to associate's degree education and then mentoring to advance to the bachelor's of science in nursing (BSN) and further, in addition to baccalaureate programs.
- The University of Louisville School of Nursing hosts a recruitment booth at the Annual Health Fair at HNC.
- Community health students and faculty now provide education at the community middle school regarding careers in nursing.
- Based on HNC's feedback to the School of Nursing, criteria for selection of students into the RN–BSN program are under scrutiny. Last year no African American student was accepted. One of HNC's mentorees missed selection by only a few points. Dialogue with faculty led to an examination of policies that resulted in the omission of minority students.
- Literally hundreds of undergraduate and graduate nursing students (from several academic institutions) have supervised learning experiences in the community. These include at least 10 undergraduate community health nursing students each semester, a class of 30 graduate nursing students enrolled in a health promotion class each year, and 2 or more NP students based in the clinic each semester. About 5 NP and 10 undergraduate students participate in a Back to School event each fall where Harambee offers school physicals and immunizations for underserved middle school students. Each year 2 to 4 graduate nursing students serve as research or program assistants and/or researchers, and nursing students in the PhD program engage in research-related projects.

Conclusion: Demographic Challenges

The nurse workforce is slowly becoming more diverse, and the proportion of racially and ethnically diverse nursing graduates has increased by 10 percent in the last two decades, growing from 12.3 to 22.5 percent (HRSA, 2010). Nonetheless, additional commitments are needed to further increase the diversity of the nurse workforce. Steps should be taken to recruit, retain, and foster the success of diverse individuals. One way to accomplish this is to increase the diversity of the nursing student body, an issue addressed in Chapter 4. The combination of age, gender, race/ethnicity, and life experiences provides individuals with unique perspectives that can contribute to advancing the nursing profession and providing better care to patients.

NEW STRUCTURES, NEW OPPORTUNITIES

The ACA will bring new opportunities to overcome some of the barriers discussed above and use nurses in new and expanded capacities. This section offers a brief look at four of the current initiatives—the accountable care organization (ACO), the medical/health home, the community health center (CHC), and the NMHC—that are designed to implement these changes at an affordable price regardless of whether the providers involved are part of a large, integrated health care organization like the VA, Geisinger, or Kaiser Permanente. All four initiatives have shown enough promise that they were selected to receive additional financial support under the ACA.

Depending on their outcomes, these exemplars may lead the way to broader changes in the health care system. Given this possibility, the creation of the new Center for Medicare and Medicaid Innovation within the Department of Health and Human Services may prove to be one of the most important provisions of the ACA (Whelan and Russell, 2010). The Center is designed "to test innovative payment and service delivery models to reduce program expenditures . . . while preserving or enhancing the quality of care."[30] CMS can expand the duration and scope of successful programs with priority given to programs that also apply to private payers. They can also terminate or modify programs that are not working well. These types of decisions had previously been allowed only after congressional action.

The committee offers no predictions as to which combination, if any, of these four exemplars—ACOs, medical/health homes, CHCs, and NMHCs—will best succeed at meeting patients' needs. However, it wishes to emphasize to the Center for Medicare and Medicaid Innovation that each of these four initiatives depends on high-functioning, interprofessional teams in which the competencies and skills of all nurses, including APRNs, can be more fully utilized. New models of care, still to be developed, may deliver care that is better and more efficient than that

---

[30] *Patient Protection and Affordable Care Act*, HR 3590 § 3021, 111th Congress.

provided by these four initiatives. Nursing, in collaboration with other professions, should be a part of the design of these initiatives by shaping and leading
solutions. Innovative solutions are most likely to emerge if researchers from the
nursing field work in partnership with other professionals in medicine, business,
technology, and law to create them.

Accountable Care Organizations

The ACO is a legally defined entity consisting of a group of primary care
providers, a hospital, and perhaps some specialists who share in the risk as well as
the rewards of providing quality care at a fixed reimbursement rate (Fisher et al.,
2009; MedPAC, 2009). (The use of the phrase "primary care ACO professionals"
in the ACA is inclusive of APRNs as well as physicians.) Payment for this set of
services, as provided for in the ACA, will move beyond the traditional fee-for-
service system and may include shared savings payments or capitated payments
for all services. The goal of this payment structure is to encourage the ACO to
improve the quality of the care it provides and increase care coordination while
containing growth. ACOs that use APRNs and other nurses to the full extent of
their education and training in such roles as health coaching, chronic disease
management, transitional care, prevention activities, and quality improvement
will most likely benefit from providing high-value and more accessible care that
patients will find to be in their best interest.

Medical/Health Homes

The concept of a medical home was first developed by pediatricians in the
late 1960s (AAP, 1967). The original impetus was to create a single place to house
all of individual children's medical records—particularly children with special
health needs who often must see multiple clinicians (Sia et al., 2004). Over the
years, however, the term "medical home" has evolved to refer to a specific type
of primary care practice that coordinates and provides comprehensive care; promotes a strong relationship between patient and provider; measures, monitors,
and improves the quality of care; and is not necessarily limited to children.

Medical homes play a prominent role in the ACA, but the law is not consistent in its terminology for them. In various places, the ACA refers to "medical
homes," "health homes," and even the above-discussed PCMH that is recognized
by NCQA. The ACA indicates that medical/health homes should be supported by
community-based interprofessional teams or "health teams" that include physicians, nurses, and other health professionals.[31]

The medical/health home concept has been adopted and adapted in several
ways. The latest phase of the broader nursing strategy at the VA, for example,

---

[31] *Patient Protection and Affordable Care Act*, HR 3590 § 3502, 111th Congress.

consists of the implementation of a medical home model with expanded roles for RNs. Previously, primary care providers (physicians and NPs) at the VA felt that they were not receiving enough professional support to do their jobs effectively. The new strategy calls for including staff nurses on the primary care teams. "This is not your typical staff nurse role in primary care settings," said Catherine Rick, chief nursing officer of the VA.[32] What the staff nurse brings to primary care that has not been there before is the provision of chronic care management, care coordination, health risk appraisal, health promotion, and disease prevention. Work on rolling out the VA's medical home model began in August 2009, and the program was officially launched in April 2010. The case study in Box 3-3 illustrates how the medical home concept is being applied in the VA health system.

Community Health Centers

CHCs have a long track records of providing high-value, quality primary and preventive care in poor and underserved parts of the United States. Many also offer dental, mental health, and substance abuse and pharmacy services as well. CHCs generally are very team oriented and depend on nurses to deliver services. Nurses provide primary care, preventive services, and home visits, and many serve in administrative and leadership positions. At present, 20 million Americans receive care at CHCs in 7,500 communities (NACHC, 2009). CHC patients are less likely to have unmet medical needs, visit the emergency department for nonurgent care, or need hospitalization relative to the general population. A 2007 report by the National Association of Community Health Centers found that medical expenses for patients who receive the majority of their care at a CHC are 41 percent lower ($1,810 per person) than those for comparable patients who receive most of their care elsewhere (NACHC et al., 2007). As a result, the organization estimates that CHCs save the health care system $9.9–$17.6 billion a year (NACHC, 2009).

In 2002, the Bush Administration began a significant expansion of the CHC program, which began in the 1960s as part of the "war on poverty." The program received another big boost in 2009 with a $2 billion investment as part of the American Recovery and Reinvestment Act. And in 2010, as part of the ACA, Congress allocated an additional $11 billion in funds to further expand the program (Whelan, 2010).

Nurse-Managed Health Centers

NMHCs have provided care for populations served by Medicare, Medicaid, and children's health insurance programs, as well as the uninsured, since the

---

[32] Personal communication, Cathy Rick, Chief Nursing Officer of the Department of Veterans Affairs, March 9, 2010.

BOX 3-3
Case Study: The Patient-Centered Medical Home

A Team Approach to Primary Care for Veterans

When a veteran with diabetes who was experiencing hyperglycemia visited the Overton Brooks VA Medical Center in Shreveport, Louisiana, a nurse practitioner (NP) made adjustments to his medications. But that visit was different from others he had made: he also talked with a team of providers about exercise, diet, and blood glucose self-monitoring, and they discussed what support he would need to make changes in these areas as well.

After 2 weeks, Helen Rasmussen, BSN, RN, CDE, a care manager in primary care at the facility, called the patient, who reported his daily blood glucose levels. An NP made further medication adjustments, and Ms. Rasmussen called again in 2 weeks. "The results were much improved, and he was very happy that he didn't have to come in to see a provider each time for these changes," she said.

Ms. Rasmussen has been a primary care nurse with the U.S. Department of Veterans Affairs (VA) for more than 12 years, and until recently, she said, she would not have had the time to make those follow-up calls; her caseload would have been too high. But in 2009 VA secretary Eric Shinseki announced a major push toward more "veteran-centered care" for the 6 million veterans using the system (VA, 2009). One element of that new initiative is the Patient-Centered Medical Home™ (PCMH).

The PCMH is not a new concept. Four decades after the American Academy of Pediatrics developed the concept of a medical home, however, its meaning has evolved. Many now think of the PCMH as a "health home"—a team approach to primary care that involves better care coordination and information systems (including the electronic health record) and gives patients greater access to care and to their providers (including e-mail exchanges). The patient is necessarily at the center of decision making.

We realized that we needed to dedicate additional services to being patient-centered, or what I prefer to call patient-driven—really engaging patients in shared decision-making, developing a plan of care that is based on their informed decisions and their individual preferences.

—Catherine Rick, MSN, RN, NEA-BC, FACHE, chief nursing officer, U.S. Department of Veterans Affairs

The VA's nearly 65,000 licensed nurses are fundamental to this approach at the VA. "We decided to have a full-time RN [registered nurse] care manager for every full-time primary care provider," said Catherine Rick, MSN, RN, NEA-BC, FACHE, the VA's chief nursing services officer. The RN care manager works with others on a four-person team—including a primary care provider (a physician or an NP) and support staff—to help veterans better manage their illnesses and coordinate transitions in care, such as hospital admission.

Another aspect of the PCMH at the VA is the clinical nurse leader— which, Ms. Rick said, "is probably one of the most transformational roles that the nursing profession has to offer the health care industry." The American Association of Colleges of Nursing has defined it as a new leadership role for nurses that is neither administrative nor managerial (AACN, 2007); rather, this nurse with a master's degree supervises the care provided by the team. At the VA, the clinical nurse leader oversees the care provided by more than one team, while the RN care manager focuses on the care provided by just his or her team. The VA intends to employ clinical nurse leaders in all of its medical centers by 2016 (ONS, 2009).

Too few support staff may prevent some facilities from implementing the PCMH, said Colette S. Torres, MSN, RN, CCM, associate director of primary care, Robert J. Dole VA Medical Center, Wichita, Kansas, until savings from reduced rates of hospitalization are realized. Also, the VA is measuring outcomes of the PCMH, but data have not yet been released.

Ms. Torres said that what she particularly appreciates about this model "is that we carry our patients through acute and chronic issues." Under the old model, when a veteran was hospitalized, the primary care providers would wait to see the patient. Now, she said, they visit a veteran in the hospital. "We go up and say, 'How are you doing? We're not here to provide your care; we're here because we're a part of your team.' And they absolutely love it."

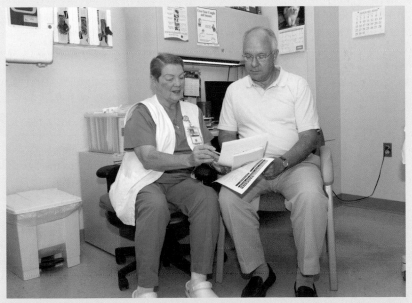

Darran E. Middleton, Medical Media

As part of Helen Rasmussen's role as a nurse care manager, she takes the time to explain health information to her patients.

1960s. There are 250 NMHCs across the United States serving 1.5 million medically underserved people, nearly half of whom are uninsured (NNCC, 2005). As the name implies, they are run by nurses—although many employ physicians, social workers, health educators, and outreach workers as members of a collaborative health team. Services generally include comprehensive primary care, family planning, prenatal services, mental/behavioral health care, and health promotion and disease prevention.

The majority of NMHCs are affiliated with a nursing school and about half with a community-based nonprofit organization (King and Hansen-Turton, 2010). NMHCs report that their clients make 15 percent fewer emergency department visits than the general population, have 35–40 percent fewer nonmaternity hospital days, and spend 25 percent less on prescriptions (NNCC, 2005). The ACA authorizes an additional $50 million in 2010 and "such sums as may be necessary for each of the fiscal years 2011 through 2014"[33] to NMHCs that offer primary care to low-income and medically underserved patients, although as of this writing, this funding specifically for NMHCs has not been allocated. The case study presented in Box 3-4 shows how an NMHC worked with community leaders to reduce health disparities in an underserved poor neighborhood in Philadelphia.

Opportunities Through Technology

There is perhaps no greater opportunity to transform practice than through technology. Information technology has long been used to support billing and payments but has become increasingly important in the provision of care as an aid to documentation and decision making. Diagnostic and monitoring machines have proven invaluable in the treatment of cancer, heart disease, and many other ailments. Examples cited by the IOM in *Crossing the Quality Chasm: A New Health System for the 21st Century* include "growing evidence that automated order entry systems can reduce errors in drug prescribing and dosing" and "improvements in timeliness through the use of Internet-based communication (i.e., e-visits, telemedicine) and immediate access to automated clinical information, diagnostic tests, and treatment results" (IOM, 2001). Since that report was published, the expanded use of online communication has resulted in so-called telehealth services that are not limited to diagnosis or treatment but also include health promotion, follow-up, and coordination of care. Delivery of telehealth services has, however, like that of APRN services, been complicated by variability in state regulations, particularly whenever online communications cross state lines.

---

[33] *Patient Protection and Affordable Care Act*, H.R. 3590 § 5208, 111th Congress.

Impact of Technology on the Design of Health Care Delivery

In 2009, the American Recovery and Reinvestment Act (ARRA) (Public Law 111-5) included provisions to create incentives for the adoption and meaningful use of health information technology (HIT). ARRA strengthened standards for maintaining the privacy and security of health information. ARRA provided grants to help state and local governments as well as health care providers in their efforts to adopt and use HIT. CMS also provided incentives, under ARRA to encourage eligible hospitals and health professionals to become "meaningful users" of certified EHRs. A definition of "meaningful use" was developed by the Secretary of HHS by official rulemaking procedures, providing opportunity for public and professional input (HHS, 2009). The meaningful use objectives will likely continue to be refined but outline core requirements that should be included in every EHR. By adopting these recommendations, users will be eligible for federal incentive payments and will be able to report information on the clinical quality of care. States can add or modify additional objectives to this definition for their Medicaid programs (CMS, 2010).

A recent article in the *New England Journal of Medicine* summarizes the meaningful use criterion as follows: "use by providers to achieve significant improvements in care" (Blumenthal and Tavenner, 2010). Given the nature of patient data collection, nurses will be integral to proper collection of meaningful use data. For example, among the first set of criteria to be measured include patient demographics, vital signs, and lists of patient's diagnoses, allergies, and active medications. As EHRs become more refined and integrated, nurses will have the opportunity to help define additional meaningful use objectives.

Implications for Time and Place of Care

Care supported by interoperable digital networks will shift in the importance of time and place. The patient/consumer will not always have to be in the same location as the provider, and the provider will not always have to interact with the patient in real time. As EHRs, computerized physician order entry systems, laboratory results, imaging systems, and pharmacies are all linked into the same network, many types of care can be provided without regard to location, as the "care grid" is available anywhere, anytime.

Remote patient monitoring is expanding exponentially. An ever-growing array of biometric devices (e.g., indwelling heart or blood sugar monitors) can collect, monitor, and report information from the patient in real time, in either an institution or the home. Some of these devices can also provide direct digitally mediated care; the automated insulin pump and implantable defibrillators are two examples.

The implications of these developments for nursing will be considerable and as yet are not fully understood (Abbott and Coenen, 2008). It is not clear

BOX 3-4
Case Study: 11th Street Family Health
Services of Drexel University

A Nurse-Managed Health Center Reduces
Health Disparities in Philadelphia

Lisa Scardigli, age 44, has suffered periodically from spasticity, a symptom of the multiple sclerosis she has lived with for more than 20 years. She had been receiving physical therapy at 11th Street Family Health Services in Philadelphia when she had a pump implanted for spinal infusion of a drug that reduces spasticity. But the pump's catheter punctured in late 2009, and she was hospitalized for several weeks. When she returned to 11th Street, she said, she got "holy heck" from the staff there; they had been worried about her. "Even the people at the front desk were up in arms over the fact that I didn't call," Ms. Scardigli said. "It went from the physical therapist to the primary care person to the security guard. I was actually missed."

This is a small story, but it illustrates a big reason for this health center's success: it not only serves its community (there were 26,000 clinical visits in 2009); it also *creates* community. And that may have something to do with the fact that it is run by nurses.

This nurse-managed health center provides primary care and other services in a neighborhood in North Philadelphia where most of the 6,000 residents are African American, have low incomes, and are medically underserved. Nurse practitioners (NPs) and social workers make up teams that are augmented as needed by physicians, nutritionists, and others.

Having been launched in 1998 in a recreation center, 11th Street is now a federally qualified health center housed in a $3.3 million, 17,000-square-foot facility, with a staff of 53.

I describe the center as a healthy-living center. And that is what the residents wanted. It's not just access to clinical services. It's providing opportunity for a neighborhood that doesn't have a lot of opportunity for people to get healthier.

—Patricia Gerrity, PhD, RN, FAAN, director, Eleventh Street Family Health Services of Drexel University, Philadelphia

---

The center's work began gradually, as a joint project of the Philadelphia Housing Authority and Drexel University's College of Nursing and Health Professions. In 1996 director Patricia Gerrity, PhD, RN, FAAN, placed a public health nurse at each of four housing developments in the neighborhood. The nurses responded to residents' immediate concerns: the need for stop signs, animal control, food assistance, and training in CPR. "Over that first year or two we gained the trust of the residents because we weren't defining the issues; they were," Dr. Gerrity said. "And it showed that we were making a long-term commitment."

From there, she met with area representatives to discover their visions for the community. They wanted a health care center, they said, one they could access regardless of their ability to pay. A community advisory board was formed, and the search for funding began. (Over the years the center has received funding from federal, state, and private sources.)

Dr. Gerrity uses the word "transdisciplinary" rather than "multidisciplinary" or "interdisciplinary" to describe the care provided at 11th Street. "Transdisciplinary means you start to break down the barriers between disciplines. Each person learns something about the other person's discipline, and it enriches their own practice," Dr. Gerrity said. For example, behavioral health care has been incorporated into every primary care visit, with NPs and social workers closely collaborating.

The range of services provided is remarkably diverse. Patients like Ms. Scardigli undergo physical therapy. Patients with diabetes join cooking classes that make use of locally grown produce. First-time mothers receive home visits through the Nurse–Family Partnership. Six to eight mother–infant pairs meet through the Centering Parenting program. A fitness center with a full-time personal trainer is on site, full dental care is available, and chronic illness management groups provide peer support.

Unpublished outcome data for patients with diabetes show that in an 18-month period, the proportion who had glycosylated hemoglobin levels below 7 percent doubled and that low-density lipoprotein cholesterol and blood pressure levels fell as well. Also seen were reductions in depression and low-birth-weight infants and increases in immunization and breast cancer screening.

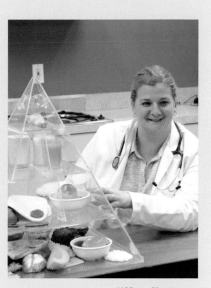

USEventPhotos.com

A nurse at 11th Street Family Health Services uses the food pyramid to educate patients about a healthy diet.

Access to payment for care coordination through medical home designation is important to the center's sustainability. Despite meeting the criteria set by the National Committee for Quality Assurance for qualifying as a Patient-Centered Medical Home™, 11th Street was denied the designation because it is led by nurses rather than physicians—an issue for the 250 nurse-managed health centers across the nation.

Lisa Scardigli is so impressed by all the center does that she now sits on the community advisory board. Recently, she brought in a neighbor of hers who needed new dentures. "She loves it," Ms Scardigli said. "She's 90, and she's from down south, so it reminds her of when the doctor used to come to your house and knew the family and sat down and broke bread."

how much of nursing care might be independent of physical location when HIT is fully implemented, but it will likely be a significant subset of care, possibly in the range of 15–35 percent of what nurses do today. That is, for this proportion of care, nurses need not be in the same locale (or even the same nation) as their patients. As new technologies impact the hospital and other settings for nursing services, this phenomenon may increase.

Implications for Nursing Practice

HIT will fundamentally change the ways in which RNs plan, deliver, document, and review clinical care. The process of obtaining and reviewing diagnostic information, making clinical decisions, communicating with patients and families, and carrying out clinical interventions will depart radically from the way these activities occur today. Moreover, the relative proportion of time RNs spend on various tasks is likely to change appreciably over the coming decades. While HIT arguably will have its greatest influence on how RNs plan and document their care, all facets of care will be mediated increasingly by digital workflow, computerized knowledge management, and decision support.

In the future, virtually every facet of nursing practice in each setting where it is rendered will have a significant digital dimension around a core EHR. Biometric data collection will increasingly be automated, and diagnostic tests, medications, and some therapies will be computer generated and managed and delivered with computer support. Patient histories and examination data will increasingly be collected by devices that interface directly with the patient and automatically stream into the EHR. Examples include automated blood pressure cuffs, personal digital assistant (PDA)–based functional status, and patient history surveys.

In HIT-supported organizations, a broader array and higher proportion of services of all types will be provided within the context of computer templates and workflows. Care and its documentation will less frequently be "free-hand." As routine aspects of care become digitally mediated and increasingly rote, RNs and other clinicians can be expected to shift and expand their focus to more complex and nuanced "high-touch" tasks that these technologies cannot readily or appropriately accomplish, such as communication with and guidance and support for patients and their families. There will likely be greater opportunities for such interventions as counseling, behavior change, and social and emotional support—interventions that lie squarely within the province of nursing practice.

Impact of Technology on Quality, Efficiency, and Outcomes

Adoption of HIT is expected to increase the efficiency and effectiveness of clinician interactions with each patient and the target population. EHRs and other HIT should lower the cost per unit of service delivered and/or improve the quality of care as measured by outcomes or achievement of other end points, such as increased adherence to optimal guidelines. HIT will lead to greater efficiency if it takes less time for a clinician to provide the same unit of service or if a lower-cost clinician practicing with extensive HIT support can deliver the same type of care as a higher-cost non-HIT-supported provider. Controlled time and motion studies that have compared clinicians performing the same task with and without HIT support have produced mixed findings on time efficiencies gained across clinicians and settings. One area with emerging evidence is hospital nursing time spent in documentation, with studies showing a 23–24 percent reduction (Poissant et al., 2005). On the other hand, these efficiency gains may be partially offset by the information demands of quality improvement initiatives and similar programs undertaken by a growing number of institutions (DesRoches et al., 2008).[34]

According to a review of the literature conducted for the committee, although research on the impact of HIT on the quality of nursing care is limited, documentation quality and accessibility generally improve after the implementation of HIT. Medication errors almost always decrease after the implementation of bar code medication administration (Waneka and Spetz, 2009). DesRoches and colleagues (2008) conducted a national survey of more than 3,436 RNs (1,392 responses) and found that hospitals with basic EHR systems were more likely to be recognized for nursing excellence (magnets/magnet-like) and to have quality improvement programs. No differences were found in time spent on patient care activities for nurses in hospitals with and without minimally functioning systems.

Technology is also used to measure patient outcomes, with varying results. While measuring outcomes is critical to the provision of 21st-century health care, complications have developed in ensuring that outcome measures from different institutions and organizations are, in fact, comparable. Even ensuring that outcome measures from different parts of the same organization are comparable can be problematic. Researchers in Colorado conducted a comprehensive review of the use of rescue agents—a Joint Commission–approved quality measure—based on the EHRs at the Children's Hospital in Aurora. They found that variations in the way information was entered in the EHRs accounted for significant variations within the institution and could be responsible for as much as a 40-fold difference in outcome measures among hospitals (Kahn and Ranade, 2010). The researchers concluded that "more detailed clinical information may result in quality measures that are not comparable across institutions due [to] institution-specific workflow."

---

[34] This paragraph draws on a paper commissioned by the committee on "Health Care System Reform and the Nursing Workforce: Matching Nursing Practice and Skills to Future Needs, Note Past Demands," prepared by Julie Sochalski, University of Pennsylvania School of Nursing, and Jonathan Weiner, Johns Hopkins University Bloomberg School of Public Health (see Appendix F on CD-ROM).

A longitudinal study of 326 hospitals found that those that had implemented more advanced EHR systems over the time period had higher costs and increased nurse staffing levels (Furukawa et al., 2010). Patient complications increased in these hospitals, while mortality for some conditions declined. It should be noted, however, that these results may be difficult to interpret because of the implementation of minimum nurse staffing regulations at the same time that the implementation of EHRs ramped up. During that time, nurse staffing rose, and thus costs per patient rose, and if there is any correlation between implementation of EHRs and increased nurse staffing due to the ratios, the results may confound the two. In addition, the study did not control for hospital ownership (e.g., nonprofit, for-profit) or system affiliation, both of which might be important.

Finally, a systematic review of the literature (fewer than 25 articles) showed that the time spent on documentation of care may increase or decrease with EHRs (Thompson et al., 2009). The increases in time however, may be compensated for by the use of EHRs in other activities, such as giving/receiving reports, reconciling medications, and planning care.

Technology Transforming Roles for Nurses

The new practice milieu—where much of nursing and medical care is mediated and supported within an interoperable "digital commons"—will support and potentially even require much more effective integration of multiple disciplines into a collaborative team focused on the patient's unique set of needs. Furthermore, interoperable EHRs linked with personal health records and shared support systems will influence how these teams work and share clinical activities. It will increasingly be possible for providers to work on digitally linked teams that will collaborate with patients and their families no longer limited by real-time contact.[35]

As the knowledge base and decision pathways that previously resided primarily in clinicians' brains are transferred to clinical decision support and CPOE modules of advanced HIT systems, some types of care most commonly provided by nurses can readily shift to personnel with less training or to patients and their families. Similarly, many types of care previously provided by physicians and other highly trained personnel can be provided effectively by APRNs and other specialty trained RNs. Furthermore, the performance of these fundamentally restructured teams will be monitored through the use of biometric, psychometric, and other types of process and outcome "e-indicators" extracted from the HIT infrastructure.

---

[35] This and the next paragraph draw on a paper commissioned by the committee on "Health Care System Reform and the Nursing Workforce: Matching Nursing Practice and Skills to Future Needs, Note Past Demands," prepared by Julie Sochalski, University of Pennsylvania School of Nursing, and Jonathan Weiner, Johns Hopkins University Bloomberg School of Public Health (see Appendix F on CD-ROM).

Increasingly, technology is allowing nurses and other health care providers to offer their services in a wider range of settings. For example, the ability of the Visiting Nurse Service of New York to tap into mobile technology, as described in Chapter 2, allowed that organization to provide ever more complex care in the home setting (IOM, 2010a).

Involving Nurses in Technology Design and Implementation

As the largest segment of the health care workforce with some of the closest, most sustained interactions with patients, nurses are often the greatest users of technology. In many instances, they may know what will work best with regard to technological solutions, but they are asked for their opinions infrequently. According to a survey of nurses at 25 leading acute care facilities across the United States, nurses find "that existing systems are often splintered, unable to interface and require multiple log-on to access or enter data. They call repeatedly for integrated systems to ease their workload and help them reach clinical transformation" (Bolton et al., 2008).

Studies show that involving nurses in the design, planning, and implementation of technology systems leads to fewer problems during implementation (Hunt et al., 2004). The TIGER Initiative (for Technology Informatics Guiding Education Reform) is a collaborative effort of 1,400 nurses from various organizations, government agencies, and vendors whose goal is "to interweave informatics and enabling technologies transparently into nursing practice" (TIGER, 2009). As leaders from the TIGER Initiative told the committee, "Regardless of the setting or environment of care, the best, most up to date information is required to support safe, effective care and promote optimal outcomes." And yet, they pointed out, "Today, health information is not shared across the various providers and stakeholder groups who provide, fund and research care." The members of the TIGER Initiative hope to help change that situation by developing the capacity of nursing students and members of the nursing workforce "to use electronic health records to improve the delivery of health care" and "engage more nurses in leading both the development of a national health care information technology (NHIT) infrastructure and health care reform." They also see the need to "accelerate adoption of smart, standards based, interoperable technology that will make health care delivery safer, more efficient, timely, accessible, and patient-centered, while also reducing the burden of nurses" (TIGER, 2009).

Nurses have also invented new technology to help them care for their patients. For instance, Barbara Medoff Cooper, professor in pediatric nursing and director of the Center for Biobehavioral Research at the University of Pennsylvania School of Nursing, developed a microchip device that is situated between the nipple and the rest of the baby bottle. It measures the sucking ability of premature neonatal babies, which has been shown to be an accurate indication of the infant's ability to feed successfully and thus survive discharge. The information thus gathered has helped guide parents and providers in better planning for the care of high-risk neonates at home (Bakewell-Sachs et al., 2009; Medoff-Cooper et al., 2009).

Another effort, called TelEmergency, brings a certified emergency room physician to 12 rural hospitals in Mississippi from the University of Mississippi via a T-1 line, but only when needed. The system is managed by a group of 35 APRNs who provide care in these rural communities, including management of the technology as a referral system. The nurses are able to handle 60 percent of all emergency care, saving the hospital consortium $72,000 per month (AAN, 2010b).

The case study in Box 3-5 shows how nurses at one institution are working to ensure that they spend their time in patient care and not on the technology associated with delivering modern health care.

CONCLUSION

The nursing profession has evolved more rapidly than the public policies that affect it. The ability of nurses to better serve the public is hampered by the constraints of outdated policies, particularly those involving nurses' scopes of practice. Evidence does not support the conclusion that APRNs are less able than physicians to provide safe, effective, and efficient care (Brown and Grimes, 1995; Fairman, 2008; Groth et al., 2010; Hatem et al., 2008; Hogan et al., 2010; Horrocks et al., 2002; Hughes et al., 2010; Laurant et al., 2004; Mundinger et al., 2000; Office of Technology Assessment, 1986). The roles of APRNs—and the roles of all nurses—are undergoing changes that will help make the transformative practice models outlined at the beginning of this chapter a more common reality. Such changes must be supported by a number of policy decisions, including efforts to remove the existing regulatory barriers to nursing practice. If the current conflicts between what nurses can do based on their education and training and what they may do according to state and federal policies and regulations are not addressed, patients will continue to experience limited access to high-quality care.

Despite the evidence demonstrating that APRNs are educated, trained, and competent to provide safe, high-quality care without the need for physician supervision, states' legislative decisions regarding legal scopes of practice range from restrictive to permissive. While medicine and a number of other professions enjoy practice regulations that are comparable across states, this goal has been elusive for nurses, particularly those working in advanced practice. With the availability now of a consensus document that offers agreed-upon standards for APRN education, training, and regulation, states that have been reluctant in the past may move toward broader scopes of practice. Such a move, however, considered by the committee to be a critical one, is not guaranteed. And while the committee defers to the rights of states to continue their regulation of health professionals, it also wishes to note why and how the federal government can play an important role in this arena.

The primary reason the federal government has a compelling interest in state regulation of health professionals is the responsibility to patients covered by federal programs such as Medicare and Medicaid. If access to care is hindered, if costs are unduly high, or if quality of care could be improved for these millions of patients through evidence-based changes to the ways in which professionals may practice, the federal government has a right to explore the options and encourage change. An additional reason is the federal government's unique perspective—somewhat removed from that of the individual states—enabling it to shed light on the value and benefit to all Americans of harmonizing practice regulations among the states.

Certain federal entities may both defer to the states in adopting their own practice regulations and encourage the adoption of regulations that are consistent with current clinical evidence and comparable across the country. Congress, CMS, OPM, and the FTC each have specific authority or responsibility for decisions that either must be made at the federal level to be consistent with state efforts to remove scope-of-practice barriers or could be made to encourage and support those efforts. While no single actor or agency can independently make a sweeping change to eliminate current barriers, the various state and federal entities can each make relevant decisions that together can lead to much-needed improvements.

In addition to regulatory barriers, cultural and organizational barriers constrain nurses' ability to identify solutions and implement them quickly, knowing that patients' lives and well-being are at stake. Moreover, an important priority in national health care reform is achieving better value for the expenditures made on health care services. Since health care is labor intensive, getting more value from the health care system will depend in large part on enhancing the productivity and effectiveness of the workforce. Nurses therefore represent a large and unexploited opportunity to achieve greater value in health care.

The committee believes that any proposed changes in the responsibilities of the nursing workforce should be evaluated against their ability to support the provision of seamless, affordable, quality care that is accessible to all. In particular, the committee argues that now is the time to finally eliminate the outdated regulations and organizational and cultural barriers that limit the ability of nurses, including APRNs, to practice to the full extent of their education, training, and competence. The committee also believes that nurses must be allowed to lead improvement and redesign efforts (see Chapter 5).

Specifically, in order that all Americans may have access to high-quality, safe health care, federal and state actions are required to update and standardize scope-of-practice regulations to take advantage of the full capacity and education of nurses. Cultural and organizational barriers should also be eliminated. States and insurance companies must follow through with specific regulatory,

BOX 3-5
Case Study: Technology at Cedars-Sinai Medical Center

Sending Alerts via Text Message Shortens
Nurses' Response Times to Critical Alarms

In January 2010 a California hospital was fined for the death of a man whose cardiac alarm had been set to an inaudible level; when his heart stopped, the emergency room nurses were unaware of it and failed to intervene (California Department of Public Health, 2009). That same month a man died in a Massachusetts hospital after his heart rate declined over a 20-minute period; nurses did not hear his cardiac alarm, investigators found, and a second alarm had been turned off (McKinney, 2010).

Nurses attend to a variety of alarms and alerts during a shift, and there is often no system in place for prioritizing urgency. Confusion and "alarm fatigue" can result, with potentially lethal consequences: the ECRI Institute lists alarm hazards as the second most serious of the top 10 technology hazards in health care for 2010 (ECRI Institute, 2010). The problem has been shown to pose a danger to patient safety (Graham and Cvach, 2010), as have problems with clinical alarms in general (ACCE Healthcare Technology Foundation, 2006). Unfortunately, nurses are rarely involved in decisions about new technologies in health care, although the patient's bedside has been identified as the area most in need of technological innovation (Bolton et al., 2008).

At a combined telemetry and medical–surgical unit at Cedars-Sinai Medical Center in Los Angeles, nurses are taking the lead in testing ways to aggregate and prioritize the alarms to which they must respond, most recently via text messages sent to nurses' and nursing assistants' BlackBerry devices. This system has replaced pagers and many bedside alarms, with promising results.

We're responding a lot faster, which hopefully translates into intervening to prevent harm and saving someone's life.

—Ray Hancock, MSN, RN, director of critical care and telemetry services, Cedars–Sinai Medical Center, Los Angeles

---

Timely, Accurate Messaging. In a unit where routine alerts might range in importance from an out-of-reach water pitcher to cardiac arrest, getting "the right message to the right person at the right time" is critical, said Joanne Pileggi, MSN, RN, the unit's nurse manager. Working with Emergin, a communications software company, the unit's nurses and nursing assistants categorized the alarms they receive—from cardiac monitors, patients' call buttons, bed alarms, code blues, and the laboratory—according to their urgency, classifying them as red (most critical), blue (moderately critical), or yellow (least critical).

For example, if a patient's cardiac monitor detects a dangerous arrhythmia, that information is sent to the unit's "command center," where a cardiac nurse sends out a red alert via text message to that patient's nurse and the charge nurse. A beep or vibration from the nurse's BlackBerry indicates that a new text message has arrived. The nurse can glance at the device, see that the alert is red, and reply immediately, eliminating several problems with overhead paging systems: the need for repeated pages, the inability of the nurse to respond, excessive noise on the unit, and delays in response.

The 30-bed unit employs nine registered nurses (RNs) on the day shift and nine on the night shift and has been testing a variety of devices for more than 2 years. Staff were involved from the beginning, Ms. Pileggi said, and everyone, including aides, received training from Emergin.

An Investment in Safety. Use of the BlackBerry devices has cut the number of overhead pages on the unit by more than half. Nurses report less alarm fatigue and faster response times to alarms, and they receive critical laboratory values 10 minutes sooner under the new system than under the old one. They also save time by not handling alarms that do not require a nurse's attention.

Darren Dworkin, chief information officer for Cedars-Sinai, said the initial costs of purchasing the devices and training the staff have paid off in more efficient and safer care. "Enabling nurses to spend more time at the bedside is a goal we want to achieve," he said, "and so if the technology achieves that, then we

are achieving our return on investment." The unit has not conducted a cost–benefit analysis.

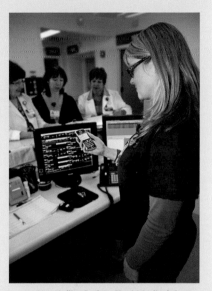

Lisa Hollis, Cedars-Sinai Medical Center

Los Angeles hospital Cedars-Sinai is a leader in using mobile devices for text message patient alerts and notifications.

Few manufacturers are designing technologies with nurses in mind, and limitations of the available technology have meant that not all ideas for improving processes can be tested. For example, the unit could not incorporate IV pump alarms into the most recent test. Still, bedside nurses and patients are quite pleased. The nurses are looking forward to a test of iPhones, which will display cardiac rhythms on screen. Said Ms. Pileggi, "We're anticipating patients' needs, so there hasn't been the need for patients to call as often."

policy, and financial changes that uphold patient-centered care as the organizing principle for a reformed health care system. The education and training of nurses support their ability to offer a wider range of services safely and effectively—as documented by numerous studies. And nurses must respond to the challenge, reinventing themselves as needed in a rapidly evolving health care system. Nursing is, of course, not the only profession to confront the need to transform itself in response to new realities; similarly disruptive challenges have been faced in other fields, such as medicine, health care, publishing, education, business, manufacturing, and the military. In the field of health care, expansion of scopes of practice to reflect the full extent of one's education and training should occur for all health professionals to maximize the contributions of each to patient care. For example, one impact of enhancing nurses' scopes of practice may be to allow the currently inadequate numbers of physicians to better use their time and skills on the most complex and challenging cases and tasks, as well as broaden the array of services they can offer as part of a collaborative team of providers (e.g., within new models of care—ACOs, medical homes, transitional care—that are part of the ACA, as well as in groups of specialty providers). To facilitate the most effective transition to team practice, as well as practice that encompasses the full extent of their scope, all providers will require continual teaching and learning to facilitate the highest level of team functioning (see Chapter 4).

Key factors that will contribute to the success of managing such a transition include technological literacy, good communication skills, adaptability to organizational changes, and a willingness to evaluate and reinvent how work is organized and accomplished (Kimball and O'Neil, 2002). Going forward under the ACA and whatever reforms may follow, the health care system is likely to change so rapidly that building the adaptive capacity of the nursing workforce to work across settings and in different types of roles in new models of care will require intentional development, expanded resources, and policy and regulatory changes.

Finally, the committee believes that if practice is to be transformed, nurses graduating with a bachelor's degree must be better prepared to enter the practice environment and confront the challenges they will encounter. Therefore, the committee concludes that nurse residency programs should be instituted to provide nurses with an appropriate transition to practice and develop a more competent nursing workforce.

REFERENCES

AACN (American Association of Colleges of Nursing). 2007. *White paper on the education and role of the clinical nurse leader.* http://www.aacn.nche.edu/Publications/WhitePapers/ClinicalNurseLeader07.pdf (accessed March 26, 2010).

AACN. 2008. *The essentials of baccalaureate education for professional nursing practice.* Washington, DC: AACN. http://www.aacn.nche.edu/education/pdf/BaccEssentials08.pdf.

AACN. 2010a. *Enhancing diversity in the nursing workforce.* http://www.aacn.nche.edu/Media/FactSheets/diversity.htm (accessed July 1, 2010).

AACN. 2010b. *Nursing faculty shortage fact sheet.* http://www.aacn.nche.edu/Media/Factsheets/facultyshortage.htm (accessed September 23, 2010).

AAMC (Association of American Medical Colleges). 2009. *Analysis in brief: The aging of full-time U.S. Medical school faculty: 1967-2007.* http://www.aamc.org/data/aib/aibissues/aibvol9_no4.pdf (accessed September 23, 2010).

AAN (American Academy of Nursing). 2010a. *Edge Runner directory: Post-baccalaureate nurse residency.* http://www.aannet.org/i4a/pages/index.cfm?pageId=3303 (accessed September 13, 2010).

AAN. 2010b. *Edge Runner directory: Telemergency: Distance emergency care using nurse practitioners.* http://www.aannet.org/custom/edgeRunner/index.cfm?pageid=3303&showTitle=1 (accessed September 13, 2010).

AAN. 2010c. *Edge Runner directory: The Harambee Nursing Center: Community-based, nurse-led health care.* http://www.aannet.org/custom/edgeRunner/index.cfm?pageid=3303&showTitle=1 (accessed May 19, 2010).

AANP (American Academy of Nurse Practitioners). 2010. *Nurse practitioner facts.* http://www.aanp.org/AANPCMS2/AboutAANP/NPFactSheet.htm (accessed July 2, 2010).

AAP (American Academy of Pediatrics). 1967. *Pediatric records and a "Medical home"* Edited by Council on Pediatric Practice, Standards of child care. Evanston, IL: AAP.

AARP. 2010a. *AARP 2010 policy supplement: Scope of practice for advanced practice registered nurses.* http://championnursing.org/sites/default/files/2010%20AARPPolicySupplementScopeofPractice.pdf (accessed September 10, 2010).

AARP. 2010b. *Consumer access & barriers to care: Physician-nurse practitioner restrictive collaboration requirements by state (map).* http://championnursing.org/aprnmap (accessed August 26, 2010).

Abbott, P. A., and A. Coenen. 2008. Globalization and advances in information and communication technologies: The impact on nursing and health. *Nursing Outlook* 56(5):238-246, e232.

Abelson, R. 2010. A health insurer pays more to save. *New York Times*, June 21.

ACCE (American College of Clinical Engineering) Healthcare Technology Foundation. 2006. *Impact of clinical alarms on patient safety.* http://www.acce-htf.org/White%20Paper.pdf (accessed March 22, 2010).

Aiken, L., and R. Cheung. 2008. *Nurse workforce challenges in the United States: Implications for policy.* OECD Health Working Paper No. 35. Available from http://www.oecd.org/dataoecd/34/9/41431864.pdf.

Aiken, L. H., R. B. Cheung, and D. M. Olds. 2009. Education policy initiatives to address the nurse shortage in the United States. *Health Affairs* 28(4):w646-w656.

AMA (American Medical Association). 2009. The AMA scope of practice data series: Nurse practitioners. Chicago, IL: AMA.

AP (Associated Press). 2010. *28 states seek to expand the role of nurse practitioners* (April 14, 2010). http://www.dallasnews.com/sharedcontent/dws/news/nation/stories/DN-drnurse_14nat.ART.State.Edition1.4c7c973.html (accessed June 27, 2010).

ASA (American Society of Anesthesiologists). 2004. *The scope of practice of nurse anesthetists.* Washington, DC: ASA.

Asch, S., E. McGlynn, M. Hogan, R. Hayward, P. Shekelle, L. Rubenstein, J. Keesey, J. Adams, and E. Kerr. 2004. Comparison of quality of care for patients in the Veterans Health Administration and patients in a national sample. *Annals of Internal Medicine* 141(12):938-945.

Bakewell-Sachs, S., B. Medoff-Cooper, J. Silber, G. Escobar, J. Silber, and S. Lorch. 2009. Infant functional status: The timing of physiologic maturation of premature infants. *Pediatrics* 123:e878-e886.

Beecroft, P. C., L. Kunzman, and C. Krozek. 2001. RN internship: Outcomes of a one-year pilot program. *Journal of Nursing Administration* 31(12):575-582.

Beecroft, P. C., L. A. Kunzman, S. Taylor, E. Devenis, and F. Guzek. 2004. Bridging the gap between school and workplace: Developing a new graduate nurse curriculum. *Journal of Nursing Administration* 34(7-8):338-345.

Benner, P., M. Sutphen, V. Leonard, and L. Day. 2009. *Educating nurses: A call for radical transformation.* San Francisco, CA: Jossey-Bass.

Blumenthal, D., and M. Tavenner. 2010. The "meaningful use" regulation for electronic health records. *New England Journal of Medicine* 636(6):501-504.

Bodenheimer, T., and H. H. Pham. 2010. Primary care: Current problems and proposed solutions. *Health Affairs* 29(5):799-805.

Bolton, L., and H. Aronow. 2009. The business case for TCAB: Estimates of cost savings with sustained improvement. *American Journal of Nursing* 109(11):77-80.

Bolton, L. B., C. A. Gassert, and P. F. Cipriano. 2008. Smart technology, enduring solutions: Technology solutions can make nursing care safer and more efficient. *Journal of Healthcare Information Management* 22(4):24-30.

Boult, C., L. Karm, and C. Groves. 2008. Improving chronic care: The "guided care" model. *The Permanente Journal* 12(1):50-54.

Brown, S. A., and D. E. Grimes. 1995. A meta-analysis of nurse practitioners and nurse midwives in primary care. *Nursing Research* 44(6):332-339.

Buerhaus, P., D. Staiger, and D. Auerbach. 2009a. *The future of the nursing workforce in the United States: Data, trends, and implications.* Boston: Jones & Bartlett.

Buerhaus, P. I., D. I. Auerbach, and D. O. Staiger. 2009b. The recent surge in nurse employment: Causes and implications. *Health Affairs* 28(4):w657-668.

Cady, D. M. 2006. *Reports of Board of Trustees.* http://www.ama-assn.org/ama1/pub/upload/mm/38/a-06bot.pdf (accessed September 21, 2010).

California Department of Public Health. 2009. *Statement of deficiencies and plan of correction.* http://www.cdph.ca.gov/certlic/facilities/Documents/HospitalAdministrativePenalties-2567Forms-LNC/2567StJudeMedicalCenter-Fullerton-EventC0IX11.pdf (accessed March 22, 2010).

Canadian Paediatric Society. 2000. Advanced practice nursing roles in neonatal care. *Paediatric Child Health* 5(3):178-182.

Cebul, R. D., J. B. Rebitzer, L. J. Taylor, and M. E. Votruba. 2008. Organizational fragmentation and care quality in the U.S healthcare system. *Journal of Economic Perspectives* 22(4):93-113.

Chapman, S. A., C. D. Wides, and J. Spetz. 2010. Payment regulations for advanced practice nurses: Implications for primary care. *Policy, Politics, & Nursing Practice* 11(2):89-98. http://ppn.sagepub.com/content/early/2010/09/08/1527154410382458.

Christian, S., C. Dower, and E. O'Neil. 2007. *Chart overview of nurse practitioner scopes of practice in the United States.* San Francisco, CA: Center for Health Professions, University of California, San Francisco.

CMS (Centers for Medicare and Medicaid Services). 2010. Medicare and Medicaid programs; electronic health record incentive program. *Federal Register* 75(144):44314-44588.

Cooper, R. 1998. Current and projected workforce of nonphysician clinicians. *JAMA* 280(9):788-794.

Cooper, R. A. 2007. New directions for nurse practitioners and physician assistants in the era of physician shortages. *Academic Medicine* 82(9):827-828.

Craven, G., and S. Ober. 2009. Massachusetts nurse practitioners step up as one solution to the primary care access problem. *Policy, Politics, & Nursing Practice* 10(2):94-100.

Croasdale, M. 2006. Physician task force confronts scope-of-practice legislation. *American Medical News*, September 21. http://www.ama-assn.org/amednews/2006/02/13/prl10213.htm.

Cunningham, R. 2010. *Tapping the potential of the health care workforce: Scope of practice and payment policies for advanced practice nurses and physician assistants* (background paper no. 76). Washington, DC: National Health Policy Forum.

Cys, J. 2000. Physicians: Medicare nurse pay too broad. *American Medical News*, July 24. http://www.ama-assn.org/amednews/2000/07/24/gvsb0724.htm.

Dall, T. M., Y. J. Chen, R. F. Seifert, P. J. Maddox, and P. F. Hogan. 2009. The economic value of professional nursing. *Medical Care* 47(1):97-104.

Daly, R. 2007. Psychiatrists, allies defeat psychology-prescribing bills. *Psychiatric News* 42(16):6.

Darves, B. 2007. *Physician employment and compensation outlook for '07.* http://www.nejmjobs.org/physician-compensation-trends.aspx (accessed September 9, 2010).

Dentzer, S. 2010. Geisinger chief Glenn Steele: Seizing health reform's potential to build a superior system. *Health Affairs* 29(6):1200-1207.

DeSanti, S. S., J. Farrell, and R. A. Feinstein. 2010. *Letter to Kentucky Cabinet for Health and Family Services*, January 28. http://www.ftc.gov/os/2010/02/100202kycomment.pdf.

DesRoches, C., K. Donelan, P. Buerhaus, and L. Zhonghe. 2008. Registered nurses use of electronic health records: Findings from a national survey. *Medscape Journal of Medicine* 10(7).

Djukic, M., and C. T. Kovner. 2010. Overlap of registered nurse and physician practice: Implications for U.S. Health care reform. *Policy, Politics, & Nursing Practice* 11(1):13-22.

Dulisse, B., and J. Cromwell. 2010. No harm found when nurse anesthetists work without supervision by physicians. *Health Affairs* 29(8):1469-1475.

ECRI Institute. 2010. *2010 top 10 technology hazards.* https://www.ecri.org/Forms/Documents/Top_Ten_Technology_Hazards_2010.pdf (accessed March 22, 2010).

Fairman, J. 2008. *Making room in the clinic: Nurse practitioners and the evolution of modern health care.* 1st ed. Piscataway, NJ: Rutgers University Press.

Fisher, E., M. McClellan, J. Bertko, S. Lieberman, J. Lee, J. Lewis, and J. Skinner. 2009. Fostering accountable health care: Moving forward in Medicare. *Health Affairs* 28:W219-W231.

Flinter, M. 2009. *Testimony submitted to inform the Forum on the Future of Nursing: Community health, public health, primary care, and long-term care.* Philadelphia, PA, December 3.

Flynn, L., D. Suh, G. Dickson, M. Xie, and C. Boyer. 2010. Effects of nursing structures and processes on med errors. Poster presented at The 2010 State of the Science Congress on Nursing Research, September 27, Washington, DC.

Fox, K. 2010. Keeping the conversation going. *ADA News Daily*, September 24. Available from http://www.ada.org/news/2769.aspx.

Freidson, E. 1970. *Profession of medicine: A study of the sociology of applied knowledge.* Chicago: University of Chicago Press.

FTC (Federal Trade Commission). 2010. *Federal Trade Commission complaint charges conspiracy to thwart competition in teeth-whitening services: North Carolina dental board charged with improperly excluding non-dentists.* http://www.ftc.gov/opa/2010/06/ncdental.shtm (accessed September 29, 2010).

Furukawa, M. F., T. S. Raghu, and B. B. M. Shao. 2010. Electronic medical records, nurse staffing, and nurse-sensitive patient outcomes: Evidence from california hospitals. *Health Services Research* 45(4):941-962.

Goode, C. J., M. R. Lynn, C. Krsek, and G. D. Bednash. 2009. Nurse residency programs: An essential requirement for nursing. *Nursing Economic$* 27(3):142-147, 159; quiz 148.

Goode, C. J., and C. A. Williams. 2004. Post-baccalaureate nurse residency program. *Journal of Nursing Administration* 34(2):71-77.

Graham, K., and M. Cvach. 2010. Monitor alarm fatigue: Standardizing use of physiological monitors and decreasing nuisance alarms. *American Journal of Critical Care* 19(1):28-34.

Groth, S. W., L. Norsen, and H. Kitzman. 2010. Long-term outcomes of advanced practice nursing. In *Nurse practitioners: Evolution and future of advanced practice.* 5th ed., edited by E. M. Sullivan-Marx, D. O. McGivern, J. A. Fairman, and S. A. Greenberg. New York: Springer. Pp. 93-110.

Halfer, D., and E. Graf. 2006. Graduate nurse perceptions of the work experience. *Nursing Economic$* 24(3):150-155.

Hansen-Turton, T., A. Ritter, H. Begun, S. L. Berkowitz, N. Rothman, and B. Valdez. 2006. Insurers' contracting policies on nurse practitioners as primary care providers: The current landscape and what needs to change. *Policy, Politics, & Nursing Practice* 7(3):216-226.

Hansen-Turton, T., A. Ritter, and R. Torgan. 2008. Insurers' contracting policies on nurse practitioners as primary care providers: Two years later. *Policy, Politics, & Nursing Practice* 9(4):241-248.

Harris Interactive. 2008. *New WSJ.com/Harris Interactive study finds satisfaction with retail-based health clinics remains high.* http://www.harrisinteractive.com/NEWS/allnewsbydate.asp?NewsID=1308 (accessed August 6, 2010).

Hatem, M., J. Sandall, D. Devane, H. Soltani, and S. Gates. 2008. Midwife-led versus other models of care for childbearing women. *Cochrane Database of Systematic Reviews* (4):CD004667.

Hayes, L. J., L. O'Brien-Pallas, C. Duffield, J. Shamian, J. Buchan, F. Hughes, H. K. Spence Laschinger, N. North, and P. W. Stone. 2006. Nurse turnover: A literature review. *International Journal of Nursing Studies* 43(2):237-263.

HHS (Department of Health and Human Services). 2009. *CMS and ONC issue regulations proposing a definition of 'meaningful use' and setting standards for electronic health record incentive program.* http://www.hhs.gov/news/press/2009pres/12/20091230a.html (accessed September 29, 2010).

Hogan, P. F., R. F. Seifert, C. S. Moore, and B. E. Simonson. 2010. Cost effectiveness analysis of anesthesia providers. *Nursing Economic$* 28(3):159-169.

Hooker, R., and L. Berlin. 2002. Trends in the supply of physician assistants and nurse practitioners in the United States. *Health Affairs* 21(5):174-181.

Horrocks, S., E. Anderson, and C. Salisbury. 2002. Systematic review of whether nurse practitioners working in primary care can provide equivalent care to doctors. *BMJ* 324(7341):819-823.

HRSA (Health Resources and Services Adminsitration). 2004. *Supply, demand, and use of licensed practical nurses.* Rockville, MD: HRSA.

HRSA. 2006. *The registered nurse population: Findings from the National Sample Survey of Registered Nurses, March 2004.* Rockville, MD: HRSA.

HRSA. 2008. *The physician workforce.* Rockville, MD: HRSA.

HRSA. 2010. *The registered nurse population: Findings from the 2008 National Sample Survey of Registered Nurses.* Rockville, MD: HRSA.

Hughes, F., S. Clarke, D. A. Sampson, J. A. Fairman, and E. M. Sullivan-Marx. 2010. Research in support of nurse practitioners. In *Nurse practitioners: Evolution and future of advanced practice.* 5th ed., edited by E. M. Sullivan-Marx, D. O. McGivern, J. A. Fairman, and S. A. Greenberg. New York: Springer. Pp. 65-92.

Huijbregts, P. A. 2007. Chiropractic legal challenges to the physical therapy scope of practice: Anybody else taking the ethical high ground? *Journal of Manual & Manipulative Therapy* 15(2):69-80.

Hunt, E., S. Sproat, and R. Kitzmiller. 2004. *The nursing informatics implementation guide,* edited by K. Hannah and M. Ball. New York: Springer-Verlag.

INQRI (The Blog of the Interdisciplinary Nursing Quality Research Initiative). 2010a. *Interrupting a nurse can lead to errors.* http://inqri.blogspot.com/2010_07_01_archive.html (accessed September 29, 2010).

INQRI. 2010b. *Lessons learned from 9 states on building successful HAI reporting programs.* http://inqri.blogspot.com/2010/08/lessons-learned-from-9-states-on.html (accessed September 29, 2010).

IOM (Institute of Medicine). 2001. *Crossing the quality chasm: A new health system for the 21st century.* Washington, DC: National Academy Press.

IOM. 2003. *Unequal treatment: Confronting racial and ethnic disparities in health care.* Washington, DC: The National Academies Press.

IOM. 2004. *In the nation's compelling interest: Ensuring diversity in the health care workforce.* Washington, DC: The National Academies Press.

IOM. 2006. *Unequal treatment: Confronting racial and ethnic disparities in health care.* Washington, DC: The National Academies Press.

IOM. 2010a. *A summary of the December 2009 Forum on the Future of Nursing: Care in the community.* Washington, DC: The National Academies Press.

IOM. 2010b. *A summary of the October 2009 Forum on the Future of Nursing: Acute care.* Washington, DC: The National Academies Press.

Jha, A., J. Perlin, K. Kizer, and R. Dudley. 2003. Effect of the transformation of the Veterans Affairs health care system on the quality of care. *New England Journal of Medicine* 348(22): 2218-2227.

Johnson, C. 2010. *Doctor shortage? 28 states May expand nurses' role with doctor shortage, 'Dr. Nurses' seek bigger role in primary care; 28 states consider* (April 13, 2010). http://abcnews. go.com/Health/wireStory?id=10363562 (accessed May 19, 2010).

Kahn, M. G., and D. Ranade. 2010. The impact of electronic medical records data sources on an adverse drug event quality measure. *Journal of the American Medical Informatics Association* 17(2):185-191.

Kerr, E., R. Gerzoff, S. Krein, J. Selby, J. Piette, J. Curb, W. Herman, D. Marrero, K. Narayan, M. Safford, T. Thompson, and C. Mangione. 2004. Diabetes care quality in the Veterans Affairs health care system and commercial managed care: The triad study. *Annals of Internal Medicine* 141(4):272-281.

Kimball, B., and E. O'Neil. 2002. *Health care's human crisis: The American nursing shortage.* Princeton, NJ: RWJF.

King, E. S., and T. Hansen-Turton. 2010. Nurse-managed health centers. In *Nurse practitioners: The evolution and future of advanced practice*, edited by E. M. Sullivan-Marx, D. O. McGivern, J. A. Fairman and S. A. Greenberg. New York: Springer Publishing Company. Pp. 183-198.

Kovner, C. T., C. S. Brewer, S. Fairchild, S. Poornima, H. Kim, and M. Djukic. 2007. Newly licensed RNs' characteristics, work attitudes, and intentions to work. *American Journal of Nursing* 107(9):58-70; quiz 70-51.

KP (Kaiser Permanente). 2010. *Fast facts about Kaiser Permanente.* http://xnet.kp.org/newscenter/ aboutkp/fastfacts.html (accessed September 29, 2010).

Krozck, C. 2008. The new graduate RN residency: Win/win/win for nurses, hospitals, and patients. *Nurse Leader* 6(5):41-44.

Krugman, M., J. Bretschneider, P. Horn, C. Krsek, R. Moutafis, and M. Smith. 2006. The national post-baccalaureate graduate nurse residency program: A model for excellence in transition to practice. *Journal for Nurses in Staff Development* 22(4):196-205.

Kurtzman, E. T., E. M. Dawson, and J. E. Johnson. 2008. The current state of nursing performance measurement, public reporting, and value-based purchasing. *Policy, Politics, & Nursing Practice* 9(3):181-191.

Labor Management Partnership. 2010. *San Diego's home health care team sees more patients, faster.* http://www.lmpartnership.org/node/344 (accessed September 29, 2010).

Laport, N., W. Sermeus, G. Vanden Boer, and P. Van Herck. 2008. Adjusting reimbursement for nursing care. *Policy, Politics, & Nursing Practice* 9(2):94-102, 103-111.

Laurant, M., D. Reeves, R. Hermens, J. Braspenning, R. Grol, and B. Sibbald. 2004. Substitution of doctors by nurses in primary care. Cochrane Database of Systematic Reviews(2):CD001271.

Lenz, E., M. Mundinger, R. Kane, S. Hopkins, and S. Lin. 2004. Primary care outcomes in patients treated by nurse practitioners or physicians: Two-year follow-up. *Medical Care Research and Review* 61(3):332-351.

The Lewin Group. 2009. *Wisdom at work: Retaining experienced RNs and their knowledge—case studies of top performing organizations.* Falls Church, VA: The Lewin Group.

Lugo, N. R., E. T. O'Grady, D. R. Hodnicki, and C. M. Hanson. 2007. Ranking state NP regulation: Practice environment and consumer healthcare choice. *American Journal for Nurse Practitioners* 11(4):8-24.

Lynaugh, J. E. 2008. Kate Hurd-Mead lecture. Nursing the great society: The impact of the Nurse Training Act of 1964. *Nursing History Review* 16:13-28.

Marsteller, J., Y.-J. Hsu, P. Pronovost, and D. Thompson. 2010 June 28. *The relationship of nursing hours to ICU central line-associated bloodstream infections and length of stay.* Poster presented at AcademyHealth Annual Research Meeting, Boston, MA.

McKinney, M. 2010. Alarm fatigue sets off bells: Mass. Incident highlights need for protocols check. *Modern Healthcare* 40(15):14.

Medoff-Cooper, B., J. Shults, and J. Kaplan. 2009. Sucking behavior of preterm neonates as a predictor of developmental outcomes. *Journal of Developmental and Behavioral Pediatrics* 30(1):16-22.

MedPAC (Medicare Payment Advisory Commission). 2006. *Report to the Congress: Increasing the value of Medicare.* Washington, DC: MedPAC.

MedPAC. 2008. *Report to the Congress: Reforming the delivery system.* Washington, DC: MedPAC.

MedPAC. 2009. *Report to the Congress: Improving incentives in the Medicare program.* Washington, DC: MedPAC.

Mehrotra, A., M. C. Wang, J. R. Lave, J. L. Adams, and E. A. McGlynn. 2008. Retail clinics, primary care physicians, and emergency departments: A comparison of patients' visits. *Health Affairs* 27(5):1272-1282.

Mundinger, M. O., R. L. Kane, E. R. Lenz, A. M. Totten, W. Y. Tsai, P. D. Cleary, W. T. Friedewald, A. L. Siu, and M. L. Shelanski. 2000. Primary care outcomes in patients treated by nurse practitioners or physicians: A randomized trial. *JAMA* 283(1):59-68.

NACHC (National Association of Community Health Centers). 2009. *America's health centers.* Bethesda, MD: NACHC.

NACHC, The Robert Graham Center, and Capital Link. 2007. *Access granted: The primary care payoff.* Washington, DC: NACHC, The Robert Graham Center, Capital Link.

Naylor, M. D., and E. T. Kurtzman. 2010. The role of nurse practitioners in reinventing primary care. *Health Affairs* 29(5):893-899.

NCSBN (National Council of State Boards of Nursing). 2008. *Toward an evidence-based regulatory model for transitioning new nurses to practice.* https://www.ncsbn.org/Pages_from_Leader-to-Leader_FALL08.pdf (accessed September 13, 2010).

NCQA (National Committee for Quality Assurance). 2010. *About NCQA.* http://www.ncqa.org/tabid/675/Default.aspx (accessed July 9, 2010).

NNCC (National Nursing Centers Consortium). 2005. Fact sheet. Philadelphia, PA: NNCC.

NRHA (National Rural Health Association). 2010. *What's different about rural health care?* http://www.ruralhealthweb.org/go/left/about-rural-health/what-s-different-about-rural-health-care (accessed September 13, 2010).

Office of Technology Assessment. 1986. *Health technology case study 37: Nurse practitioners, physician assistants, and certified nurse-midwives: A policy analysis.* Washington, DC: U.S. Government Printing Office.

Ohlhausen, M. K., M. R. Baye, J. Schmidt, and L. B. Parnes. 2007. Letter to Louann Stanton, September 27. Available from http://www.ftc.gov/os/2007/10/v070015massclinic.pdf.

Ohlhausen, M. K., M. R. Baye, J. Schmidt, and L. B. Parnes. 2008. Letter to Elaine Nekritz, May 29. Available from http://www.ftc.gov/os/2008/06/V080013letter.pdf.

ONS (Office of Nursing Services, Department of Veterans Affairs). 2009. *VA nursing: Connecting all the pieces of the puzzle to transform care for veterans.* http://www1.va.gov/NURSING/docs/OfficeofNursingServices-ONS_Annual_Report_2009-WEB.pdf (accessed March 27, 2010).

Pearson, L. 2010. *The Pearson report: A national overview of nurse practitioner legislation and healthcare issues.* http://www.pearsonreport.com/ (accessed June 26, 2010).

Pennsylvania Governor's Office. 2009. *Governor Rendell thanks "pioneers" for making Pennsylvania the national leader on chronic care management and creating patient-centered medi-*

cal homes. http://www.portal.state.pa.us/portal/server.pt?open=512&objID=3053&PageID=
431159&mode=2&contentid=http://pubcontent.state.pa.us/publishedcontent/publish/global/
news_releases/governor_s_office/news_releases/governor_rendell_thanks__pioneers__for_
making_pennsylvania_the_national_leader_on_chronic_care_management_and_creating_
patient_centered_medical_homes.html (accessed July 1, 2010).

Phillips, R., L. Green, G. Fryer, and S. Dovey. 2001. Trumping professional roles: Collaboration
of nurse practitioners and physicians for a better U.S. health care system. *American Family
Physician* 64(8):1325.

Phillips, S. 2010. 22nd annual legislative update: Regulatory and legislative successes for APNs.
Nursing Practice 35(1):24-47.

Poissant, L., J. Pereira, R. Tamblyn, and Y. Kawasumi. 2005. The impact of electronic health records
on time efficiency of physicians and nurses: A systematic review. *Journal of the American Medical Informatics Association* 12(5):505-516.

Roberts, K., and G. Hayes. 2005. The Harambee Nursing Center. *Kentucky Nurse* Oct-Dec. http://
findarticles.com/p/articles/mi_qa4084/is_200510/ai_n15716986/.

Rosenstein, A. H., and M. O'Daniel. 2005. Disruptive behavior and clinical outcomes: Perceptions of
nurses and physicians. *American Journal of Nursing* 105(1):54-64; quiz 64-55.

Rosenstein, A. H., and M. O'Daniel. 2008. A survey of the impact of disruptive behaviors and communication defects on patient safety. *Joint Commission Journal on Quality and Patient Safety*
34(8):464-471.

Rostant, D. M., and D. M. Cady. 1999. *Liability issues in perinatal nursing.* Philadelphia, PA: Lip-
pincott Williams & Wilkins.

Rudavsky, R., C. E. Pollack, and A. Mehrotra. 2009. The geographic distribution, ownership, prices,
and scope of practice at retail clinics. *Annals of Internal Medicine* 151(5):315-320.

RWJF (Robert Wood Johnson Foundation). 2010a. *Map of the number of nurse practritioners per
primary care doctor by county, 2009.* http://thefutureofnursing.org/NursingResearchNetwork1
(accessed December 15, 2010).

RWJF. 2010b. *Map of the number of physician assistants per primary care doctor by county, 2009.*
http://thefutureofnursing.org/NursingResearchNetwork2 (accessed December 6, 2010)

RWJF. 2010c. *Nurse practitioners and physician assistants in the United States: Current patterns
of distribution and recent trends.* http://thefutureofnursing.org/NursingResearchNetwork7 (accessed December 6, 2010)

RWJF. 2010d. *Sermo.com physicians' opinions about the impact of allowing NPs to practice independently.* http://thefutureofnursing.org/NursingResearchNetwork4 (accessed December 6, 2010)

RWJF. 2010e. *Sermo.Com survey data on physicians' opinions of nurse practitioners and nurses'
educational preparation.* http://thefutureofnursing.org/NursingResearchNetwork8 (accessed
December 6, 2010)

Safriet, B. J. 2010. *Federal options for maximizing the value of advanced practice nurses in providing
quality, cost-effective health care.* Paper commissioned by the Committee on the RWJF Initiative on the Future of Nursing, at the IOM (see Appendix H on CD-ROM).

Sermo.com. 2009. *Survey of U.S. Physicians indicates AMA no longer represents them.* http://
www.sermo.com/about-us/pr/07/july/3/sermo-survey-us-physicians-indicates-ama-no-longer-
represents-them (accessed September 23, 2010).

Sia, C., T. Tonniges, E. Osterhus, and S. Taba. 2004. History of the medical home concept. *Pediatrics*
113(5):1473-1478.

Sorbel, A. L. 2010. *Calif. doctors sue to ensure nurse anesthetists are supervised.* http://www.ama-
assn.org/amednews/2010/02/22/prsa0222.htm (accessed September 10, 2010).

Staiger, D., D. Auerbach, and P. Buerhaus. 2000. Expanding career opportunities for women and the
declining interest in nursing as a career. *Nursing Economic$* 18(5):230-236.

Staiger, D. O., D. I. Auerbach, and P. I. Buerhaus. 2009. Comparison of physician workforce estimates
and supply projections. *JAMA* 302(15):1674-1680.

Steinwald, B. 2008. *Primary care professionals: Recent supply trends, projections, and valuation of services.* Washington, DC: GAO.

Stevens, R. 1999. *In sickness and wealth, American hospitals in the twentieth century.* Baltimore, MD: The Johns Hopkins University Press.

Sullivan-Marx, E. M. 2008. Lessons learned from advanced practice nursing payment. *Policy, Politics, & Nursing Practice* 9(2):121-126.

Tai, T. W., S. I. Bame, and C. D. Robinson. 1998. Review of nursing turnover research, 1977-1996. *Social Science and Medicine* 47(12):1905-1924.

Thompson, D., P. Johnston, and C. Spurr. 2009. The impact of electronic medical records on nursing efficiency. *Journal of Nursing Administration* 39(10):444-451.

TIGER (Technology Informatics Guiding Education Reform). 2009. *Testimony submitted to inform the Forum on the Future of Nursing: Community health, public health, primary care, and long-term care.* Philadelphia, PA, December 3.

UHC (University HealthSystem Consortium). 2009. *The UHC/AACN residency program.* Oak Brook, IL: UHC. Available from https://www.uhc.edu/docs/003733604_NRP_brochure.pdf.

U.S. Census Bureau. 2010. *State & county quickfacts.* http://quickfacts.census.gov/qfd/states/00000. html (accessed August 19, 2010).

VA (Department of Veterans Affairs). 2007. *VA employment brochures: Advanced practice nursing.* http://www.vacareers.va.gov/Resources_Download/APN_Brochure_021210.txt (accessed September 29, 2010).

VA. 2009. *Remarks by Secretary Eric K. Shinseki: Veterans Health Administration national leadership board strategic planning summit, Annapolis, MD, April 22, 2009.* http://www1.va.gov/opa/speeches/2009/09_0422.asp (accessed March 27, 2010).

VA. 2010. *VA benefits & health care utilization.* http://www1.va.gov/VETDATA/Pocket-Card/4X6_summer10_sharepoint.pdf (accessed August 19, 2010).

Versant. 2010. *The versant RN residency solution.* http://www.versant.org/item.asp?id=81 (accessed September 29, 2010).

VHA (Veterans Health Administration). 2003. *VHA vision 2020.* http://purl.access.gpo.gov/GPO/LPS35526 (accessed September 29, 2010).

VHA. 2009. *Quality initiatives undertaken by the Veterans Health Administration.* http://www.cbo.gov/doc.cfm?index=10453&zzz=39420 (accessed March 25, 2010).

Waneka, R., and J. Spetz. 2009. *2007-2008 annual school report: Data summary and historical trend analysis.* Sacramento, CA: California Board of Registered Nursing.

Whelan, E.-M. 2010. *The importance of community health centers: Engines of economic activity and job creation.* http://www.americanprogress.org/issues/2010/08/community_health_centers.html (accessed September 13, 2010).

Whelan, E., and L. Russell. 2010. *Better health care at lower costs why health care reform will drive better models of health care delivery.* http://www.americanprogress.org/issues/2010/03/health_delivery.html (accessed July 9, 2010).

White House. 2009. *Remarks by the President to a joint session of Congress on health care on September 9, 2009.* http://www.whitehouse.gov/the-press-office/remarks-president-a-joint-session-congress-health-care (accessed September 29, 2010).

White House. 2010. *Remarks by the President to the American Nurses Association.* http://www.whitehouse.gov/the-press-office/remarks-president-a-joint-session-congress-health-care (accessed June 26, 2010).

Williams, C. A., C. J. Goode, C. Krsek, G. D. Bednash, and M. R. Lynn. 2007. Postbaccalaureate nurse residency 1-year outcomes. *Journal of Nursing Administration* 37(7/8):357-365.

Yin, J. C., and K. P. Yang. 2002. Nursing turnover in Taiwan: A meta-analysis of related factors. *International Journal of Nursing Studies* 39(6):573-581.

Zysberg, L., and D. M. Berry. 2005. Gender and students' vocational choices in entering the field of nursing. *Nursing Outlook* 53(4):193-198.

ANNEX 3-1
STATE PRACTICE REGULATIONS
FOR NURSE PRACTITIONERS

TABLE 3-A1 State-by-State Regulatory Requirements for Physician
Involvement in Care Provided by Nurse Practitioners

State	Physician Involvement Requirement (for Prescription)	On-Site Oversight Requirement	Quantitative Requirements for Physician Chart Review	Maximum NP-to-Physician Ratio
Alabama	MD Collaboration Required	10% of the time	10% of all charts, all adverse outcomes	1 MD - 3 full-time NPs or max. total of 120 hours/week
Alaska	None	None	No	N/A
Arizona	None	None	No	N/A
Arkansas	MD Collaboration Required	None	No	None stated
California	MD Supervision Required	None	No	4 prescribing NPs - 1 MD
Colorado	None (although preceptor and mentoring period required for prescribing during the first 3,600 hours of prescriptive practice)	None	No	5 NPs - 1 MD; board may waive restriction
Connecticut	MD Collaboration Required	None	No	None stated
Delaware	MD Collaboration Required	None	No	None stated
Florida	MD Supervision Required	None	No	1 MD - no more than 4 offices in addition to MD's primary practice location (If MD provides primary health care services)

continued

TABLE 3-A1 *continued*

State	Physician Involvement Requirement (for Prescription)	On-Site Oversight Requirement	Quantitative Requirements for Physician Chart Review	Maximum NP-to-Physician Ratio
Georgia	MD Delegation Required	None	All controlled substance Rx w/in 3 mos of issuance of Rx, all adverse outcomes w/in 30 days of discovery, 10% of all other charts at least annually	4 NPs - 1 MD
Hawaii	MD Collaboration Required*	None	No	None stated
Idaho	None	None	No	N/A
Illinois	MD Delegation Required	At least once per month (no duration specified)	Yes, periodic review required for Rx orders	None stated
Indiana	MD Collaboration Required	None	Yes, at least 5% random sample of charts and medications prescribed for patients	None stated
Iowa	None	None	No	N/A
Kansas	MD Collaboration Required	None	No	None stated
Kentucky	MD Collaboration Required	None	No	None stated
Louisiana	MD Collaboration Required	None	No	None stated
Maine	None (although supervision by a physician or nurse practitioner is required for first 24 months of NP practice)	None	No	N/A
Maryland	MD Collaboration Required	None	Yes (percentage left to MD & NP discretion)	None stated

TABLE 3-A1 *continued*

State	Physician Involvement Requirement (for Prescription)	On-Site Oversight Requirement	Quantitative Requirements for Physician Chart Review	Maximum NP-to-Physician Ratio
Massachusetts	MD Supervision Required	None	Yes (for Rx only - once every 3 months, percentage left to MD & NP discretion)	None stated
Michigan	MD Delegation Required	None	No	None stated
Minnesota	MD Delegation Required	None	No	None stated
Mississippi	MD Collaboration Required	At least once every 3 months	Yes - a representative sample of either 10% or 20 charts, whichever is less, every month	None stated
Missouri	MD Delegation Required	NP must first practice for at least one month at same location of collaborating MD, after which time MD must be on-site once every 2 weeks	Yes - once every 2 weeks	3 FTE NPs - 1 MD
Montana	None	None	15 or 5% of charts, whichever is less, reviewed quarterly (may be reviewed by MD or NP peer)	None stated
Nebraska	MD Collaboration Required	None	No	None stated
Nevada	MD Collaboration Required	Part of a day, once a month	Yes (percentage left to MD & NP discretion)	3 NPs - 1 MD
New Hampshire	None	None	No	N/A
New Jersey	MD Collaboration Required	None	Yes - periodic review (percentage left to MD & NP discretion)	None stated
New Mexico	None	None	No	N/A

continued

TABLE 3-A1 *continued*

State	Physician Involvement Requirement (for Prescription)	On-Site Oversight Requirement	Quantitative Requirements for Physician Chart Review	Maximum NP-to-Physician Ratio
New York	MD Collaboration Required	None	Yes at least once every 3 months (percentage left to MD & NP discretion)	4:1 NPs to physicians (only applies if more than 4 NPs practice off-site)
North Carolina	MD Supervision Required	None	Yes (for initial 6 months of collaboration, must be review and countersigning by MD w/in 7 days of NP-patient contact & meetings of NP-MD on weekly basis for first month, & then at least monthly for next 5 months)	None stated
North Dakota	MD Collaboration Required	None	No	None stated
Ohio	MD Collaboration Required	None	Yes - periodic review (annually, percentage left to MD & NP discretion)	3 NPs - 1 MD
Oklahoma	MD Supervision Required	None	No	2 FTE NPs or max 4 PT NPs - 1 MD
Oregon	None	None	No	N/A
Pennsylvania	MD Collaboration Required	None	Yes (percentage left to MD & NP discretion)	4 NPs - 1 MD
Rhode Island	MD Collaboration Required	None	No	None stated
South Carolina	MD Delegation Required	None	No	3 NPs - 1 MD
South Dakota	MD Collaboration Required	No less than one half day a week or 10% of the time	Yes (percentage left to MD & NP discretion)	4 NPs - 1 MD
Tennessee	MD Supervision Required	Once every 30 days (no duration specified)	20% of all charts every 30 days	None stated

TABLE 3-A1 *continued*

State	Physician Involvement Requirement (for Prescription)	On-Site Oversight Requirement	Quantitative Requirements for Physician Chart Review	Maximum NP-to-Physician Ratio
Texas	MD Delegation Required	For sites serving medically underserved populations: at least once every 10 days (no duration specified). 10% for designated alternative practice sites.	10% of all charts	3 NPs or FTE - 1 MD (for alternative practice sites, 4 - 1; can be waived up to 6 - 1)
Utah	MD Collaboration Required**	None	No	None stated
Vermont	MD Collaboration Required	None	Yes (percentage left to MD & NP discretion)	None stated
Virginia	MD Supervision Required	MD must "regularly practice" at location where NP practices	Yes - periodic review (percentage left to MD & NP discretion)	4 NPs - 1 MD
Washington	None	None	No	N/A
West Virginia	MD Collaboration Required	None	Periodic and joint review of Rx practice (no percentage specified)	None stated
Wisconsin	MD Collaboration Required	None	No	None stated
Wyoming	None	None	No	None stated

NOTES: For the purposes of this chart, "collaboration" includes all collaboration-like requirements (such as "collegial relationship," etc.).
FTE = full-time equivalent; MD = medical doctor; NP = nurse practitioner; PT = part time; Rx = prescription.
* This requirement will be altered pending new rules in 2011.
** For controlled substance schedules II-III only.
SOURCE: NNCC, 2009. Reprinted with permission from Tine Hansen-Turton, NNCC. Copyright 2009 NNCC.

REFERENCE

NNCC. 2009. *NNCC's state-by-state guide to regulations regarding nurse practitioner and physician practice 2009.* http://www.nncc.us/research/ContractingToolkit/contractingtoolkitgrid.pdf (accessed December 6, 2010).

4

Transforming Education

Key Message #2: Nurses should achieve higher levels of education and training through an improved education system that promotes seamless academic progression.

Major changes in the U.S. health care system and practice environments will require equally profound changes in the education of nurses both before and after they receive their licenses. Nursing education at all levels needs to provide a better understanding of and experience in care management, quality improvement methods, systems-level change management, and the reconceptualized roles of nurses in a reformed health care system. Nursing education should serve as a platform for continued lifelong learning and include opportunities for seamless transition to higher degree programs. Accrediting, licensing, and certifying organizations need to mandate demonstrated mastery of core skills and competencies to complement the completion of degree programs and written board examinations. To respond to the underrepresentation of racial and ethnic minority groups and men in the nursing workforce, the nursing student body must become more diverse. Finally, nurses should be educated with physicians and other health professionals as students and throughout their careers.

Major changes in the U.S. health care system and practice environments will require equally profound changes in the education of nurses both before and after they receive their licenses. In Chapter 1, the committee set forth a vision of health care that depends on a transformation of the roles and responsibilities of nurses. This chapter outlines the fundamental transformation of nurse education that must occur if this vision is to be realized.

The primary goals of nursing education remain the same: nurses must be prepared to meet diverse patients' needs; function as leaders; and advance science that benefits patients and the capacity of health professionals to deliver safe, quality patient care. At the same time, nursing education needs to be transformed in a number of ways to prepare nursing graduates to work collaboratively and effectively with other health professionals in a complex and evolving health care system in a variety of settings (see Chapter 3). Entry-level nurses, for example, need to be able to transition smoothly from their academic preparation to a range of practice environments, with an increased emphasis on community and public health settings. And advanced practice registered nurses (APRNs) need graduate programs that can prepare them to assume their roles in primary care, acute care, long-term care, and other settings, as well as specialty practices.

This chapter addresses key message #2 set forth in Chapter 1: Nurses should achieve higher levels of education and training through an improved education system that promotes seamless academic progression. The chapter begins by focusing on nurses' undergraduate education, emphasizing the need for a greater number of nurses to enter the workforce with a baccalaureate degree or to progress to this degree early in their career. This section also outlines some of the challenges to meeting undergraduate educational needs. The chapter then turns to graduate nursing education, stressing the need to increase significantly the numbers and preparation of nurse faculty and researchers at the doctoral level. The third section explores the need to establish, maintain, and expand new competencies throughout a nurse's education and career. The chapter next addresses the challenge of underrepresentation of racial and ethnic minority groups and men in the nursing profession and argues that meeting this challenge will require increasing the diversity of the nursing student body. The fifth section describes some creative solutions that have been devised for addressing concerns about educational capacity and the need to transform nursing curricula. The final section presents the committee's conclusions regarding the improvements needed to transform nursing education.

The committee could have devoted this entire report to the topic of nursing education—the subject is rich and widely debated. However, the committee's statement of task required that it examine a range of issues in the field, rather than delving deeply into the many challenges involved in and solutions required to advance the nursing education system. Several comprehensive reports and analyses addressing nursing education have recently been published. They include a 2009 report from the Carnegie Foundation that calls for a "radical transformation" of nursing education (Benner et al., 2009); a 2010 report from a conference sponsored by the Macy Foundation that charts a course for "life-long learning" that is assessed by the "demonstration of competency [as opposed to written assessment] in both academic programs and in continuing education" (AACN and AAMC, 2010); two consensus reports from the Institute of Medicine (IOM) that call for greater interprofessional education of physicians, nurses, and other health professionals, as well as new methods of improving and demonstrating competency throughout one's career (IOM, 2003b, 2009); and other articles and reports on necessary curriculum changes, faculty development, and new partnerships in education (Erickson, 2002; Lasater and Nielsen, 2009; Mitchell et al., 2006; Orsolini-Hain and Waters, 2009; Tanner et al., 2008). Additionally, in February 2009, the committee hosted a forum on the future of nursing in Houston, Texas, that focused on nursing education. Discussion during that forum informed the committee's deliberations and this chapter; a summary of that forum is included on the CD-ROM in the back of this report.[1] Finally, Appendix A highlights other recent reports relevant to the nursing profession. The committee refers readers wishing to explore the subject of nursing education in greater depth to these publications.

UNDERGRADUATE EDUCATION

This section begins with an overview of current undergraduate nursing education, including educational pathways, the distribution of undergraduate degrees, the licensing exam, and costs (see Appendix E for additional background information on undergraduate education). The discussion then focuses on the need for more nurses prepared at the baccalaureate level. Finally, barriers to meeting undergraduate educational needs are reviewed.

Overview of Current Undergraduate Education

Educational Pathways

Nursing is unique among the health care professions in the United States in that it has multiple educational pathways leading to an entry-level license to practice (see the annexes to Chapter 1 and Appendix E). For the past four decades, nursing students have been able to pursue three different educational pathways to become registered nurses (RNs): the bachelor's of science in nursing (BSN), the associate's degree in nursing (ADN), and the diploma in nursing. More recently, an accelerated, second-degree bachelor's program for students who possess a baccalaureate degree in another field has become a popular option. This multiplicity of options has fragmented the nursing community and has created

---

[1] The summary also can be downloaded at http://www.iom.edu.

confusion among the public and other health professionals about the expectations for these educational options. However, these pathways also provide numerous opportunities for women and men of modest means and diverse backgrounds to access careers in an economically stable field.

In addition to the BSN, ADN, or diploma received by RNs, another under-graduate-level program available is the licensed practical/vocational diploma in nursing. Licensed practical/vocational nurses (LPNs/LVNs) are especially impor-tant because of their contributions to care in long-term care facilities and nursing homes.[2] LPNs/LVNs receive a diploma after completion of a 12-month program. They are not educated or licensed for independent decision making for complex care, but obtain basic training in anatomy and physiology, nutrition, and nursing techniques. Some LPNs/LVNs continue their education to become RNs; in fact, approximately 17.9 percent of RNs were once licensed as LPNs/LVNs (HRSA, 2010b). While most LPNs/LVNs have an interest in advancing their education, a number of barriers to their doing so have been cited, including financial con-cerns, lack of capacity and difficulty getting into ADN and BSN programs, and family commitments (HRSA, 2004). Although this chapter focuses primarily on the education of RNs and APRNs, the committee recognizes the contributions of LPNs/LVNs in improving the quality of health care. The committee also recog-nizes the opportunity the LPN/LVN diploma creates as a possible pathway toward further education along the RN and APRN tracks for the diverse individuals who hold that diploma.

Distribution of Undergraduate Degrees

At present, the most common way to become an RN is to pursue an ADN at a community college. Associate's degree programs in nursing were launched in the mid-20th century in response to the nursing shortage that followed World War II (Lynaugh, 2008; Lynaugh and Brush, 1996). The next most common undergradu-ate nursing degree is the BSN, a 4-year degree typically offered at a university. Baccalaureate nursing programs emphasize liberal arts, advanced sciences, and nursing coursework across a wider range of settings than are addressed by ADN programs, along with formal coursework that emphasizes both the acquisition of leadership development and the exposure to community and public health com-petencies. The least common route to becoming an RN currently is the diploma program, which is offered at a hospital-based school and generally lasts 3 years. During the 20th century, as nursing gained a stronger theoretical foundation and other types of nursing programs increased in number, the number of diploma programs declined remarkably except in a few states, such as New Jersey, Ohio,

---

[2] While titles for LPNs and LVNs vary from state to state, their responsibilities and education are relatively consistent. LPNs/LVNs are required to pass the National Council Licensure Examination for Practical Nurses (NCLEX-PN) to secure a license to practice.

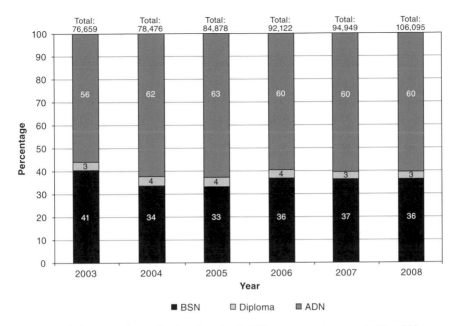

FIGURE 4-1 Trends in graduation from basic RN programs, by type, 2002–2008.
SOURCE: NLN, 2010b.

and Pennsylvania. Figure 4-1 gives an overview of trends in the distribution of nursing graduates by initial nursing degree.

Entry into Practice: The Licensing Exam[3]

Regardless of which educational pathway nursing students pursue, those working toward an RN must ultimately pass the National Council Licensure Examination for Registered Nurses (NCLEX-RN), which is administered by the National Council of State Boards of Nursing (NCSBN), before they are granted a license to practice. Rates of success on the NCLEX-RN are often used for rating schools or for marketing to potential students. As with many entry-level licensing exams, however, the NCLEX-RN uses multiple-choice, computer-based methods to test the minimum competency required to practice nursing safely. The exam is administered on a pass/fail basis and, although rigorous, is not meant to be a test of optimal performance. Following passage of the exam, individual state boards of nursing grant nurses their license to practice.

The content of the NCLEX-RN is based on surveys of what new nurses need to know to begin their practice. As with most entry-level licensing exams, the

---

[3] See https://www.ncsbn.org/nclex.htm.

content of the NCLEX-RN directly influences the curricula used to educate nursing students. Currently, the exam is skewed toward acute care settings because this is where the majority of nurses are first employed and where most work throughout their careers. To keep pace with the changing demands of the health care system and patient populations, including the shift toward increasing care in community settings (see Chapter 2), the focus of the exam will need to shift as well. Greater emphasis must be placed on competencies related to community health, public health, primary care, geriatrics, disease prevention, health promotion, and other topics beyond the provision of nursing care in acute care settings to ensure that nurses are ready to practice in an evolving health care system.

Costs of Nursing Education

Although a limited number of educational grants and scholarships are available, most of individuals seeking nursing education must finance their own education at any level of preparation. Costs vary based on the pathway selected for basic preparation and through to doctoral preparation. The LPN degree is the least expensive to attain, followed by the ADN, BSN (accelerated program), BSN, master's of science in nursing (MSN), and PhD/doctor of nursing practice (DNP) degrees. It is no surprise that educational costs and living expenses play a major role in determining which degree is pursued and the numbers of nurses who seek advanced degrees.

To better understand the costs of nursing education, the committee asked the Robert Wood Johnson Foundation (RWJF) Nursing Research Network to estimate the various costs associated with pursuing nursing education, specifically at the advanced practice level, in comparison with those for a medical doctor (MD) or doctor of osteopathy (DO). The RWJF Nursing Research Network produced several comparison charts in an attempt to convey accurately the differences in costs between alternative nursing degrees and the MD or DO degree. This task required making assumptions about public versus private and proprietary/for-profit education options, prerequisites for entry, and years required to complete each degree. An area of particular difficulty arose in assessing costs associated with obtaining an ADN degree. In most non–health care disciplines, the associate's degree takes 2 years to complete. In nursing, however, surveys have found that it takes students 3 to 4 years to complete an ADN program because of the need to fulfill prerequisites necessary to prepare students for entry into degree programs and the lack of adequate faculty, which lead to long waiting lists for many programs and classes (Orsolini-Hain, 2008). Box 4-1 illustrates the challenges of this task by outlining the difficulty of comparing the cost of becoming a physician with the cost of becoming an APRN. The task of comparing the increasing "sticker costs" of nursing and medical education was complicated further because much of the data needed to compute those costs is either missing or drawn from incomparable years. In the end, the committee decided not to include detailed discussion of the costs of nursing education in this report.

BOX 4-1
Costs of Health Professional Education

Depending on the method used, the number of advanced practice registered nurses (APRNs) that can be trained for the cost of training 1 physician is between 3 and 14. Assessing the costs of education is a multidimensional problem. Manno (1998) has suggested that costs for higher education can be measured in at least four ways:

- "the production cost of delivering education to students;
- the 'sticker price' that students/families are asked to pay;
- the cost to students to attend college, including room and board, books and supplies, transportation, tuition, and fees; and
- the net price paid by students after financial aid awards" (Starck, 2005).

While the first of these measures, the production cost to the institution, is the most complete, it is the most complex to derive. One study attempted to compare the educational cost for various health professions. This study, sponsored by the Association of Academic Health Centers (Gonyea, 1998), used the 1994 methodology of Valberg and colleagues, which included 80 percent essential education and 20 percent complementary research and service (Valberg et al., 1994). The conclusion reached was that for every 1 physician (4 years), 14 advanced nurse practitioners or 12 physician assistants could be produced (Starck, 2005).

If one examines simply the cost to students of postsecondary training (the "sticker price"), the differences among professions are slightly less dramatic. The cost to students is defined as the tuition and fees students/families pay. This measure does not include costs associated with room and board, books, transportation, and other living expenses. Nor does it include those costs incurred by the educational programs that may be beyond what is covered by tuition revenues. Residency programs for physicians are not included in this estimate because students do not pay them.

Medical residencies are funded largely by Medicare, and in 2008, totaled approximately $9 billion per year ($100,000 on average for each of about 90,000 residents) for graduate medical education (MedPAC, 2009). Some of the Medicare expenditures are for indirect costs, such as the greater costs associated with operating a teaching hospital. Estimates of the average cost per resident for the federal government are difficult to establish because of the wide variation in payments by specialty and type of hospital. In addition, residency costs vary significantly by year, with the early years requiring more supervision than the later years.

Why More BSN-Prepared Nurses Are Needed

The qualifications and level of education required for entry into the nursing profession have been widely debated by nurses, nursing organizations, academics, and a host of other stakeholders for more than 40 years (NLN, 2007). The causal relationship between the academic degree obtained by RNs and patient outcomes is not conclusive in the research literature. However, several studies support a significant association between the educational level of RNs and outcomes for patients in the acute care setting, including mortality rates (Aiken et al., 2003; Estabrooks et al., 2005; Friese et al., 2008; Tourangeau et al., 2007; Van den Heede et al., 2009). Other studies argue that clinical experience, qualifications before entering a nursing program (e.g., SAT scores), and the number of BSN-prepared RNs that received an earlier degree confound the value added through the 4-year educational program. One study found that the level of experience of nurses was more important than their education level in mitigating medication errors in hospitals (Blegen et al., 2001). Another study performed within the Department of Veterans Affairs (VA) system found no significant association between the proportion of RNs with a baccalaureate degree and patient outcomes at the hospital level (Sales et al., 2008).

This debate aside, an all-BSN workforce at the entry level would provide a more uniform foundation for the reconceptualized roles for nurses and new models of care that are envisioned in Chapters 1 and 2. Although a BSN education is not a panacea for all that is expected of nurses in the future, it does, relative to other educational pathways, introduce students to a wider range of competencies in such arenas as health policy and health care financing, leadership, quality improvement, and systems thinking. One study found that new BSN graduates reported significantly higher levels of preparation in evidence-based practice, research skills, and assessment of gaps in areas such as teamwork, collaboration, and practice (Kovner et al., 2010)—other important competencies for a future nursing workforce. Moreover, as more nurses are being called on to lead care coordination efforts, they should have the competencies requisite for this task, many of which are included in the American Association of Colleges of Nursing's (AACN's) *Essentials of Baccalaureate Education for Professional Nursing Practice*.[4]

Care within the hospital setting continues to grow more complex, and nurses must make critical decisions associated with care for sicker, frailer patients. Care in this setting depends on sophisticated, life-saving technology coupled with complex information management systems that require skills in analysis and synthesis. Care outside the hospital is becoming more complex as well. Nurses are being called upon to coordinate care among a variety of clinicians and community agencies; to help patients manage chronic illnesses, thereby preventing acute care episodes and disease progression; and to use a variety of technological tools to improve the quality and effectiveness of care. A more educated nursing workforce would be better equipped to meet these demands.

An all-BSN workforce would also be poised to achieve higher levels of education at the master's and doctoral levels, required for nurses to serve as primary care providers, nurse researchers, and nurse faculty—positions currently in great demand as discussed later in this chapter. Shortages of nurses in these positions continue to be a barrier to advancing the profession and improving the delivery of care to patients.

---

[4] See http://www.aacn.nche.edu/education/pdf/BaccEssentials08.pdf.

Some health care organizations in the United States are already leading the way by requiring more BSN-prepared nurses for entry-level positions. A growing number of hospitals, particularly teaching and children's hospitals and those that have been recognized by the American Nurses Credentialing Center Magnet Recognition Program (see Chapter 5), favor the BSN for employment (Aiken, 2010). Depending on the type of hospital, the goal for the proportion of BSN-prepared nurses varies; for example, teaching hospitals aim for 90 percent, whereas community hospitals seek at least 50 percent (Goode et al., 2001). Absent a nursing shortage, then, nurses holding a baccalaureate degree are usually the preferred new-graduate hires in acute care settings (Cronenwett, 2010). Likewise, in a recent survey of 100 physician members of Sermo.com (see Chapter 3 for more information on this online community), conducted by the RWJF Nursing Research Network, 76 percent of physicians strongly or somewhat agreed that nurses with a BSN are more competent than those with an ADN. Seventy percent of the physicians surveyed also either strongly or somewhat agreed that all nurses who provide care in a hospital should hold a BSN, although when asked about the characteristics they most value in nurses they work with, the physicians placed a significantly higher value on compassion, efficiency, and experience than on years of nursing education and caliber of nursing school (RWJF, 2010c).

In community and public health settings, the BSN has long been the preferred minimum requirement for nurses, given the competencies, knowledge of community-based interventions, and skills that are needed in these settings (ACHNE, 2009; ASTDN, 2003). The U.S. military and the VA also are taking steps to ensure that the nurses making up their respective workforces are more highly educated. The U.S. Army, Navy, and Air Force require all active duty RNs to have a baccalaureate degree to practice, and the U.S. Public Health Service has the same requirement for its Commissioned Officers. Additionally, as the largest employer of RNs in the country, the VA has established a requirement that nurses must have a BSN to be considered for promotion beyond entry level (AACN, 2010c). As Table 4-1 shows, however, the average earnings of BSN-prepared nurses are not substantially higher than those of ADN- or diploma-prepared nurses.

Decades of "blue ribbon panels" and reports to Congress on the health care workforce have found that there is a significant shortage of nurses with baccalaureate and higher degrees to respond to the nation's health needs (Aiken, 2010). Almost 15 years ago, the National Advisory Council on Nurse Education and Practice, which advises Congress and the secretary of Health and Human Services on areas relevant to nursing, called for the development of policy actions that would ensure a minimum of 66 percent of RNs who work as nurses would have a BSN or higher degree by 2010 (Aiken et al., 2009). The result of policy efforts of the past decade has been a workforce in which approximately 50 percent of RNs hold a BSN degree or higher, a figure that includes ADN- and diploma-educated RNs who have gone on to obtain a BSN (HRSA, 2010b). Of significant note, the Tri-Council for Nursing, which consists of the American Nurses Association, American Organization of Nurse Executives, National

TABLE 4-1 Average Earnings of Full-Time RNs, by Highest Nursing or Nursing-Related Education and Job Title

Position	Earnings				
	Diploma ($)	Associate's Degree ($)	Bachelor's Degree ($)	Master's/ Doctoral Degree ($)	Overall Average ($)
All nurses	65,349	60,890	66,316	87,363	66,973
Staff nurse	63,027	59,310	63,382	69,616	61,706
First-line management	68,089	66,138	75,144	85,473	72,006
Senior/middle management	74,090	69,871	79,878	101,730	81,391
Patient coordinator	62,693	60,240	64,068	71,516	62,978

NOTE: Only those who provided earnings information to surveyors are included in the calculations used for this table.
SOURCE: HRSA, 2010b.

League for Nursing (NLN), and AACN, recently released a consensus policy statement calling for a more highly educated nursing workforce, citing the need to increase the number of BSN-prepared nurses to deliver safer and more effective care (AACN, 2010a).

In sum, an increase in the percentage of nurses with a BSN is imperative as the scope of what the public needs from nurses grows, expectations surrounding quality heighten, and the settings where nurses are needed proliferate and become more complex. The formal education associated with obtaining the BSN is desirable for a variety of reasons, including ensuring that the next generation of nurses will master more than basic knowledge of patient care, providing a stronger foundation for the expansion of nursing science, and imparting the tools nurses need to be effective change agents and to adapt to evolving models of care. As discussed later in this chapter, the committee's recommendation for a more highly educated nursing workforce must be paired with overall improvements to the education system and must include competencies in such areas as leadership, basic health policy, evidence-based care, quality improvement, and systems thinking. Moreover, even as the breadth and depth of content increase within prelicensure curricula, the caring essence and human connectedness nurses bring to patient care must be preserved. Nurses need to continue to provide holistic, patient-centered care that goes beyond physical health needs to recognize and respond to the social, mental, and spiritual needs of patients and their families. Other fundamental elements of nursing education, such as ethics and integrity, need to remain intact as well.

The Goal and a Plan for Achieving It

In the committee's view, increasing the percentage of the current nursing workforce holding a BSN from 50 to 100 percent in the near term is neither practical nor achievable. Setting a goal of increasing the percentage to 80 percent by 2020 is, however, bold, achievable, and necessary to move the nursing workforce to an expanded set of competencies, especially in the domains of community and public health, leadership, systems improvement and change, research, and health policy.

The committee believes achieving the goal of 80 percent of the nursing workforce having a BSN is possible in part because much of the educational capacity needed to meet this goal exists. RNs with an ADN or diploma degree have a number of options for completing the BSN, as presented below. The combination of these options and others yet to be developed will be needed to meet the 80 percent goal—no one strategy will provide a universal solution. Technologies, such as the use of simulation and distance learning through online courses, will have to play a key role as well. Above all, what is needed to achieve this goal is the will of nurses to return to higher education, support from nursing employers and others to help fund nursing education, the elevation of educational standards, an education system that recognizes the experience and previous learning of returning students, and regional collaboratives of schools of nursing and employers to share financial and human resources.

While there are challenges associated with shortages of nurse faculty and clinical education sites (discussed below), these challenges are less problematic for licensed RNs pursuing a BSN than for prelicensure students, who require more intense oversight and monitoring by faculty. Additionally, most of what ADN-prepared nurses need to move on to a baccalaureate degree can be taught in a classroom or online, with additional tailored clinical experience. Online education creates flexibility and provides an additional skill set to students who will use technology into the future to retrieve and manage information.

Over the course of its deliberations and during the forum on education held in Houston, the committee learned about several pathways that are available to achieve the goal of 80 percent of the nursing workforce having a BSN (additional innovations discussed at the forum on education can be found in the forum summary on the CD-ROM in the back of this report). For RNs returning to obtain their BSN, a number of options are possible, including traditional RN-to-BSN programs. Many hospitals also have joint arrangements with local universities and colleges to offer onsite classes. Hospitals generally provide stipends to employees as an incentive to continue their education. Online education programs make courses available to all students regardless of where they live. For prospective nursing students, there are traditional 4-year BSN programs at a university, but there are also community colleges now offering 4-year baccalaureate degrees in some states (see the next section). Educational collaboratives between universities and community colleges, such as the Oregon Consortium for Nursing Education (described in Box 4-2), allow for automatic and seamless transition from an ADN to a BSN program, with all schools sharing curriculum, simulation facilities, and faculty. As described below, this type of model is goes beyond the conventional articulation agreement between community colleges and universities. Beyond traditional nursing schools, new providers of nursing education are entering the

BOX 4-2
Case Study: The Oregon Consortium
for Nursing Education (OCNE)

Sharing Resources to Prepare the Next Generation of Nurses

I n 2006, when Basilia Basin, BSN, RN, entered nursing school at Mount Hood Community College in Gresham, Oregon, near Portland, she was not sure whether she would pursue a bachelor's degree. A paycheck was important, she thought, and if she could obtain an associate's degree and a license after 3 years of schooling, why stay on for a fourth year to get her bachelor's? She took her time answering the question, but in the end she went for "the opportunity for professional development," she said.

Ms. Basin was in the first class of nursing students affiliated with the Oregon Consortium for Nursing Education (OCNE; www.ocne.org), a partnership, formed in 2003, between the five geographically dispersed campuses of Oregon Health & Science University (OHSU) and eight community colleges across Oregon. The 13 campuses share a standard, competency-based curriculum that was developed by faculty at full-partner community colleges and the university. The model makes the best

OCNE is an outgrowth of a great need in Oregon for a new kind of nurse. That new nurse is capable of independent decision making while practicing in acute care settings and able to marshal the best available evidence while providing leadership within changing systems.

—Christine A. Tanner, PhD, RN, A. B. Youmans-Spaulding distinguished professor, School of Nursing, Oregon Health & Science University, Portland, Oregon

use of scarce resources by pooling faculty, classrooms, and clinical education resources in a state with urban, rural, and frontier settings (Gubrud-Howe et al., 2003; Tanner et al., 2008). Community college nursing students can obtain their associate's degree in 3 years and continue for another year at OHSU to receive their baccalaureate without leaving their rural communities. This is facilitated through a seamless co-enrollment process across types of schools and financial aid transfers from the community college to the

market, such as proprietary/for-profit schools. These programs are offering new models and alternatives for delivering curriculum and reaching RNs and prospective students, although each of these schools should be evaluated for its ability to meet nursing accreditation standards, including the provision of clinical experiences required to advance the profession.

Two other important programs designed to facilitate academic progression to higher levels of education are the LPN-to-BSN and ADN-to-MSN programs.

university. The overarching goal is twofold: to broaden and strengthen the professional competency of new nurses like Ms. Basin and to use scarce resources wisely to address the nursing shortage.

Ms. Basin took her nursing licensure examination after she attained her associate's degree, remaining dually enrolled at Mount Hood and OHSU. "It was quite a unique experience," she said, "working as a nurse and being in school to become a nurse."

That experience is one that Christine A. Tanner, PhD, RN, FAAN, would like to make less unique for nursing students in her state. "We created a system that makes the best use of faculty resources, clinical training sites, and the strengths of the community college systems and the university," said Dr. Tanner, A. B. Youmans-Spaulding distinguished professor at OHSU's nursing school. Using resources more efficiently was not her sole aim, however. The nation needs "a new kind of nurse," she said, one competent in the skills needed for care in the 21st century. But only 21 percent of nurses receiving an associate's degree nationwide go on to obtain a bachelor's degree (HRSA, 2006), leaving the nation with an insufficient supply of nurses who can become faculty, advanced practice registered nurses, or clinicians prepared for a future

health care system that emphasizes community-based care.

Dr. Tanner knew that nursing schools needed a new kind of curriculum. She and her OHSU colleagues met with representatives of the community colleges and agreed to craft a single nursing curriculum that would span all 13 campuses. The first course in the program, after prerequisites, is health promotion. It introduces students to clinical decision making and nursing leadership—"learning to think like a nurse," as Dr. Tanner put it—as they relate to prevention and wellness. Students then move on to courses in chronic illness management and acute care. Those who remain enrolled for the bachelor's take courses in population-based care, epidemiology, leadership, and outcome management.

Although the number of nursing students per faculty member in Oregon nearly doubled between 2001 and 2008 (Oregon Center for Nursing, 2009), 95 to 100 percent of graduates of OCNE schools pass the nursing licensure exam (the national average is 88 percent [NCSBN, 2009]). Of students in the OCNE system who attain an associate's degree, 45 percent receive a bachelor's degree. One important result is that nurses with a baccalaureate are becoming more widely distributed in rural areas.

Dr. Tanner is working on edu-

continued

The ADN-to-MSN program, in particular, is establishing a significant pathway to advanced practice and faculty positions, especially at the community college level. Financial support to help build capacity for these programs will be important, including funding for grants and scholarships for nurses wishing to pursue these pathways. By the same token, the committee believes that diploma programs should be phased out over the next 10 years and should consolidate their resources with those of community college or preferably university programs

BOX 4-2 *continued*

cational redesign with the Center to Champion Nursing in America, funded by the Robert Wood Johnson Foundation, and its state partnerships of nursing and other stakeholders concerned about the nursing shortage. Ten state partnerships have committed to adopting the model; five states—Hawaii, New York, North Carolina, California, and New Mexico—have already begun. Dr. Tanner is consulting with faculty members in at least ten other states, and the nation's largest urban public university system,

the City University of New York, is adopting the model as well.

Robyn Alper, MA, BSN, RN, an OCNE graduate now working as a nurse for a county in northern Oregon, may personify the OCNE ideal. "The students coming out of OCNE have the skill to practice anywhere, but with an eye toward being a leader in the profession," Ms. Alper said. "I feel I can go out into the community—not with every skill perfectly honed, but I know how to find what I need to get my job done."

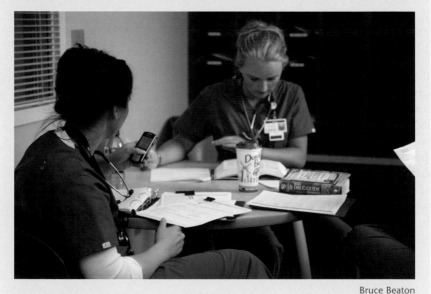

Bruce Beaton

Nursing students study together. OCNE provides a supportive environment and opportunities for students to progress seamlessly to a BSN degree.

offering the baccalaureate degree. Additionally, there are federal resources currently being used to support diploma schools that could better be used to expand baccalaureate and higher education programs.

The committee anticipates that it will take a few years to build the educational capacity needed to achieve the goal of 80 percent of the nursing workforce being BSN-prepared by 2020, but also emphasizes that existing BSN completion programs have capacity that is far from exhausted. Regional networks of schools working together, along with health care organizations, may best facilitate reaching this goal. Moreover, the committee believes this clearly defined goal will stimulate stakeholders to take action. Examples of such action include academic and health care organizations/employers partnering to achieve strategic alignment around workforce development; government and foundations introducing funding opportunities for scholarships to build faculty and provide tuition relief; state boards of nursing increasing the use of earmarks on licensure fees to offset the cost of education; and states developing statewide policy agendas and political action plans with identified leaders in nursing, government, and business to adopt measures to meet the goal.

The Role of Community Colleges

Community colleges play a key role in attracting students to the nursing education pipeline. Specifically, they provide an opportunity for students who may not have access to traditional university baccalaureate programs because of those programs' lack of enrollment capacity, distance, or cost.

Community colleges have an important role to play in ensuring that more BSN-prepared nurses are available in all regions of the United States and that nursing education at the associate level is high quality and affordable and prepares ADN nurses to move on to higher levels of education. Currently, ADN- and BSN-prepared nurses are not evenly distributed nationwide. BSN-prepared RNs are found more commonly in urban areas, while many rural and other medically underserved communities depend heavily on nurses with associate's degrees to staff their hospitals, clinics, and long-term care facilities (Cronenwett, 2010). Figure 4-2 shows the highest nursing or nursing-related education by urban/rural residence. According to a study by the Urban Institute, "medical personnel, including nurses, tend to work near where they were trained" (Bovjberg, 2009; see Figure 4-3). This suggests that state and community investments in nursing education (e.g., building nursing school capacity, building infrastructure to support that capacity, funding the purchase of technology, and offering scholarships) may be an effective way to reduce local and regional shortages. Community colleges are the predominant educational institutions in rural and medically underserved areas. Therefore, they must either join educational collaboratives or develop innovative and easily accessible programs that seamlessly connect students to schools offering the BSN and higher degrees, or they must develop their own BSN programs (if feasible within state laws and regulations). Community colleges must foster a culture that promotes and values academic progression and should encourage their students to continue their education through strategies that include making them aware of the full range of educational pathways and opportunities available to them (e.g., ADN-to-MSN and online RN-to-BSN programs). Box 4-3 describes a community college in Florida where nursing students can take advantage of lower costs and online classes to receive a BSN degree.

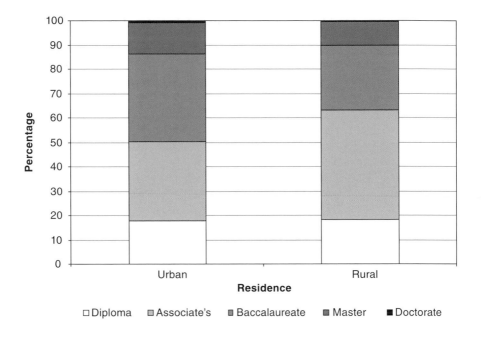

FIGURE 4-2 Highest nursing or nursing-related education by urban/rural residence.
SOURCE: Calculations performed using the data and documentation for the 2004 National Sample of Registered Nurses, available from the Health Resources and Services Administration's Geospatial Data Warehouse (HRSA, 2010a).

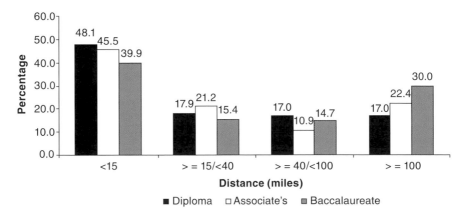

FIGURE 4-3 Distance between nursing education program and workplace for early-career nurses (graduated 2007–2008).
SOURCE: RWJF, 2010a. Reprinted with permission from Lori Melichar, RWJF.

Barriers to Meeting Undergraduate Educational Needs

Although the committee believes the capacity needed to ensure a nursing workforce that is 80 percent BSN-prepared by 2020 can be attained using the approaches outlined above, getting there will not be easy. Nursing schools across the United States collectively turn away tens of thousands of qualified applicants each year because of a lack of capacity (Kovner and Djukic, 2009)—a situation that makes filling projected needs for more and different types of nurses difficult. Figure 4-4 shows the breakdown of numbers of qualified applicants who are turned away from ADN and BSN programs.

An examination of the root causes of the education system's insufficient capacity to meet undergraduate educational needs reveals four major barriers: (1) the aging and shortage of nursing faculty; (2) insufficient clinical placement opportunities of the right kind or duration for prelicensure nurses to learn their profession; (3) nursing education curricula that fail to impart relevant competencies needed to meet the future needs of patients and to prepare nurses adequately for academic progression to higher degrees; and (4) inadequate workforce planning, which stems from a lack of the communications, data sources, and information systems needed to align educational capacity with market demands. This final root cause—inadequate workforce planning—affects all levels of nursing education and is the subject of Chapter 6.

Aging and Shortage of Nursing Faculty

There are not enough nursing faculty to teach the current number of nursing students, let alone the number of qualified applicants who wish to pursue nursing. The same forces that are leading to deficits in the numbers and competencies of bedside nurses affect the capacity of nursing faculty as well (Allan and Aldebron, 2008). According to a survey by the NLN, 84 percent of U.S. nursing schools tried to hire new faculty in the 2007–2008 academic year; of those, four out of five found it "difficult"[5] to recruit faculty, and one out of three found it "very difficult." The principal difficulties included "not enough qualified candidates" (cited by 46 percent) and the inability to offer competitive salaries (cited by 38 percent). The survey concluded that "post-licensure programs were much more likely to cite a shortage of faculty, whereas pre-licensure programs reported that lack of clinical placement settings were [sic] the biggest impediment to admitting more students. Specifically, almost two thirds (64 percent) of doctoral programs and one half of RN-BSN and master's programs identified an insufficient faculty pool to draw from as the major constraint to expansion, in contrast to one third of prelicensure programs" (NLN, 2010a).

---

[5] "Difficult" is the sum of schools responding either "somewhat difficult" or "very difficult." Personal communication, Kathy A. Kaufman, Senior Research Scientist, Public Policy, National League for Nursing, September 8, 2010.

BOX 4-3
Case Study: Community Colleges Offering the BSN

The College of Nursing at St. Petersburg College and Others
Open the Door to the Bachelor's Degree in Nursing

Tamela Monroe was 33 and working in sales in 1997 when she decided to pursue a career in nursing. She looked into the associate's degree program at a campus of St. Petersburg Junior College about a mile from her home in Palm Harbor, Florida. She did not consider the bachelor's of science in nursing (BSN) program at the University of South Florida (USF) in Tampa; she had started working as a nurse's aide and felt she could not give up her job to go to school full time. "I was just starting out in nursing," she said. "And to lose any more money would not have been a good thing." She earned her associate's degree in 2001.

When St. Petersburg Junior College changed its name to St. Petersburg College in 2002 and became the first baccalaureate-granting community college in Florida, Ms. Monroe pursued the BSN there. She was a licensed registered nurse (RN) working in a cardiac progressive care unit; classes were held in the community hospital where she worked. She received her bachelor's degree in 2004, and went on to USF to obtain her master's degree in 2006. Now 46, she is a clinical nurse leader in an orthopedic and neuroscience unit in a Tampa-area facility, as well as an adjunct instructor in nursing at Saint Petersburg College.

The more education a nurse has, the better the patient outcomes you're going to see.

—Jean Wortock, PhD, MSN, ARNP, dean and professor, College of Nursing at St. Petersburg College, St. Petersburg, Florida

---

The first community college in Florida to grant baccalaureate degrees, St. Petersburg College enrolled the first students in its BSN program in 2002. Now, its 613 BSN students and 687 associate's degree in nursing students can take classes on campus or online. Nine community colleges in Florida offer the BSN, and at least three other states are working on allowing their community colleges to offer baccalaureates, including BSNs.

Ms. Monroe is grateful to have earned a BSN at a cost 20 percent lower than the university's tuition, and she sees this as an important development in nursing education. "It presents an opportunity for nurses in this area who might not have the finances or the time to travel all the way to a larger campus," she said.

Some critics argue that in granting baccalaureates, community colleges are reaching beyond the bounds of their original mission of granting 2-year degrees as a stepping stone to a university education. Other opponents say that community college enrollments—and funds—are already stretched to the limit. In Michigan, for instance, critics say that community college tuition for the BSN will have to rise to avoid the need for more state funding (Lane, 2009).

Still, many nurses are praising the quality, convenience, flexibility, and affordability of the BSN programs available at community colleges. Jean Wortock, PhD, MSN, ARNP, dean and professor of nursing at Saint Petersburg College, said her school's BSN program is opening up an important channel for Florida nurses to advance their education in a state where 46 percent of qualified applicants to BSN programs were turned away in 2009 because of faculty shortages and other factors (Florida Center for Nursing, 2010). "We strongly encourage all of our baccalaureate graduates to go on for master's degrees," she said. "And a number of ours have."

Dr. Wortock said that St. Petersburg College and USF have worked closely in the past 9 years to determine the degrees each institution would offer: "We're offering some that they prefer not to offer so that they can focus more on master's programs in a particular field." St. Petersburg College now offers 22 bachelor's degrees, and even though both institutions have RN-to-BSN programs, the St. Petersburg nursing

school has had high enough enrollments to allow the hiring of eight full-time faculty members with doctorates to teach in its BSN program.

Dr. Wortock has talked to nurses at community colleges in California, Washington, and Michigan about how her school took the lead in offering the BSN in Florida. And while she acknowledged that the movement is controversial, it is a movement nonetheless. "It will give us a cadre of graduates and nurses that are much more prepared for research and evidence-based practice," she said.

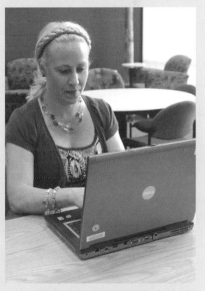

Casey Feldkamp, Institutional Advancement, St. Petersburg College

Nursing instructor Tamela Monroe, herself a former BSN student at St. Petersburg college, teaches nursing students in a virtual classroom.

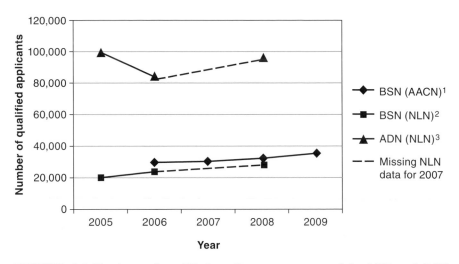

FIGURE 4-4 Numbers of qualified applicants not accepted in ADN and BSN programs.

NOTES:

[1] Number of qualified applicants not accepted in baccalaureate generic RN programs, based on AACN data in *Enrollment and Graduations in Baccalaureate and Graduate Programs in Nursing* (2006-07, Table 37; 2007-08, Table 39; 2008-09, Table 38; 2009-2010, Table 39).

[2] Number of qualified applicants not accepted in baccalaureate generic RN and RN-to-BSN programs, based on National League for Nursing data in *Nursing Data Review* (2004-05, Tables 3 & 6; 2005-06, Tables 2 & 5; 2007-08; Tables 2 & 5).

[3] Number of qualified applicants not accepted in associate's degree RN programs, based on National League for Nursing data in *Nursing Data Review* (2004-05, Tables 3 & 6; 2005-06, Tables 2 & 5; 2007-08; Tables 2 & 5).

The definition of "qualified" varies from nursing program to nursing program and is based on each program's admission requirements and completion standards at the schools that were surveyed.

SOURCE: RWJF, 2010b. Reprinted with permission from Lori Melichar, RWJF.

Age is also a contributing factor to faculty shortages. Nursing faculty tend to be older than clinical nurses because they must meet requirements for an advanced degree in order to teach. Figure 4-5 shows that the average age of nurses who work as faculty as their principal nursing position—the position in which a nurse spends the majority of his or her working hours[6]—is 50 to 54. By contrast, the median age of the total RN workforce is 46. More than 19 percent of RNs whose principal position is faculty are aged 60 or older, while only 8.7 percent

---

[6] Personal communication, Joanne Spetz, Professor, Community Health Systems, University of California, San Francisco, September 2, 2010.

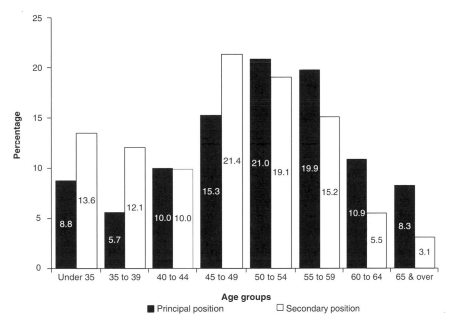

FIGURE 4-5 Age distribution of nurses who work as faculty.
SOURCE: HRSA, 2010b.

of nurses who have a secondary position as faculty—those who hold a nonfaculty
(e.g., clinical) principal position—are aged 60 or older. Nurses who work as faculty as their secondary position tend to be younger; among nurses under age 50,
more work as faculty as their secondary than as their principal position (HRSA,
2010b). Moreover, the average retirement age for nursing faculty is 62.5 (Berlin
and Sechrist, 2002); as a result, many full-time faculty will be ready to retire
soon. Given the landscape of the health care system and the fragmented nursing
education system, the current pipeline cannot easily replenish this loss, let alone
meet the potential demand for more educators. In addition to the innovative strategies of the Veterans Affairs Nursing Academy (VANA) and Gulf Coast Health
Services Steering Committee for responding to faculty shortages (discussed later
in this chapter), a potential opportunity to relieve faculty shortages could involve
the creation of programs that would allow MSN, DNP, and PhD students to teach
as nursing faculty interns, with mentoring by full-time faculty. Box 4-4 presents
a nurse profile of one assistant professor and her experience moving into an
academic career.

Effects of the first degree at entry into the profession Nurses who enter the
profession with an associate's degree are less likely than those who enter with a

BOX 4-4
Nurse Profile: Jennifer Wenzel*

Pursuing an Academic Career

Although she believes that "all nurses make a difference, wherever we practice, whatever we do," Jennifer Wenzel, PhD, RN, CCM, said that her primary motivation in choosing an academic career, one that combined research with teaching, was that it gave her a way "to have a wider, broader impact."

She's an assistant professor of nursing at Johns Hopkins University in Baltimore, the manager of the Center for Collaborative Intervention Research, and the principal investigator or co-investigator on 17 research projects in the past decade. In her research Dr. Wenzel has explored, among other topics, rural African Americans with cancer and self-care in patients with diabetes. She has also studied "professional bereavement" and resilience in oncology nurses—how nurses cope with the recurring loss of patients—with lead researcher Sharon Krumm, PhD, RN. Dr. Wenzel said that one not-so-surprising finding has been a discussion of "some of the pressures and demands that nurses place on themselves and on each other."

What she finds exciting about her work, whether with students or with research subjects, she said, is "the opportunity for sustainability. I'm trying to build something that has a lasting effect. That's always been my dream—what can we give people that will help them, not just in the situation that they're in, but in future situations, as well?"

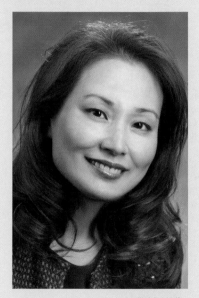

Keith Weller

Jennifer Wenzel, PhD, RN, CCM

---

*This nurse profile was inadvertently omitted from the prepublication version of this report.

bachelor's degree to advance to the graduate level over the course of their career (Cleary et al., 2009). Figure 4-6 gives an overview of the highest educational degree obtained by women and men who hold the RN license. It includes RNs who are working as nurses and those who have retired, have changed professions, or are no longer working. According to an analysis by Aiken and colleagues (2009),

The "broader impact," the "lasting effect": these are the goals of a woman reared in a tradition of service. An adopted child, she grew up in San Diego in a military family that valued hard work, education, and helping others. And even though neither of her parents finished college, they supported her decision to enter a "two-plus-two" nursing program at Southern Adventist University in Collegedale, Tennessee, in the 1980s.

She went through a bit of culture shock there. As an Asian American, she didn't look like most of her patients; as a Californian, she didn't sound like them, either. There were times it became clear that her patients had no idea what she was saying: "I would overhear somebody say to another, 'Is she speaking English? Can you tell?'" Dr. Wenzel said that it taught a lesson that has served her well as a teacher and a researcher: in order to be understood, you have to listen.

She earned an associate's degree after two years and went on to complete the bachelor's in two more years while working as a staff nurse in endocrinology at a Chattanooga hospital, supporting not only her own education but also her sister's. "There had always been this idea that it's important to give back, that society doesn't necessarily owe you anything," Dr. Wenzel said of her family's values.

After completing her bachelor's, she taught a clinical course at a Chattanooga community college. She enjoyed it but felt more drawn to clinical practice and worked as a case manager at a Georgia facility. Her first real immersion in education came at the University of Virginia, where as a doctoral student she was asked to teach a clinical group on inpatient oncology. Other offers soon followed, and she discovered that nurses with advanced degrees always have options.

I challenged a tradition by starting my PhD at a fairly young age. With the critical shortage of faculty, we cannot afford to lose candidates for faculty positions. We probably need them sooner than we can get them.

—Jennifer Wenzel, PhD, RN, CCM, assistant professor of nursing, Johns Hopkins University, Baltimore

---

That's the message she's getting as a Robert Wood Johnson Foundation Nurse Faculty Scholar, as well. The national program aids junior nursing faculty in becoming academic leaders, skilled teachers, and productive scholars. And it's what she tries to impart to her students, too. She tells them: "'I know that many of you have the ability to [get a doctorate] if you want to do it. And don't let anyone tell you that you can't.'" That sort of determination continues to fuel her career. "It's a real pleasure to see people who are starting out doing something that you love," said Dr. Wenzel. "Seeing their excitement about it reenergizes you and helps to remind you what drew you to the profession."

nurses whose initial degree is the ADN are just as likely as BSN-prepared nurses to seek another degree. Approximately 80 percent of the time, however, ADN graduates fail to move beyond a BSN. Therefore, the greatest number of nurses with a master's or doctorate, a prerequisite for serving as faculty, received a BSN as their initial degree. Since two-thirds of current RNs received the ADN as their

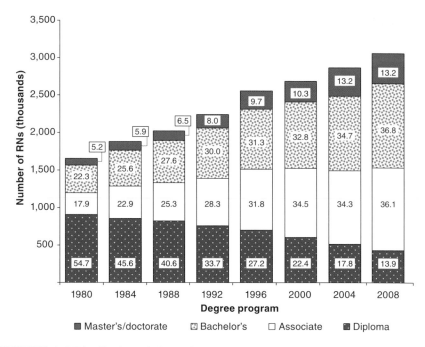

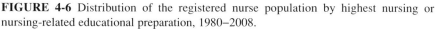

FIGURE 4-6 Distribution of the registered nurse population by highest nursing or nursing-related educational preparation, 1980–2008.

NOTES: The totals in each bar may not equal the estimated numbers for RNs in each survey year because of incomplete information provided by respondents and the effect of rounding. Only those who provided information on initial RN educational preparation to surveyors were included in the calculations used for this figure.

SOURCE: HRSA, 2010b.

initial degree, Aiken's analysis suggests that currently "having enough faculty (and other master's prepared nurses) to enable nursing schools to expand enrollment is a mathematical improbability" (Aiken et al., 2009). A separate analysis of North Carolina nurses led to a similar conclusion (Bevill et al., 2007). Table 4-2 shows the length of time it takes those nurses who do move on to higher levels of education to progress from completing initial nursing education to completing the highest nursing degree achieved.

Salary disparities   Another factor that contributes to the current nursing faculty shortage is salary disparities between nurses working in education and those working in clinical service (Gilliss, 2010). As shown in Table 4-3, the average annual earnings of nurses who work full time as faculty (most with either a master's or doctoral degree) total $63,949. By contrast, nurse practitioners (NPs) (with

TABLE 4-2 Years Between Completion of Initial and Highest RN Degrees

Initial RN Education	Highest Nursing or Nursing-Related Degree		
	Bachelor's	Master's	Doctorate
Diploma	10.5	13.9	15.6
Associate's	7.5	11.5	12.5
Bachelor's	—	8.2	12.4

NOTE: Average years between diploma and ADN not calculated due to larger than average rates of missing data. Too few cases to report estimated percent (fewer than 30 respondents).
SOURCE: HRSA, 2010b.

TABLE 4-3 Average Annual Earnings of Nurses Who Work Full Time as Faculty in Their Principal Nursing Position, 2008

	Annual Earnings ($)
All Faculty	63,985
Earnings by type of program	
Faculty in diploma/ADN programs	62,689
Faculty in BSN programs	64,789
Earnings by faculty job title	
Instructor/lecturer	54,944
Professor	69,691

SOURCE: HRSA, 2010b.
NOTE: Only registered nurses who provided earnings information were included in the calculations used for this table.

either a master's or doctoral degree) average just over $85,000 (see Table 4-4). Section 5311 of the Affordable Care Act (ACA) offers an incentive designed to offset lower faculty salaries by providing up to $35,000 in loan repayments and scholarships for eligible nurses who complete an advanced nursing degree and serve "as a full-time member of the faculty of an accredited school of nursing, for a total period, in the aggregate, of at least 4 years."[7] However, the ACA does not provide incentives for nurses to develop the specific educational and clinical competencies required to teach.

Projections of future faculty demand To establish a better understanding of future needs, the committee asked the RWJF Nursing Research Network to proj-

---

[7] *Patient Protection and Affordable Care Act*, HR 3590 § 5311, 111th Congress.

TABLE 4-4 Average Earnings by Job Title of Principal
Position for Nurses Working Full Time

Position Title	Average Annual Earnings ($)
Staff nurse	61,706
Management/administration	78,356
First-line management	72,006
Middle management	74,799
Senior management	96,735
Nurse anesthetist	154,221
Clinical nurse specialist	72,856
Nurse midwife	82,111
Nurse practitioner	85,025
Patient educator	59,421
Instructor	65,844
Patient coordinator	62,978
Informatics nurse	75,242
Consultant	76,473
Researcher	67,491
Surveyor/auditor/regulator	65,009
Other*	64,003
Total	66,973

NOTE: *Other position title includes nurses for whom position title is
unknown.
Only registered nurses who provided earnings and job title information are
included in the calculations used for this table.
SOURCE: HRSA, 2010b.

ect faculty demand for the next 15 years. After reviewing data from the AACN[8]
and the NLN (Kovner et al., 2006), the network estimated that between 5,000
and 5,500 faculty positions will remain unfilled in associate's, baccalaureate,
and higher degree programs. This projection is based on historical nurse faculty
retirement rates and on graduation trends in research-focused nursing PhD programs. Although a doctoral degree is often required or preferred for all current
faculty vacancies, some of these positions can be filled with faculty holding DNP
or master's degrees.

If faculty retirement rates decrease and/or new faculty positions are created
to meet future demands (resulting, for example, from provisions for loan repayment in the ACA), these factors will affect the shortage estimates. Additionally,
the faculty supply may be affected positively by growing numbers of graduates
with a DNP degree (discussed later in this chapter) who, as noted above, may be
eligible for faculty positions in some academic institutions.

---

[8] Personal communication, Di Fang, Director of Research and Data Services, AACN, March 3,
2010.

Insufficient Clinical Placement Opportunities

As nursing education has moved out of hospital-based programs and into mainstream colleges and universities, integrating opportunities for clinical experience into coursework has become more difficult (Cronenwett, 2010). Nursing leaders continue to confront challenges associated with the separation of the academic and practice worlds in ensuring that nursing students develop the competencies required to enter the workforce and function effectively in health care settings (Cronenwett and Redman, 2003; Fagin, 1986). While efforts are being made to expand placements in the community and more care is being delivered in community settings, the bulk of clinical education for students still occurs in acute care settings.

The required number of clinical hours varies widely from one program to another, and most state boards of nursing do not specify a minimum number of clinical hours in prelicensure programs (NCSBN, 2008). It is likely, moreover, that many of the clinical hours fail to result in productive learning. Students spend much of their clinical time performing routine care tasks repeatedly, which may not contribute significantly to increased learning. Faculty report spending most of their time supervising students in hands-on procedures, leaving little time focused on fostering the development of clinical reasoning skills (McNelis and Ironside, 2009).[9]

Some advances in clinical education have been made through strong academic–service partnerships. An example of such partnerships in community settings is nurse-managed health centers (discussed in Chapter 3), which serve a dual role as safety net practices and clinical education sites. Another, commonly used model is having skilled and experienced practitioners in the field oversee student clinical experiences. According to a recent integrative review, using these skilled practitioners, called preceptors, in a clinical setting is at least as effective as traditional approaches while conserving scarce faculty resources (Udlis, 2006). A variety of other clinical partnerships have been designed to increase capacity in the face of nursing faculty shortages (Baxter, 2007; DeLunas and Rooda, 2009; Kowalski et al., 2007; Kreulen et al., 2008; Kruger et al., 2010).

In addition to academic–service partnerships and preceptor models, the use of high-fidelity simulation offers a potential solution to the problem of limited opportunities for clinical experience, with early studies suggesting the effectiveness of this approach (Harder, 2010). The NLN, for example, has established an online community called the Simulation Innovation Resource Center, where nurse faculty can learn how to "design, implement, and evaluate the use of simulation" in

---

[9] This paragraph, and the three that follow, were adapted from a paper commissioned by the committee on "Transforming Pre-Licensure Nursing Education: Preparing the New Nurse to Meet Emerging Health Care Needs," prepared by Christine A. Tanner, Oregon Health & Science University School of Nursing (see Appendix I on CD-ROM).

their curriculum.[10] However, there is little evidence that simulation expands faculty capacity, and no data exist to define what portion of clinical experience it can replace. To establish uniform guidelines for educators, accreditation requirements should be evaluated and revised to allow simulation to fulfill the requirement for a standard number of clinical hours. The use of simulation in relationship to the promotion of interprofessional education is discussed below.

Increased attention is being focused on the dedicated education unit (DEU) as a viable alternative for expanding clinical education capacity (Moscato et al., 2007). In this model, health care units are dedicated to the instruction of students from one program. Staff nurses who want to serve as clinical instructors are prepared to do so, and faculty expertise is used to support their development and comfort in this role. DEUs were developed in Australia and launched in the United States at the University of Portland in Oregon in 2003. Since then, the University of Portland has helped at least a dozen other U.S. nursing schools establish DEUs. In programs that offer DEUs, students perform two 6-week rotations per semester, each instructor/staff nurse teaches no more than two students at a time, and a university faculty member oversees the instruction. Early results suggest the DEU can dramatically increase capacity and have a positive effect on satisfaction among students and nursing staff. A multisite study funded by RWJF is currently under way to evaluate outcomes of the DEU model.

DEUs offer benefits for the nursing schools, the hospitals, the faculty, and the students. Because the hospital employs the clinical instructors, the nursing school can increase its enrollment without increasing costs. The hospital benefits by training students it can hire after their graduation and licensure. Students benefit by having consistent clinical instructors each day, something not guaranteed under the traditional preceptorship model. As the case study in Box 4-5 shows, the benefits of DEUs extend beyond the academic environment to the practice setting as well.

Need for Updated and Adaptive Curricula

A look at the way nursing students are educated at the prelicensure level[11] shows that most schools are not providing enough nurses with the required competencies in such areas as geriatrics and culturally relevant care to meet the changing health needs of the U.S. population (as outlined in Chapter 2) (AACN and Hartford, 2000). The majority of nursing schools still educate students primarily for acute care rather than community settings, including public health and long-term care. Most curricula are organized around traditional medical specialties (e.g., maternal–child, pediatrics, medical–surgical, or adult health) (McNelis

---

[10] See http://sirc.nln.org/.

[11] Available evidence is based on evaluation of BSN programs and curricula. Evidence was not available for ADN or diploma programs.

and Ironside, 2009). The intricacies of care coordination are not adequately addressed in most prelicensure programs. Nursing students may gain exposure to leading health care disciplines and know something about basic health policy and available health and social service programs, such as Medicaid. However, their education often does not promote the skills needed to negotiate with the health care team, navigate the regulatory and access stipulations that determine patients' eligibility for enrollment in health and social service programs, or understand how these programs and health policies impact health outcomes. Nursing curricula need to be reexamined and updated. They need to be adaptive enough to undergo continuous evaluation and improvement based on new evidence and a changing science base, changes and advances in technology, and changes in the needs of patients and the health care system.

Many nursing schools have dealt with the rapid growth of health research and knowledge by adding layers of content that require more instruction (Ironside, 2004). A wide range of new competencies also are being incorporated into requirements for accreditation (CCNE, 2009; NLNAC, 2008). For example, new competencies have been promulgated to address quality and patient safety goals (Cronenwett et al., 2007; IOM, 2003a). Greater emphasis on prevention, wellness, and improved health outcomes has led to new competency requirements as well (Allan et al., 2005). New models of care being promulgated as a result of health care reform will need to be introduced into students' experiences and will require competencies in such areas as care coordination. These models, many of which could be focused in alternative settings such as schools and workplaces, will create new student placement options that will need to be tested for scalability and compared for effectiveness with more traditional care settings. (See also the discussion of competencies later in the chapter.)

The explosion of knowledge and decision-science technology also is changing the way health professionals access, process, and use information. No longer is rote memorization an option. There simply are not enough hours in the day or years in an undergraduate program to continue compressing all available information into the curriculum. New approaches must be developed for evaluating curricula and presenting fundamental concepts that can be applied in many different situations rather than requiring students to memorize different lists of facts and information for each situation.

Just as curricula must be assessed and rethought, so, too, must teaching–learning strategies. Most nurse faculty initially learned to be nurses through highly structured curricula that were laden with content (NLN Board of Governors, 2003), and too few have received advanced formal preparation in curriculum development, instructional design, or performance assessment. Faculty, tending to teach as they were taught, focus on covering content (Benner et al., 2009; Duchscher, 2003). They also see curriculum-related requirements as a barrier to the creation of learning environments that are both engaging and student-centered (Schaefer and Zygmont, 2003; Tanner, 2007).

BOX 4-5
Case Study: The Dedicated Education Unit

A New Model of Education to Increase
Enrollment Without Raising Costs

Jamie Sharp, a 21-year-old University of Portland (UP) nursing student who has performed clinical rotations in a variety of units, remembers a particularly unpleasant experience in a psychiatric unit where she felt she was "in the way" of her nurse preceptors. This was in stark contrast to her experience on a neurovascular unit at Providence St. Vincent Medical Center, where she had just one clinical instructor, a nurse who was eager to teach her.

That neurovascular unit was a dedicated education unit (DEU). Created in Australia in the late 1990s and launched in the United States at UP in 2003, the DEU model joins a school of nursing with units at local hospitals, where experienced staff nurses become clinical instructors of juniors and seniors in the bachelor's degree program. Each instructor teaches no more than two students at a time, but the DEU can be used around the clock.

With a DEU, a nursing school can "cultivate a unit" as an excellent learning environment, said UP's dean of nursing, Joanne Warner, PhD, RN, FAAN. Most important, she added, is "the expertise of the nurses there—they know the clinical procedures, the current medications, the policies of the hospital." The DEU differs from a usual clinical rotation in the relationship that develops between instructor and student, something that cannot take place when a preceptor has eight students that change from week to week. The instructor gets to know the strengths and weaknesses of the student and supports the student in building confidence and relevant knowledge and skills.

Our clinical instructors want the patients to go home with the best outcomes and the students to leave here with the best learning experiences. These students will be the ones taking care of us in the future, and we want them to be very well prepared.

—Cindy Lorion, MSN, RN, nurse manager, neurovascular and orthopedic units, Providence St. Vincent Medical Center, Portland, Oregon

---

Ms. Sharp was paired with Cathy Mead, ADN, RN, a nurse with 25 years of experience in the unit who received clinical instructor training from the nursing school. Her instruction is overseen by both a university faculty member and the unit's nurse manager.

Dr. Warner said that the benefits to her school and to students are quite tangible: "We have tripled our enrollment. If we had a traditional model I would not have the budget to hire the clinical faculty needed." The number of students on clinical rotations increased from 227 in 14 units in 2002, before the DEUs were implemented, to 333 in 6 units in 2006, after the DEUs were instituted (Moscato et al., 2007). Now, up to 60 percent of a UP nursing student's clinical rotations take place in DEUs. But equally important, the students report learning more in DEUs and are seeking clinical placements on them.

It might appear that the university profits far more than the hospital—especially since nearly 40,000 qualified applicants were turned away from baccalaureate nursing programs in 2009 because of shortages of faculty and clinical teaching sites (AACN, 2009c)—but that is not the case, said Cindy Lorion, MSN, RN, nurse manager of the neurovascular and orthopedic units at Providence St. Vincent Medical Center. The clinical instructors are enthusiastic about their new role. They receive adjunct faculty appointments at UP, gaining such benefits as library access but no additional pay from the university (some but not all facilities increase a clinical instructor's salary).

Ms. Lorion has seen an increase in evidence-based practice and in the retention of nurses, as well as better-prepared graduates, many of whom seek jobs at the hospital. She also said that "a village" grows around the students, with everyone from physicians to nurses' aides taking part in "raising" them.

The partnership has led to changes in teaching and in clinical care. After a student made an error by injecting a medication into the wrong tube, the hospital changed its policy on syringe placement, and the school added a "tubes lab" to its courses.

A limited number of available clinical training sites in some areas may hamper widespread use of the model, and some units may take students on reluctantly, requiring a change in organizational culture. Nonetheless, more than 100 schools of nursing participated in an international symposium on DEUs in 2007, and more than 20 are developing their own DEUs.

After 25 years as a nurse, Ms. Mead is pursuing her bachelor's degree. "I definitely have to keep it fresh," she said of the challenge of working with students like Ms. Sharp. "And not everyone can say that after being on the same unit for years."

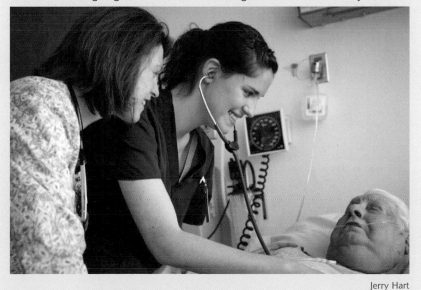

Jerry Hart

Seasoned nurse and clinical instructor Cathy Meade provides guidance as student Jamie Sharp examines a patient.

GRADUATE NURSING EDUCATION

Even absent passage of the ACA, the need for APRNs, nurse faculty, and nurse researchers would have increased dramatically under any scenario (Cronenwett, 2010). Not only must schools of nursing build their capacity to prepare more students at the graduate level, but they must do so in a way that fosters a unified, competency-based approach with the highest possible standards. Therefore, building the science of nursing education research, or how best to teach students, is an important emphasis for the field of nursing education. For APRNs, graduate education should ensure that they can contribute to primary care and help respond to shortages, especially for those populations who are most underserved. For nurse researchers, a focus on fundamental improvements in the delivery of nursing care to improve patient safety and quality is key.

Numbers and Distribution of Graduate-Level Nurses

As of 2008, more than 375,000 women and men in the workforce had received a master's degree in nursing or a nursing-related field, and more than 28,000 had gone on to receive either a doctorate in nursing or a nursing-related doctoral degree in a field such as public health, public administration, sociology, or education[12] (see Table 4-5) (HRSA, 2010b). Master's degrees prepare RNs for roles in nursing administration and clinical leadership or for work in advanced practice roles (discussed below) (AARP, 2010 [see Annex 1-1]). Many nursing faculty, particularly clinical instructors, are prepared at the master's level. Doctoral degrees include the DNP and PhD. A PhD in nursing is a research-oriented degree designed to educate nurses in a wide range of scientific areas that may include clinical science, social science, policy, and education. Traditionally, PhD-educated nurses teach in university settings and conduct research to expand knowledge and improve care, although they can also work in clinical settings and assume leadership and administrative roles in health care systems and academic settings.

The DNP is the complement to other practice doctorates, such as the MD, PharmD, doctorate of physical therapy, and others that require highly rigorous clinical training. Nurses with DNPs are clinical scholars who have the capacity to translate research, shape systems of care, potentiate individual care into care needed to serve populations, and ask the clinical questions that influence organizational-level research to improve performance using informatics and quality improvement models. The DNP is a relatively new degree that offers nurses an opportunity to become practice scholars in such areas as clinical practice, leadership, quality improvement, and health policy. The core curriculum for DNPs is

---

[12] Nursing-related doctoral degrees are defined by the National Sample Survey of Registered Nurses as non-nursing degrees that are directly related to a nurse's career in the nursing profession. "Nursing-related degrees include public health, health administration, social work, education, and other fields" (HRSA, 2010b).

TABLE 4-5 Estimated Distribution of Master's and Doctoral Degrees as Highest Nursing or Nursing-Related Educational Preparation, 2000–2008

Degree	Estimated Distribution		
	2000	2004	2008
Master's	257,812	350,801	375,794
Master's of science in nursing (MSN)	202,639	256,415	290,084
Nursing-related master's degree	55,173	94,386	85,709
Percent of master's degrees that are nursing (MSN)	78.6	73.1	77.2
Doctoral	17,256	26,100	28,369
Doctorate in nursing	8,435	11,548	13,140
Nursing-related doctoral degree	8,821	14,552	15,229
Percent of doctorates that are nursing	48.9	44.2	46.3

SOURCE: HRSA, 2010b.

guided by the AACN's *Essentials of Doctoral Education for Advanced Nursing Practice*.[13]

Schools of nursing have been developing DNP programs since 2002, but only in the last 5 years have the numbers of graduates approached a substantial level (Raines, 2010). Between 2004 and 2008 the number of programs offering the degree increased by nearly 40 percent, as is shown in Figure 4-7. At this point, more evidence is needed to examine the impact DNP nurses will have on patient outcomes, costs, quality of care, and access in clinical settings. It is also difficult to discern how DNP nurses could affect the provision of nursing education and whether they will play a significant role in easing faculty shortages. While the DNP provides a promising opportunity to advance the nursing profession, and some nursing organizations are promoting this degree as the next step for APRNs, the committee cannot comment directly on the potential role of DNP nurses because of the current lack of evidence on outcomes.

Although 13 percent of nurses hold a graduate degree, fewer than 1 percent (28,369 nurses) have a doctoral degree in nursing or a nursing-related field, the qualification needed to conduct independent research (HRSA, 2010b). In fact, only 555 students graduated with a PhD in nursing in 2009, a number that has remained constant for the past decade (AACN, 2009a). As noted, key roles for PhD nurses include teaching future generations of nurses and conducting research that becomes the basis for improvements in nursing practice. As the need for nursing education and research and for nurses to engage with interprofessional research teams has grown, the numbers of nurses with a PhD in nursing or a related field have not kept pace (see Figure 4-7 for trends in the various nursing programs). The main reasons for this lag are (1) an inadequate pool of nurses

---

[13] See http://www.aacn.nche.edu/dnp/pdf/essentials.pdf.

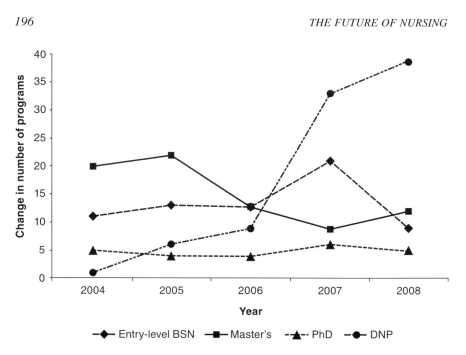

FIGURE 4-7 Growth trends in different nursing programs.
NOTE: BSN = bachelor's of science in nursing; DNP = doctor of nursing practice.
SOURCES: AACN, 2005, 2006, 2007, 2008a, 2009b.

with advanced nursing degrees to draw upon, (2) faculty salaries and benefits that are not comparable to those of nurses with advanced nursing degrees working in clinical settings, and (3) a culture that promotes obtaining clinical experience prior to continuing graduate education.

Preparation of Advanced Practice Registered Nurses

Nurses prepared at the graduate level to provide advanced practice services include those with master's and doctoral degrees. APRNs serve as NPs, certified nurse midwives (CNMs), clinical nurse specialists (CNSs), and certified registered nurse anesthetists (CRNAs). To gain certification in one of these advanced practice areas, nurses must take specialized courses in addition to a basic core curriculum. Credit requirements vary from program to program and from specialty to specialty, but typically range from a minimum of 40 credits for a master's to more than 80 credits for a DNP. Upon completion of required coursework and clinical hours, students must take a certification exam that is administered by a credentialing organization relevant to the specific specialization, such as the American Nursing Credentialing Center (for NPs and CNSs), the American Midwifery Certification Board (for CNMs), or the National Board on Certification and Recertification of Nurse Anesthetists (for CRNAs).

Nurses who receive certification, including those serving in all advanced practice roles, provide added assurance to the public that they have acquired the specialized professional development, training, and competencies required to provide safe, quality care for specific patient populations. For example, NPs and CNSs may qualify for certification after completing a master's degree, post-master's coursework, or doctoral degree through an accredited nursing program, with specific advanced coursework in areas such as health assessment, pharmacology, and pathophysiology; additional content in health promotion, disease prevention, differential diagnosis, and disease management; and at least 500 hours of faculty-supervised clinical training within a program of study (ANCC, 2010a, 2010c).

Certification is time-limited, and maintenance of certification requires ongoing acquisition of both knowledge and experience in practice. For example, most advanced practice certification must be renewed every 5 years (NPs, CNSs); requirements include a minimum of 1,000 practice hours in the specific certification role and population/specialty. These requirements must be fulfilled within the 5 years preceding submission of the renewal application (ANCC, 2010b). CRNAs are recertified every 2 years and must be substantially engaged in the practice of nurse anesthesia during those years, in addition to completing continuing education credits (NBCRNA, 2009). Recertification for CNMs is shifting from 8 to 5 years and also involves a continuing education requirement (AMCB, 2009).

As the health care system grows in complexity, expectations are that APRNs will have competence in expanding areas such as technology, genetics, quality improvement, and geriatrics. Coursework and clinical experience requirements are increasing to keep pace with these changes. Jean Johnson, Dean of the School of Nursing at The George Washington University, notes that in terms of education, this is a time of major transition for APRNs.[14] With the DNP, some nursing education institutions are now able to offer professional parity with other health disciplines that are shifting, or have already shifted, to require doctorates in their areas of practice, such as pharmacy, occupational and physical therapy, and speech pathology. As discussed above, DNP programs allow nurses to hone their expertise in roles related to nurse executive practice, health policy, informatics, and other practice specialties. (It should be noted, however, that throughout this report, the discussion of APRNs does not distinguish between those with master's and DNP degrees who have graduated from an accredited program.)

Research Roles

Graduate-level education produces nurses who can assume roles in advanced practice, leadership, teaching, and research. For the latter role, a doctoral degree is required, yet as noted above, fewer than 1 percent of nurses have achieved

---

[14] Personal communication, Jean Johnson, Dean, School of Nursing, George Washington University, September 3, 2010.

this level of education. This number is insufficient to meet the crucial need for research in two key areas: nursing education and nursing science.

Research on Nursing Education

At no time in recent history has there been a greater need for research on nursing education. As health care reform progresses, basic and advanced nursing practices are being defined by the new competencies alluded to above and discussed in the next section, yet virtually no evidence exists to support the teaching approaches used in nursing education.[15]

Additionally, little research has focused on clinical education models or clinical experiences that can help students achieve these competencies, even though clinical education constitutes the largest portion of nurses' educational costs. Likewise, little evidence supports appropriate student/faculty ratios. Yet current clinical education models and student/faculty ratios are limiting capacity at a time when the need for new nurses is projected to increase. The paucity of evidence in nursing education and pedagogy calls for additional research and funding to ascertain the efficiency and effectiveness of approaches to nursing education, advancing evidence-based teaching and interprofessional knowledge. Chapter 7 outlines specific research priorities that could shape improvements to nursing education.

In a recent editorial, Broome (2009) highlighted the need for three critical changes required to "systematically build a . . . science that could guide nurse educators to develop high quality, relevant, and cost-effective models of education that produce graduates who can make a difference in the health system":

- funding to support nursing education research, potentially via mechanisms through the Health Resources and Services Administration;
- multidisciplinary research training programs, including postdoctoral training to prepare a cadre of nurses dedicated to developing the science of nursing education; and
- efforts to foster the development of PhD programs that have faculty expertise to mentor a new generation of nursing education researchers.

Research on Nursing Science

The expansion of knowledge about the science of nursing is key to providing better patient care, improving health, and evaluating outcomes. Along with an adequate supply of qualified nurses, meeting the nation's growing health care needs

---

[15] Some faculty development programs and training opportunities are offered through universities and professional organizations, such as the AACN and the NLN. Additionally, the NLN offers a certification program for nurse educators, who can publically confirm knowledge in the areas of pedagogy, learning, and the complex encounter between educator and student. This certification program can provide a basis for innovation and the continuous quality improvement of nursing education.

requires continued growth in the science of delivering effective care for people and populations and designing health systems. Nurse scientists are a critical link in the discovery and translation of knowledge that can be generated by nurses and other health scientists. To carry out this crucial work, a sustainable supply of and support for nurse scientists will be necessary (IOM, 2010).

The research conducted by nurse scientists has led to many fundamental improvements in the provision of care. Advances have been realized, for example, in the prevention of pressure ulcers; the reduction of high blood pressure among African American males; and the models described elsewhere in this report for providing transitional care after hospital discharge and for promoting health and well-being among young, disadvantaged mothers and their newborns. Yet nursing's research capacity has been largely overlooked in the development of strategies for responding to the shortage of nurses or effecting the necessary transformation of the nursing profession. The result has been a serious mismatch between the urgent need for knowledge and innovation to improve care and the nursing profession's ability to respond to that need, as well as a limitation on what nursing schools can include in their curricula and what is disseminated in the clinical settings where nurses engage.

A chapter of the National Research Council's 2005 report, *Advancing the Nation's Health Needs: NIH's Research Training Program*, focuses on nursing research; it identified factors that would likely influence its future, for example: an aging cadre of nursing science researchers, longer times required to complete doctoral degrees, increasing demands on nursing faculty to also meet workforce demands, and the emergence of clinical doctoral programs (NRC, 2005). Evaluating these and other factors will be essential to achieving the transformation of the nursing profession that this report argues is essential to a transformed health care system.

COMPETENCY-BASED EDUCATION

Competencies that are well known to the nursing profession, such as care management and coordination, patient education, public health intervention, and transitional care, are likely to dominate in a reformed health care system. As Edward O'Neil, Director, Center for the Health Professions at the University of California, San Francisco, pointed out however, "these traditional competencies must be reinterpreted for students into the settings of the emergent care system, not the one that is being left behind. This will require faculty to not only teach to these competencies but also creatively apply them to health environments that are only now emerging" (O'Neil, 2009). Emerging new competencies in decision making, quality improvement, systems thinking, and team leadership must become part of every nurse's professional formation from the prelicensure through the doctoral level.

A review of medical school education found that evidence in favor of competency-based education is limited but growing (Carraccio et al., 2002). Nursing schools also have embraced the notion of competency-based education, as noted earlier in the chapter in the case study on the Oregon Consortium for Nursing Education (Box 4-2). In addition, Western Governors University uses competency-based education exclusively, allowing nursing students to move through their program of study at their own pace. Mastery of the competency is achieved to the satisfaction of the faculty without the normal time-bound semester structure (IOM, 2010).

Defining Core Competencies

The value of competency-based education in nursing is that it can be strongly linked to clinically based performance expectations. It should be noted that "competencies" here denotes not task-based proficiencies but higher-level competencies that represent the ability to demonstrate mastery over care management knowledge domains and that provide a foundation for decision-making skills under variety of clinical situations across all care settings.

Numerous sets of core competencies for nursing education are available from a variety of sources. It has proven difficult to establish a single set of competencies that cover all clinical situations, across all settings, for all levels of students. However, there is significant overlap among the core competencies that exist because many of them are derived from such landmark reports as *Recreating Health Professional Practice for a New Century* (O'Neil and Pew Health Professions Commission, 1998) and *Health Professions Education: A Bridge to Quality* (IOM, 2003b). The competencies in these reports focus on aspects of professional behavior (e.g., ethical standards, cultural competency) and emphasize areas of care (e.g., prevention, primary care), with overarching goals of (1) providing patient-centered care, (2) applying quality improvement principles, (3) working in interprofessional teams, (4) using evidence-based practices, and (5) using health information technologies.

Two examples of sets of core competencies come from the Oregon Consortium for Nursing Education[16] and the AACN. The former set features competencies that promote nurses' abilities in such areas as clinical judgment and critical thinking; evidence-based practice; relationship-centered care; interprofessional collaboration; leadership; assistance to individuals and families in self-care practices for promotion of health and management of chronic illness; and teaching, delegation, and supervision of caregivers. The AACN's set of competencies is outlined in *Essentials for Baccalaureate Education* and highlights such areas as "patient-centered care, interprofessional teams, evidence-based practice, quality improvement, patient safety, informatics, clinical reasoning/critical thinking, genetics and genomics, cultural sensitivity, professionalism, practice across the lifespan, and end-of-life care" (AACN, 2008b). While students appear to gradu-

---

[16] See http://www.ocne.org/.

ate with ample factual knowledge of these types of core competencies, however, they often appear to have little sense of how the competencies can be applied or integrated into real-world practice situations (Benner et al., 2009).

Imparting emerging competencies, such as quality improvement and systems thinking, is also key to developing a more highly educated workforce. Doing so will require performing a thorough evaluation and redesign of educational content, not just adding content to existing curricula. An exploration of the educational changes required to teach all the emerging competencies required to meet the needs of diverse patient populations is beyond the scope of this report.

Defining an agreed-upon set of core competencies across health professions could lead to better communication and coordination among disciplines (see the discussion of the Interprofessional Education Collaborative below for an example of one such effort). Additionally, the committee supports the development of a unified set of core competencies across the nursing profession and believes it would help provide direction for standards across nursing education. Defining these core competencies must be a collaborative effort among nurse educators, professional organizations, and health care organizations and providers. This effort should be ongoing and should inform regular updates of nursing curricula to ensure that graduates at all levels are prepared to meet the current and future health needs of the population.

Assessing Competencies

Changes in the way competencies are assessed are also needed. In 2003, the IOM's *Health Professions Education: A Bridge to Quality* called for systemwide changes in the education of health professionals, including a move on the part of accrediting and certifying organizations for all health professionals toward mandating a competency-based approach to education (IOM, 2003a). Steps are already being taken to establish competency-based assessments in medical education. In its 2009 report to Congress on *Improving Incentives in the Medicare Program*, the Medicare Payment Advisory Commission highlighted an initiative of the Accreditation Council for Graduate Medical Education to require greater competency-based assessment of all residency programs that train physicians in the United States (MedPAC, 2009). The NCSBN has considered various challenges related to competency assessment and is considering approaches to ensure that RNs can demonstrate competence in the full range of areas that are required for the practice of nursing.[17]

A competency-based approach to education strives to make the competencies for a particular course explicit to students and requires them to demonstrate mastery of those competencies (Harden, 2002). Performance-based assessment then shows whether students have both a theoretical grasp of what they have learned

---

[17] Personal communication, Kathy Apple, CEO, NCSBN, May 30, 2010.

and the ability to apply that knowledge in a real-world or realistically simulated situation. The transition-to-practice or nurse residency programs discussed in Chapter 3 could offer an extended opportunity to reinforce and test core competencies in real-world settings that are both safe and monitored.

Lifelong Learning and Continuing Competence

Many professions, such as nursing, that depend heavily on knowledge are becoming increasingly technical and complex (The Lewin Group, 2009). No individual can know all there is to know about providing safe and effective care, which is why nurses must be integral members of teams that include other health professionals. Nor can a single initial degree provide a nurse with all she or he will need to know over an entire career. Creating an expectation and culture of lifelong learning for nurses is therefore essential.

From Continuing Education to Continuing Competence

Nurses, physicians, and other health professionals have long depended on continuing education programs to maintain and develop new competencies over the course of their careers. Yet the 2009 IOM study *Redesigning Continuing Education in the Health Professions* cites "major flaws in the way [continuing education] is conducted, financed, regulated, and evaluated" and states that the evidence base underlying current continuing education programs is "fragmented and undeveloped." These shortcomings, the report suggests, have hindered the identification of effective educational methods and their integration into coordinated, comprehensive programs that meet the needs of all health professionals (IOM, 2009). Likewise, the NCSBN has found that there is no clear link between continuing education requirements and continued competency.[18] A new vision of professional development is needed that enables learning both individually and from a collaborative, team perspective and ensures that "all health professionals engage effectively in a process of lifelong learning aimed squarely at improving patient care and population health" (IOM, 2009).

This new comprehensive vision is often termed "continuing competence." The practice setting, like the academic setting, is challenged by the need to integrate traditional and emerging competencies. Therefore, building the capacity for lifelong learning—which encompasses both continuing competence and advanced degrees—requires ingenuity on the part of employers, businesses, schools, community and government leaders, and philanthropies. The case study in Box 4-6 describes a program that extends the careers of nurses by training them to transition from the acute care to the community setting.

---

[18] Personal communication, Kathy Apple, CEO, NCSBN, May 30, 2010.

Interprofessional Education

The importance of interprofessional collaboration and education has been recognized since the 1970s (Alberto and Herth, 2009). What is new is the introduction of simulation and web-based learning—solutions that can be used to can break down traditional barriers to learning together, such as the conflicting schedules of medical and APRN students or their lack of joint clinical learning opportunities. Simulation technology offers a safe environment in which to learn (and make mistakes), while web-based learning makes schedule conflicts more manageable and content more repeatable. If all nursing and medical students are educated in aspects of interprofessional collaboration, such as knowledge of professional roles and responsibilities, effective communication, conflict resolution, and shared decision making, and are exposed to working with other health professional students through simulation and web-based training, they may be more likely to engage in collaboration in future work settings. Further, national quality and safety agendas, including requirements set by the Joint Commission, the Commission on Collegiate Nursing Education, the NLN, and the Association of American Medical Colleges (AAMC), along with studies that link disruptive behavior between RNs and MDs to negative patient and worker outcomes (Rosenstein and O'Daniel, 2005, 2008), create a strong incentive to not just talk about but actually work on implementing interprofessional collaboration.

England, Canada, and the United States have made strides to improve interprofessional education by bringing students together from academic health science universities and medical centers (e.g., students of nursing, medicine, pharmacy, social work, physical therapy, and public health, among others) in shared learning environments (Tilden, 2010). Defined as "occasions when two or more professions learn with, from, and about each other to improve collaboration and the quality of care" (Barr et al., 2005), such education is based on the premise that students' greater familiarity with each other's roles, competencies, nomenclatures, and scopes of practice will result in more collaborative graduates. It is expected that graduates of programs with interprofessional education will be ready to work effectively in patient-centered teams where miscommunication and undermining behaviors are minimized or eliminated, resulting in safer, more effective care and greater clinician and patient satisfaction. Interprofessional education is thought to foster collaboration in implementing policies and improving services, prepare students to solve problems that exceed the capacity of any one profession, improve future job satisfaction, create a more flexible workforce, modify negative attitudes and perceptions, and remedy failures of trust and communication (Barr, 2002).[19]

---

[19] This paragraph draws upon a paper commissioned by the committee on "The Future of Nursing Education," prepared by Virginia Tilden, University of Nebraska Medical Center College of Nursing (see Appendix I on CD-ROM).

BOX 4-6
Case Study: Nursing for Life—The RN
Career Transition Program

A New Program Extends the Working Life of Aging Nurses
By Training Them to Work in Community Settings

At age 62 Jackie Tibbetts, MS, RN, CAGS, was thinking, naturally, about retirement. She was nearing the end of a 39-year teaching career when a close friend became ill, and her proximity to her friend's care and eventual death made her realize she still had a great deal to offer. She felt compelled to return to nursing, her first profession.

Ms. Tibbetts now provides skilled nursing care at a retirement community in a suburb of Boston. She made the move to long-term care through the Nursing for Life: RN Career Transition program at Michigan State University (MSU) College of Nursing, an outgrowth of a 2002 online refresher course the school offered. Because she had maintained her registered nurse (RN) license, she was eligible for the course, and with a background in rehabilitation she determined that the long-term care setting would be a good fit. Ms. Tibbetts received online education and performed a clinical practicum near her Massachusetts home. Now 64, she plans to work as a nurse "as long as I'm able," she said.

In 2006 the Blue Cross Blue Shield of Michigan Foundation, in concert with the College of Nursing at MSU, set out to broaden the opportunities for Michigan's, and the nation's, aging nursing workforce. "We began to think about some of the needs of mid-to-late-career nurses still working in acute care and looking to move away from that work, for the physical intensity of it," said Terrie Wehrwein, PhD, RN, NEA-BC, associate professor at the school. The Blue Cross Blue Shield of Michigan Foundation and the College of Nursing at MSU were among the first recipients of a grant from Partners Investing in Nursing's Future, a joint venture of the Northwest Health Foundation and The Robert Wood Johnson Foundation. The program began in 2008 as a pilot project to train licensed RNs to work in four community settings that may be less physically demanding than acute care—home care, long-term care, hospice, and ambulatory care—and that are open to any licensed nurse, not just those in Michigan. (Two new tracks, in case management and quality and safety management, are being developed.)

I still have a tremendous amount to offer here. I can see myself working well into my 60s.

—Sheri Morris, MN, RN, graduate of Nursing for Life, Lambertville, Michigan

The program has two components: an online, self-paced didactic course has seven core modules, plus seven modules specific to each specialty, and an 80-hour clinical practicum pairs the nurse, ideally, with a single preceptor in the area of study. Nurses have 1 year to finish the online course and are encouraged to complete the practicum within 5 weeks.

The program has attracted not only aging nurses but also younger ones wanting to change work settings. And Michigan is not the only state that benefits; of the 28 nurses who have completed the program, about 10 percent live out of state. (Michigan residents who cannot afford the $1250 tuition may be eligible for aid through the state's No Worker Left Behind program. Other states may provide similar assistance.)

After receiving a bachelor's degree in nursing in 1974 and a master's in 1982, Shari Morris, MN, RN, left the profession in 1990 to home-school her four sons. She took a Minnesota refresher course in 2006, when she was 54, and got a job in a pediatrician's office. She realized she would need further training to advance in ambulatory care and enrolled in Nursing for Life. For her clinical practicum she chose two pediatric clinics in a nearby hospital.

When asked what impact the program has had on her ability to remain a nurse, she said, "I think, probably, courage." The course gave her the self-assurance to apply for a job in teaching when she could not find an opening in ambulatory care; she is now an instructor in nursing at a Michigan community college.

"I felt confident to step out of the first setting I'd been in 17 years and go into another arena, without any difficulties," Ms. Morris said.

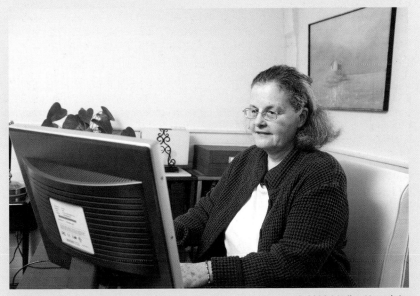

© 2010 Marilyn Humphries

The online education Jackie Tibbetts received through the Nursing for Life: RN Career Transition program helped her shift back to a nursing career after almost four decades as a teacher.

The AAMC, the American of Association of Colleges of Osteopathic Medicine, the American Dental Education Association, the American Association of Colleges of Pharmacy, the Association of Schools of Public Health, and the AACN recently formed a partnership called the Interprofessional Education Collaborative. This collaborative is committed to the development of models of collaboration that will provide the members' individual communities with the standards and tools needed to achieve productive interprofessional education practices. These organizations are committed to fulfilling the social contract that every nursing, pharmacy, dental, public health, and medical graduate is proficient in the core competencies required for interprofessional, team-based care, including preventive, acute, chronic, and catastrophic care. The collaborative is also committed to facilitating the identification, development, and deployment of the resources essential to achieving this vision. As a first step, the collaborative is developing a shared and mutually endorsed set of core competencies that will frame the education of the six represented health professions.[20]

Efforts have been made to evaluate the effectiveness of interprofessional education in improving outcomes, including increased student satisfaction, modified negative stereotypes of other disciplines, increased collaborative behavior, and improved patient outcomes. However, the effect of interprofessional education is not easily verified since control group designs are expensive, reliable measures are few, and time lapses can be long between interprofessional education and the behavior of graduates. Barr and colleagues (2005) reviewed 107 evaluations of interprofessional education in published reports and found support for three outcomes: interprofessional education creates positive interaction among students and faculty; encourages collaboration between professions; and results in improvements in aspects of patient care, such as more targeted health promotion advice, higher immunization rates, and reduced blood pressure for patients with chronic heart disease. Reeves and colleagues (2008) reviewed six later studies of varying designs. Four of the studies found that interprofessional education improved aspects of how clinicians worked together, while the remaining two found that it had no effect (Reeves et al., 2008). Although empirical evidence is mixed, widespread theoretical agreement and anecdotal evidence suggest that students who demonstrate teamwork skills in the simulation laboratory or in a clinical education environment with patients will apply those skills beyond the confines of their academic programs.[21]

---

[20] Personal communication, Geraldine Bednash, CEO, AACN, August 12, 2010.

[21] This paragraph draws upon a paper commissioned by the committee on "The Future of Nursing Education," prepared by Virginia Tilden, University of Nebraska Medical Center College of Nursing (see Appendix I on CD-ROM).

THE NEED TO INCREASE THE DIVERSITY
OF THE NURSING WORKFORCE

Chapter 3 highlighted a variety of challenges facing the nursing profession in meeting the changing needs of patients and the health care system. A major challenge for the nursing workforce is the underrepresentation of racial and ethnic minority groups and men in the profession. To better meet the current and future health needs of the public and to provide more culturally relevant care, the nursing workforce will need to grow more diverse. And to meet this need, efforts to increase nurses' levels of educational attainment must emphasize increasing the diversity of the student body. This is a crucial concern that needs to be addressed across all levels of nursing education.

Racial and Ethnic Diversity

Although the composition of the nursing student body is more racially and ethnically diverse than that of the current workforce, diversity continues to be a challenge. Figure 4-8 shows the distribution of minority students enrolled in nursing programs by race/ethnicity and by program type. Their underrepresentation is greatest for pathways associated with higher levels of education. In academic year 2008–2009, for example, ethnic minority groups made up 28.2 percent of ADN, 23.6 percent of BSN, 24.4 percent of master's, and 20.3 percent of doctoral students (NLN, 2009). Even less evidence of diversity is present among nurses in faculty positions (AACN, 2010b).

In 2003, the Sullivan Commission on Diversity in the Healthcare Workforce was established to develop recommendations that would "bring about systemic change . . . [to] address the scarcity of minorities in our health professions." The commission's report, *Missing Persons: Minorities in the Health Professions* (Sullivan Commission on Diversity in the Healthcare Workforce, 2004), offered strategies to increase the diversity of the medical, nursing, and dentistry professions and included recommendations designed to remove barriers to health professions education for underrepresented minority students. The commission's 37 recommendations called for leadership, commitment, and accountability among a wide range of stakeholders—from institutions responsible for educating health professionals, to professional organizations and health systems, to state and federal agencies and Congress. The recommendations focused on expediting strategies to increase the number of minorities in health professions, improving the education pipeline for health professionals, financing education for minority students, and establishing leadership and accountability to realize the commission's vision of increasing the diversity of health professionals. The committee believes the implementation of these recommendations holds promise for ensuring a more diverse health care workforce in the future.

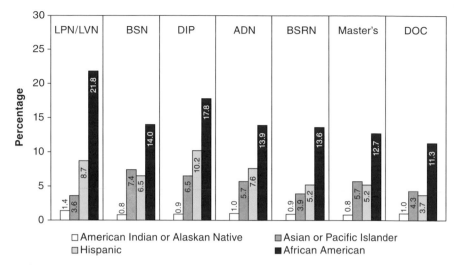

FIGURE 4-8 Percentage of minority students enrolled in nursing programs by race/ethnicity and program type, 2008–2009.
NOTE: ADN = associate's degree programs; BSN = bachelor's of science programs; BSRN = RN-to-BSN programs; DIP = diploma nursing programs; DOC = nursing school programs offering doctoral degrees; LPN = licensed practical nursing programs; LVN = licensed vocational nursing programs.
SOURCE: NLN, 2010c. Reprinted with Permission from the National League for Nursing.

In the nursing profession, creating bridge programs and educational pathways between undergraduate and graduate programs—specifically programs such as LPN to BSN, ADN to BSN, and ADN to MSN—appears to be one way of increasing the overall diversity of the student body and nurse faculty with respect to not only race/ethnicity, but also geography, background, and personal experience. Mentoring programs that support minority nursing students are another promising approach. One example of such a program is the National Coalition of Ethnic Minority Nursing Associations, a group made up of five ethnic minority nursing associations that aims to build the cadre and preparation of ethnic minority nurses and promote equity in health care across ethnic minority populations (NCEMNA, 2010). This program is described at greater length in Chapter 5. Another example of a successful program that has promoted racial and ethnic diversity is the ANA Minority Fellowship Program,[22] started in 1974 under the leadership of Dr. Hattie Bessent. This program has played a crucial role in supporting minority nurses with predoctoral and postdoctoral fellowships to advance research and clinical

---

[22] See http://www.emfp.org/.

practice (Minority Fellowship Program, 2010). Programs to recruit and retain more individuals from racial and ethnic minority groups in nursing education programs are needed. A necessary first step toward accomplishing this goal is to create policies that increase the overall educational attainment of ethnic minorities (Coffman et al., 2001).

Gender Diversity

As noted in Chapter 3, the nursing workforce historically has been composed predominantly of women. While the number of men who become nurses has grown dramatically in the last two decades, men still make up just 7 percent of all RNs (HRSA, 2010b). While most disciplines within the health professional workforce have become more gender balanced, the same has not been true for nursing. For example, in 2009 nearly half of medical school graduates were female (The Kaiser Family Foundation—statehealthfacts.org, 2010), a significant achievement of gender parity in a traditionally male-dominated profession. Stereotypes, academic acceptance, and role support are challenges for men entering the nursing profession. These barriers must be overcome if men are to be recruited in larger numbers to help offset the shortage of nurses and fill advanced and expanded nursing roles. Compounding the gender diversity problem of the nursing profession is the fact that fewer men in general are enrolling in higher education programs (Mather and Adams, 2007). While more men are being drawn to nursing, especially as a second career, the profession needs to continue efforts to recruit men; their unique perspectives and skills are important to the profession and will help contribute additional diversity to the workforce.

One professional organization that works to encourage men to join the nursing profession and supports men who do so is the American Assembly for Men in Nursing (AAMN).[23] To increase opportunities for men interested in joining the profession, the AAMN Foundation, in partnership with Johnson & Johnson, has awarded more than $50,000 in scholarships to undergraduate and graduate male nursing students since 2004 (AAMN, 2010b). Additionally, each year the AAMN recognizes the best school or college of nursing for men; in 2009, the honor was given to Monterey Peninsula College in Monterey, California, and Excelsior College in Albany, New York, for their "efforts in recruiting and retaining men in nursing, in providing men a supportive educational environment, and in educating faculty, students and the community about the contributions men have and do make to the nursing profession" (AAMN, 2010a).

---

[23] See http://www.aamn.org/.

SOLUTIONS FROM THE FIELD

This chapter has outlined a number of challenges facing nursing education. These challenges have been the subject of much documentation, analysis, and debate (Benner et al., 2009; Erickson, 2002; IOM, 2003a, 2009; Lasater and Nielsen, 2009; Mitchell et al., 2006; Orsolini-Hain and Waters, 2009; Tanner et al., 2008). Various approaches to responding to these challenges and transforming curricula have been proposed, and several are being tested. The committee reviewed the literature on educational capacity and redesign, heard testimony about various challenges and potential solutions at the public forum in Houston, and chose a number of exemplars for closer examination. Three of these models are described in this section. The committee found that each of these models provided important insight into creative approaches to maximizing faculty resources, encouraging the establishment and funding of new faculty positions, maximizing the effectiveness of clinical education, and redesigning nursing curricula.

Veterans Affairs Nursing Academy

In 2007, the VA launched the VANA—a 5-year, $40 million pilot program—with the primary goals of developing partnerships with academic nursing institutes; expanding the number of faculty for baccalaureate programs; establishing partnerships to enhance faculty development; and increasing baccalaureate enrollment to increase the supply of nurses, not solely for the VA, but for the country at large. VANA also was aimed at encouraging interprofessional programs and increasing the retention and recruitment of VA nurses.[24]

Since the program's inception, three cycles of requests for proposals have been sent to more than 600 colleges and schools of nursing, as well as to institutions within the VA system. Fifteen geographically and demographically diverse pilot sites were selected to participate in VANA based on the strength of their proposals.

Each funded VANA partnership is required to have a rigorous evaluation plan to measure outcomes. Outcomes are expected to include increased staff, patient, student, and faculty satisfaction; greater scholarly output; enhanced professional development; better continuity and coordination of care; more reliance on evidence-based practice; and enhanced interprofessional learning. Each selected school is also expected to increase enrollment by at least 20 students a year.

The program has already resulted in 2,700 new students, with 620 receiving the majority of their clinical rotation experiences at the VA. The graduates of this program may include students who have pursued a traditional prelicensure

---

[24] This paragraph, and the three that follow, draw upon a presentation made by Cathy Rick, chief nursing officer for the VA, at the Forum on the Future of Nursing: Education, held in Houston, TX on February 22, 2010 (see Appendix C) and published in *A Summary of the February 2010 Forum on the Future of Nursing: Education* (IOM, 2010).

BSN, a BSN through a second-degree program, or a BSN through an RN-to-BSN program. The number of nursing school faculty has increased by 176 and the number of VA faculty by 264.

In addition to the new nurses and faculty, educational innovations have encompassed curriculum revision, including quality and safety standards; DEUs (described earlier in Box 4-4); and a postgraduate baccalaureate nurse residency (see Chapter 3). Other changes include interprofessional simulation training and the development of evidence-based practice committees and programs. Beyond these specific changes and accomplishments, the VANA faculty has worked to develop the program into a single community of learning and to prepare students in a genuinely collaborative practice environment with clinically proficient staff and educators.

Carondolet Health Network

The Carondolet Health Network of Tucson, Arizona, is an example of how employers can offer educational benefits that improve both patient outcomes and the bottom line. Carondelet, which includes four hospitals and other facilities and employs approximately 1,650 nurses, is featured as one of seven cases studies in the Lewin Group's 2009 report *Wisdom at Work: Retaining Experienced RNs and Their Knowledge—Case Studies of Top Performing Organizations.*

After Carondelet became part of Ascension Health in 2002, the Tucson organization embarked on a strategic plan to recruit and retain more nurses. Arizona faces some of the severest nursing shortages in the nation, and most nurses prefer to live and work in higher-paying markets, such as Phoenix or southern California. When Carondelet instituted an on-site BSN program, which it subsidized in exchange for a 2-year work commitment, the response was dramatic. Instead of an anticipated class size of 20 nurses in the first semester of the program, it enrolled 104. Of interest, it was the business case—the opportunity to decrease the amount of money the organization was spending on costly temporary nurses—that tipped the balance in favor of action (The Lewin Group, 2009).

Hospital Employee Education and Training

The Hospital Employee Education and Training (HEET) program was developed through a joint effort of the 1199NW local affiliate of the Service Employees International Union and the Washington State Hospital Association Work Force Institute to help address shortages in nursing and nursing-related positions through education and upgrading of incumbent workers. The program is administered through the Washington State Board for Community and Technical Colleges. Across the state, HEET-funded programs support industry-based reform of the education system and include preparation and completion of nursing career ladder programs. HEET seeks to develop educational opportunities that support both employer needs and the career aspirations of health care workers. It features cohort-based programs, distance learning, worksite classes, use of a simulation laboratory for nursing prerequisites, case management, tutoring support for those reentering academia, and nontraditional scheduling of classes to enable working adults to attend and address employee barriers to education.

The findings for this union-inspired initiative demonstrate its potential to increase racial/ethnic diversity in the nursing population. HEET participants represent a pool of potential nurses who are more diverse than the current nursing workforce. Providing on-site classes at hospitals appears to support the participation of working adults who are enrolled in nursing school while continuing to work at least part time. Workers participating in the HEET program have had lower attrition rates and higher rates of course completion compared with community college students in nursing career tracks. The curriculum also blends academic preparation with health care career education, thereby opening the doors of college to workers who might not otherwise enroll or succeed (Moss and Weinstein, 2009).

CONCLUSION

The future of access to basic primary care and nursing education will depend on increasing the number of BSN-prepared nurses. Unless this goal is met, the committee's recommendations for greater access to primary care; enhanced, expanded, and reconceptualized roles for nurses; and updated nursing scopes of practice (see Chapter 7) cannot be achieved. The committee believes that increasing the proportion of the nursing workforce with a BSN from the current 50 percent to 80 percent by 2020 is bold but achievable. Achieving this target will help meet future demand for nurses qualified for advanced practice positions and possessing competencies in such areas as community care, public health, health policy, evidence-based practice, research, and leadership. The committee concludes further that the number of nurses holding a doctorate must be increased to produce a greater pool of nurses prepared to assume faculty and research positions. The committee believes a target of doubling the number of nurses with a doctorate by 2020 would meet this need and is achievable.

To achieve these targets, however, will require overcoming a number of barriers. The numbers of educators and clinical placements are insufficient for all the qualified applicants who wish to enter nursing school. There also is a shortage of faculty to teach nurses at all levels. Incentives for nurses at any level to pursue further education are few, and there are active disincentives against advanced education. Nurses and physicians—not to mention pharmacists and social workers—typically are not educated together and yet are increasingly required to cooperate and collaborate more closely in the delivery of care.

To address these barriers, innovative new programs to attract nursing faculty and provide a wider range of clinical education placements must clear long-standing bottlenecks. To this end, market-based salary adjustments must be made for faculty, and more scholarships must be provided to help nursing students advance their education. Accrediting and certifying organizations must mandate demonstrated mastery of clinical skills, managerial competencies, and professional development at all levels. Mandated skills, competencies, and professional development milestones must be updated on a more timely basis to keep pace with the rapidly changing demands of health care. All health professionals should receive more of their education in concert with students from other disciplines. Efforts also must be made to increase the diversity of the nursing workforce.

The nursing profession must adopt a framework of continuous lifelong learning that includes basic education, academic progression, and continuing competencies. More nurses must receive a solid education in how to manage complex conditions and coordinate care with multiple health professionals. They must demonstrate new competencies in systems thinking, quality improvement, and care management and a basic understanding of health care policy. Graduate-level nurses must develop an even deeper understanding of care coordination, quality improvement, systems thinking, and policy.

The committee emphasizes further that, as discussed in Chapter 2, the ACA is likely to accelerate the shift in care from the hospital to the community setting. This transition will have a particularly strong impact on nurses, more than 60 percent of whom are currently employed in hospitals (HRSA, 2010b). Nurses may turn to already available positions in primary or chronic care or in public or community health, or they may pursue entirely new careers in emerging fields that they help create. Continuing and graduate education programs must support the transition to a future that rewards flexibility. In addition, the curriculum at many nursing schools, which places heavy emphasis on preparing students for employment in the acute care setting, will need to be rethought (Benner et al., 2009).

REFERENCES

AACN (American Association of Colleges of Nursing). 2005. *Enrollment and graduations in baccalaureate and graduate programs in nursing, 2004-05.* Washington, DC: AACN.

AACN. 2006. *Enrollment and graduations in baccalaureate and graduate programs in nursing, 2005-06.* Washington, DC: AACN.

AACN. 2007. *Enrollment and graduations in baccalaureate and graduate programs in nursing, 2006-07.* Washington, DC: AACN.

AACN. 2008a. *Enrollment and graduations in baccalaureate and graduate programs in nursing, 2007-08.* Washington, DC: AACN.

AACN. 2008b. *The essentials of baccalaureate education for professional nursing practice.* Washington, DC: AACN. Available from http://www.aacn.nche.edu/education/pdf/BaccEssentials08.pdf.

AACN. 2009a. *Advancing higher education in nursing: 2009 annual report.* Washington, DC: AACN.

AACN. 2009b. *Enrollment and graduations in baccalaureate and graduate programs in nursing, 2008-09.* Washington, DC: AACN.

AACN. 2009c. *Student enrollment expands at U.S. Nursing colleges and universities for the 9th year despite financial challenges and capacity restraints.* http://www.aacn.nche.edu/Media/NewsReleases/2009/StudentEnrollment.html (accessed March 13, 2010).

AACN. 2010a. *Education policy: New policy statement from the Tri-Council for Nursing on the educational advancement of registered nurses.* http://www.aacn.nche.edu/Education/ (accessed September 7, 2010).

AACN. 2010b. *Enhancing diversity in the nursing workforce: Fact sheet updated March 2010.* http://www.aacn.nche.edu/Media/FactSheets/diversity.htm (accessed July 1, 2010).

AACN. 2010c. *The impact of education on nursing practice.* http://www.aacn.nche.edu/media/factsheets/impactednp.htm (accessed September 7, 2010).

AACN and AAMC (Association of American Medical Colleges). 2010. *Lifelong learning in medicine and nursing: Final conference report.* Washington, DC: AACN and AAMC.

AACN and Hartford (The John A. Hartford Foundation Institute for Geriatric Nursing). 2000. *Older adults: Recommended baccalaureate competencies and curricular guidelines for geriatric nursing care.* Washington, DC and New York: AACN and The John A. Hartford Foundation Institute for Geriatric Nursing.

AAMN (American Assembly for Men in Nursing). 2010a. *Awards: Best nursing school/college for men in nursing.* http://www.aamn.org/awschool.html (accessed September 10, 2010).

AAMN. 2010b. *Scholarships.* http://www.aamn.org/scholarships.html (accessed September 10, 2010).

AARP. 2010. *Preparation and roles of nursing care providers in America.* http://championnursing.org/resources/preparation-and-roles-nursing-care-providers-america (accessed August 17, 2010).

ACHNE (Association of Community Health Nursing Educators). 2009. *Essentials of baccalaureate nursing education for entry level community/public health nursing.* Wheat Ridge, CO: ACHNE.

Aiken, L. H. 2010. *Nursing education policy priorities.* Paper commissioned by the Committee on the RWJF Initiative on the Future of Nursing, at the IOM (see Appendix I on CD-ROM).

Aiken, L. H., S. P. Clarke, R. B. Cheung, D. M. Sloane, and J. H. Silber. 2003. Educational levels of hospital nurses and surgical patient mortality. *JAMA* 290(12):1617-1623.

Aiken, L. H., R. B. Cheung, and D. M. Olds. 2009. Education policy initiatives to address the nurse shortage in the United States. *Health Affairs* 28(4):w646-w656.

Alberto, J., and K. Herth. 2009. Interprofessional collaboration within faculty roles: Teaching, service, and research. *OJIN: The Online Journal of Issues in Nursing* 14(2).

Allan, J., and J. Aldebron. 2008. A systematic assessment of strategies to address the nursing faculty shortage, U.S. *Nursing Outlook* 56(6):286-297.

Allan, J., J. Stanley, M. Crabtree, K. Werner, and M. Swenson. 2005. Clinical prevention and population health curriculum framework: The nursing perspective. *Journal of Professional Nursing* 21(5):259-267.

AMCB (American Midwifery Certification Board). 2009. *Letter to certified nurse-midwives and certified midwives from B.W. Graves, president, AMCB.* http://www.amcbmidwife.org/assets/documents/FINAL%20CMP%20LETTER3.pdf (accessed September 27, 2010).

ANCC (American Nurses Credentialing Center). 2010a. *Adult nurse practitioner certification eligibility criteria.* http://www.nursecredentialing.org/Eligibility/AdultNPEligibility.aspx (accessed September 27, 2010).

ANCC. 2010b. *ANCC nurse certification.* http://www.nursecredentialing.org/Certification.aspx (accessed September 8, 2010).

ANCC. 2010c. *Clinical nurse specialist in adult health certification eligibility criteria.* http://www.nursecredentialing.org/Eligibility/AdultHealthCNSEligibility.aspx (accessed September 27, 2010).

ASTDN (Association of State and Territorial Directors of Nursing). 2003. *Quad council PHN competencies.* http://www.astdn.org/publication_quad_council_phn_competencies.htm (accessed September 7, 2010).

Barr, H. 2002. *Interprofessional education today, yesterday and tomorrow: A review.* London: LTSN Hs&P.

Barr, H., I. Koppel, S. Reeves, M. Hammick, and D. Freeth. 2005. *Effective interprofessional education: Argument, assumption & evidence.* Oxford, England: Blackwell Publishing, Ltd.

Baxter, P. 2007. The CCARE model of clinical supervision: Bridging the theory-practice gap. *Nurse Education in Practice* 7:103-111.

Benner, P., M. Sutphen, V. Leonard, and L. Day. 2009. *Educating nurses: A call for radical transformation.* San Francisco, CA: Jossey-Bass.

Berlin, L. E., and K. R. Sechrist. 2002. The shortage of doctorally prepared nursing faculty: A dire situation. *Nursing Outlook* 50(2):50-56.

Bevill, J. W., Jr., B. L. Cleary, L. M. Lacey, and J. G. Nooney. 2007. Educational mobility of RNs in North Carolina: Who will teach tomorrow's nurses? A report on the first study to longitudinally examine educational mobility among nurses. *American Journal of Nursing* 107(5):60-70; quiz 71.

Blegen, M. A., T. E. Vaughn, and C. J. Goode. 2001. Nurse experience and education: Effect on quality of care. *Journal of Nursing Administration* 31(1):33-39.

Bovjberg, R. 2009. *The nursing workforce challenge: Public policy for a dynamic and complex market.* Washington, DC: Urban Institute.

Broome, M. E. 2009. Building the science for nursing education: Vision or improbable dream. *Nursing Outlook* 57(4):177-179.

Carraccio, C. M. D., S. D. M. D. Wolfsthal, R. M. D. M. P. H. Englander, K. M. D. Ferentz, and C. P. Martin. 2002. Shifting paradigms: From Flexner to competencies. *Academic Medicine* 77(5):361-367.

CCNE (Commission on Collegiate Nursing Education). 2009. *Standards for accreditation of baccalaureate and graduate degree nursing programs.* Washington, DC: CCNE.

Cleary, B. L., A. B. McBride, M. L. McClure, and S. C. Reinhard. 2009. Expanding the capacity of nursing education. *Health Affairs* 28(4):w634-w645.

Coffman, J. M., E. Rosenoff, and K. Grumbach. 2001. Racial/ethnic disparities in nursing. *Health Affairs* 20(3):263-272.

Cronenwett, L. R. 2010. *The future of nursing education.* Paper commissioned by the Committee on the RWJF Initiative on the Future of Nursing, at the IOM (see Appendix I on CD-ROM).

Cronenwett, L. R., and R. Redman. 2003. Partners in action: Nursing education and nursing practice. *Journal of Nursing Administration* 33(3):131-133.

Cronenwett, L., G. Sherwood, J. Barnsteiner, J. Disch, J. Johnson, and P. Mitchell. 2007. Quality and safety education for nurses. *Nursing Outlook* 55(3):122-131.

DeLunas, L. R., and L. A. Rooda. 2009. A new model for the clinical instruction of undergraduate nursing students. *Nursing Education Perspectives* 30(6):377-380.

Duchscher, J. E. 2003. Critical thinking: Perceptions of newly graduated female baccalaureate nurses. *Journal of Nursing Education* 42(1):14-27.

Erickson, H. 2002. *Concept-based curriculum and instruction: Teaching beyond the facts.* Thousand Oaks, CA: Corwin Press.

Estabrooks, C. A., W. K. Midodzi, G. G. Cummings, K. L. Ricker, and P. Giovannetti. 2005. The impact of hospital nursing characteristics on 30-day mortality. *Nursing Research* 54(2):74-84.

Fagin, C. M. 1986. Institutionalizing faculty practice. *Nursing Outlook* 34(3):140-144.

Florida Center for Nursing. 2010. *Florida nursing education capacity and nurse faculty supply/demand: 2007-2009 trends.* http://www.flcenterfornursing.org/files/2010_Education_Report.pdf (accessed March 29, 2010).

Friese, C. R., E. T. Lake, L. H. Aiken, J. H. Silber, and J. Sochalski. 2008. Hospital nurse practice environments and outcomes for surgical oncology patients. *Health Services Research* 43(4):1145-1163.

Gilliss, C. L. 2010. *Nursing education: Leading into the future.* Cronenwett, L. R. 2010. *The future of nursing education.* Paper commissioned by the Committee on the RWJF Initiative on the Future of Nursing, at the IOM (see Appendix I on CD-ROM).

Gonyea, M. A. 1998. Assessing resource requirements and financing for health professions education. In *Mission management: A new synthesis*, edited by E. R. Rubin. Washington, DC: Association of Academic Health Centers. Pp. 217-233.

Goode, C. J., S. Pinkerton, M. P. McCausland, P. Southard, R. Graham, and C. Krsek. 2001. Documenting chief nursing officers' preference for BSN-prepared nurses. *Journal of Nursing Administration* 31(2):55-59.

Gubrud-Howe, P., K. Shaver, C. Tanner, J. Bennett-Stillmaker, S. Davidson, M. Flaherty-Robb, K. Goudreau, L. Hardham, C. Hayden, S. Hendy, S. Omel, K. Potempa, L. Shores, S. Theis, and P. Wheeler. 2003. A challenge to meet the future: Nursing education in Oregon, 2010. *Journal of Nursing Education* 42(4):163-167.

Harden, R. M. 2002. Developments in outcome-based education. *Medical Teacher* 24 (2):117-120.

Harder, B. N. 2010. Use of simulation in teaching and learning in health sciences: A systematic review. *Journal of Nursing Education* 49(1):23-28.

HRSA (Health Resources and Services Administration). 2004. *Supply, demand, and use of licensed practical nurses.* Rockville, MD: HRSA.

HRSA. 2006. *The registered nurse population: Findings from the National Sample Survey of Registered Nurses, March 2004.* Rockville, MD: HRSA.

HRSA. 2010a. *HRSA Geospatial Data Warehouse (HGDW).* http://datawarehouse.hrsa.gov/nursing-survey.aspx (accessed September 2, 2010).

HRSA. 2010b. *The registered nurse population: Findings from the 2008 National Sample Survey of Registered Nurses.* Rockville, MD: HRSA.

IOM (Institute of Medicine). 2003a. *Health professions education: A bridge to quality.* Washington, DC: The National Academies Press.

IOM. 2003b. *Health professions education: A bridge to quality.* Washington, DC: The National Academies Press.

IOM. 2009. *Redesigning continuing education in the health professions.* Washington, DC: The National Academies Press.

IOM. 2010. *A summary of the February 2010 Forum on the Future of Nursing: Education.* Washington, DC: The National Academies Press.

Ironside, P. 2004. "Covering content" and teaching thinking: Deconstructing the additive curriculum. *Journal of Nursing Education* 43(1):5-12.

The Kaiser Family Foundation—statehealthfacts.org. 2010. *Distribution of medical school graduates by gender, 2009.* http://www.statehealthfacts.org/comparetable.jsp?ind=435&cat=8&sub=101&yr=92&typ=1 (accessed September 10, 2010).

Kovner, C., and M. Djukic. 2009. The nursing career process from application through the first 2 years of employment. *Journal of Professional Nursing* 25(4):197-203.

Kovner, C. T., S. Fairchild, and L. Jacobson. 2006. *Nurse educators 2006: A report of the faculty census survey of RN and graduate programs.* Washington, DC: NLN.

Kovner, C. T., C. S. Brewer, S. Yingrengreung, and S. Fairchild. 2010. New nurses' views of quality improvement education. *Joint Commission Journal on Quality and Patient Safety* 36(1):29-35.

Kowalski, K., M. Horner, K. Carroll, D. Center, K. Foss, and S. Jarrett. 2007. Nursing clinical faculty revisited: The benefits of developing staff nurses as clinical scholars. *Journal of Continuing Education in Nursing* 38:69-75.

Kreulen, G. J., P. K. Bednarz, T. Wehrwein, and J. Davis. 2008. Clinical education partnership: A model for school district and college of nursing collaboration. *The Journal of School Nursing* 24(6):360-369.

Kruger, B. J., C. Roush, B. J. Olinzock, and K. Bloom. 2010. Engaging nursing students in long-term relationships with a home-base community. *Journal of Nursing Education* 49(1):10-16.

Lane, A. 2009. *Battle of degrees heats up: Universities, community colleges spar over four-year programs.* http://www.crainsdetroit.com/article/20091129/FREE/311299958 (accessed November 29, 2009).

Lasater, K., and A. Nielsen. 2009. The influence of concept-based learning activities on students' clinical judgment development *Journal of Nursing Education* 48(8):441-446.

The Lewin Group. 2009. *Wisdom at work: Retaining experienced RNs and their knowledge—case studies of top performing organizations.* Falls Church, VA.

Lynaugh, J. E. 2008. Kate Hurd-Mead lecture. Nursing the great society: The impact of the Nurse Training Act of 1964. *Nursing History Review* 16:13-28.

Lynaugh, J. E., and B. L. Brush. 1996. *American nursing: From hospitals to health systems.* Cambridge, MA and Oxford, U.K.: Blackwell Press.

Manno, B. V. 1998. Vocabulary lesson: Cost, price, and subsidy in American higher education. *Business Officer* 31(10):22-25.

Mather, M., and D. Adams. 2007. *The crossover in female-male college enrollment rates.* http://www.prb.org/articles/2007/crossoverinfemalemalecollegeenrollmentrates.aspx (accessed September 10, 2010).

McNelis, A. M., and P. M. Ironside. 2009. National survey on clinical education in prelicensure nursing education programs. In *Clinical nursing education: Current reflections,* edited by N. Ard and T. M. Valiga. New York: National League for Nursing.

MedPAC (Medicare Payment Advisory Commission). 2009. *Report to the Congress: Improving incentives in the Medicare program.* Washington, DC: MedPAC.

Minority Fellowship Program. 2010. *Background.* http://www.emfp.org/MainMenuCategory/About-MFP/Background.aspx (accessed September 8, 2010).

Mitchell, P. H., B. Belza, D. C. Schaad, L. S. Robins, F. J. Gianola, P. S. Odegard, D. Kartin, and R. A. Ballweg. 2006. Working across the boundaries of health professions disciplines in education, research, and service: The University of Washington experience. *Academic Medicine* 81(10):891-896.

Moscato, S. R., J. Miller, K. Logsdon, S. Weinberg, and L. Chorpenning. 2007. Dedicated education unit: An innovative clinical partner education model. *Nursing Outlook* 55(1):31-37.

Moss, H., and M. Weinstein. 2009. *Addressing the skills shortage in healthcare through the development of incumbent employees: Hospital employee education and training (HEET) program.* Eugene, OR: University of Oregon Labor Education and Research Center.

NBCRNA (National Board on Certification and Recertification of Nurse Anesthetists). 2009. *Recertification.* http://www.nbcrna.com/recertification.html (accessed September 28, 2010).

NCEMNA (National Coalition of Ethnic Minority Nurse Associations). 2010. *About NCEMNA.* http://www.ncemna.org/about.asp (accessed July 2, 2010).

NCSBN (National Council of State Boards of Nursing). 2008. *Member board profiles National Council of State Boards of Nursing.* https://www.ncsbn.org/MBP_PDF.pdf (accessed September 3, 2010).

NCSBN. 2009. *NCLEX examination pass rates, 2009.* https://www.ncsbn.org/Table_of_Pass_Rates_2009.pdf (accessed March 30, 2010).

NLN (National League for Nursing). 2007. *Reflection & dialogue: Academic/professional progression in nursing.* http://www.nln.org/aboutnln/reflection_dialogue/refl_dial_2.htm (accessed September 8, 2010).

NLN. 2009. *Annual survey of schools of nursing academic year 2008-2009.* New York: NLN.

NLN. 2010a. *2010 NLN nurse educator shortage fact sheet.* http://www.nln.org/governmentaffairs/pdf/NurseFacultyShortage.pdf (accessed July 2, 2010).

NLN. 2010b. *Nursing education research: Graduations from RN programs.* http://www.nln.org/research/slides/topic_graduations_rn.htm (accessed September 8, 2010).

NLN. 2010c. *Percentage of minority students enrolled in nursing programs by race-ethnicity and program type, 2008-2009.* http://www.nln.org/research/slides/pdf/AS0809_F14.pdf (accessed September 5, 2010.

NLN Board of Governors. 2003. *Position statement: Innovation in nursing education: A call to reform.* http://www.nln.org/aboutnln/positionstatements/innovation082203.pdf (accessed September 27, 2010).

NLNAC (National League for Nursing Accrediting Commission). 2008. *NLNAC 2008 standards and criteria.* http://www.nlnac.org/manuals/SC2008.htm (accessed March 11, 2010).

NRC (National Research Council). 2005. *Advancing the nation's health needs: NIH research training programs.* Washington, DC: National Academy of Sciences.

O'Neil, E. H., and Pew Health Professions Commission. 1998. *Recreating health professional practice for a new century: The fourth report of the Pew Health Professions Commission.* San Francisco: CA.

O'Neil, E. 2009. Four factors that guarantee health care change. *Journal of Professional Nursing* 25(6):317-321

Oregon Center for Nursing. 2009. *Oregon's nurse faculty workforce: A report from the oregon center for nursing.* http://www.oregoncenterfornursing.org/documents/OCN%20Nurse%20Faculty%20Workforce%20Report%202009.pdf (accessed March 22, 2010).

Orsolini-Hain, L. 2008. An interpretive phenomenological study on the influences on associate degree prepared nurses to return to school to earn a higher degree in nursing, Department of Nursing, University of California, San Francisco.

Orsolini-Hain, L., and V. Waters. 2009. Education evolution: A historical perspective of associate degree nursing. *Journal of Nursing Education* 48(5):266-271.

Raines, C. F. 2010. *The doctor of nursing practice: A report on progress.* Paper presented at AACN Spring Annual Meeting 2010.

Reeves, S., M. Zwarenstein, J. Goldman, H. Barr, D. Freeth, M. Hammick, and I. Koppel. 2008. Interprofessional education: Effects on professional practice and health care outcomes. *Cochrane Database of Systematic Reviews* (1):CD002213.

Rosenstein, A. H., and M. O'Daniel. 2005. Disruptive behavior and clinical outcomes: Perceptions of nurses and physicians. *American Journal of Nursing* 105(1):54-64; quiz 64-55.

Rosenstein, A. H., and M. O'Daniel. 2008. A survey of the impact of disruptive behaviors and communication defects on patient safety. *Joint Commission Journal on Quality and Patient Safety* 34(8):464-471.

RWJF (Robert Wood Johnson Foundation). 2010a. *Distance between nursing education program and workplace for early career nurses (graduated 2007-2008).* http://thefutureofnursing.org/NursingResearchNetwork5 (accessed December 6, 2010).

RWJF. 2010b. *Qualified applicants not accepted in Associate (AD) and Baccalaureate (BS) RN programs.* http://thefutureofnursing.org/NursingResearchNetwork6 (accessed December 15, 2010).

RWJF. 2010c. *Sermo.Com survey data on physicians' opinions of nurse practitioners and nurses' educational preparation.* http://thefutureofnursing.org/NursingResearchNetwork8 (accessed December 15, 2010).

Sales, A., N. Sharp, Y. F. Li, E. Lowy, G. Greiner, C. F. Liu, A. Alt-White, C. Rick, J. Sochalski, P. H. Mitchell, G. Rosenthal, C. Stetler, P. Cournoyer, and J. Needleman. 2008. The association between nursing factors and patient mortality in the Veterans Health Administration: The view from the nursing unit level. *Medical Care* 46(9):938-945.

Schaefer, K. M., and D. Zygmont. 2003. Analyzing the teaching style of nursing faculty. Does it promote a student-centered or teacher-centered learning environment? *Nursing Education Perspectives* 24(5):238-245.

Starck, P. L. 2005. The cost of doing business in nursing education. *Journal of Professional Nursing* 21(3):183-190.

Sullivan Commission on Diversity in the Healthcare Workforce. 2004. *Missing persons: Minorities in the health professions: A report of the Sullivan Commission on Diversity in the Healthcare Workforce.* Washington, DC: The Sullivan Commission.

Tanner, C. A. 2007. The curriculum revolution revisited. *Journal of Nursing Education* 46(2):51-52.

Tanner, C. A., P. Gubrud-Howe, and L. Shores. 2008. The Oregon Consortium for Nursing Education: A response to the nursing shortage. *Policy, Politics & Nursing Practice* 9(3):203-209.

Tilden, V. 2010. *The future of nursing education.* Paper commissioned by the Committee on the RWJF Initiative on the Future of Nursing, at the IOM (see Appendix I on CD-ROM).

Tourangeau, A. E., D. M. Doran, L. McGillis Hall, L. O'Brien Pallas, D. Pringle, J. V. Tu, and L. A. Cranley. 2007. Impact of hospital nursing care on 30-day mortality for acute medical patients. *Journal of Advanced Nursing* 57(1):32-44.

Udlis, K. A. 2006. Preceptorship in undergraduate nursing education: An intergrative review. *Journal of Nursing Education* 47(1):20-29.

Valberg, L. S., M. A. Gonyea, D. G. Sinclair, and J. Wade. 1994. Planning the future academic medical centre. *Canadian Medical Association Journal* 151(11):1581-1587.

Van den Heede, K., E. Lesaffre, L. Diya, A. Vleugels, S. P. Clarke, L. H. Aiken, and W. Sermeus. 2009. The relationship between inpatient cardiac surgery mortality and nurse numbers and educational level: Analysis of administrative data. *International Journal of Nursing Studies* 46(6):796-803.

5

Transforming Leadership

Key Message #3: Nurses should be full partners, with physicians and other health professionals, in redesigning health care in the United States.

Strong leadership is critical if the vision of a transformed health care system is to be realized. Yet not all nurses begin their career with thoughts of becoming a leader. The nursing profession must produce leaders throughout the health care system, from the bedside to the boardroom, who can serve as full partners with other health professionals and be accountable for their own contributions to delivering high-quality care while working collaboratively with leaders from other health professions.

In addition to changes in nursing practice and education, discussed in Chapters 3 and 4, respectively, strong leadership will be required to realize the vision of a transformed health care system. Although the public is not used to viewing nurses as leaders, and not all nurses begin their career with thoughts of becoming a leader, all nurses must be leaders in the design, implementation, and evaluation of, as well as advocacy for, the ongoing reforms to the system that will be needed. Additionally, nurses will need leadership skills and competencies to act as full partners with physicians and other health professionals in redesign and reform efforts across the health care system. Nursing research and practice must continue to identify and develop evidence-based improvements to care, and these improvements must be tested and adopted through policy changes across the health care system. Nursing leaders must translate new research findings to the practice environment and into nursing education and from nursing education into practice and policy.

Being a full partner transcends all levels of the nursing profession and requires leadership skills and competencies that must be applied both within the profession and in collaboration with other health professionals. In care environments, being a full partner involves taking responsibility for identifying problems and areas of waste, devising and implementing a plan for improvement, tracking improvement over time, and making necessary adjustments to realize established goals. Serving as strong patient advocates, nurses must be involved in decision making about how to improve the delivery of care.

Being a full partner translates more broadly to the health policy arena. To be effective in reconceptualized roles and to be seen and accepted as leaders, nurses must see policy as something they can shape and develop rather than something that happens to them, whether at the local organizational level or the national level. They must speak the language of policy and engage in the political process effectively, and work cohesively as a profession. Nurses should have a voice in health policy decision making, as well as being engaged in implementation efforts related to health care reform. Nurses also should serve actively on advisory committees, commissions, and boards where policy decisions are made to advance health systems to improve patient care. Nurses must build new partnerships with other clinicians, business owners, philanthropists, elected officials, and the public to help realize these improvements.

This chapter focuses on key message #3 set forth in Chapter 1: Nurses should be full partners, with physicians and other health professionals, in redesigning health care in the United States. The chapter begins by considering the new style of leadership that is needed. It then issues a call to nurses to respond to the challenge. The third section describes three avenues—leadership programs for nurses, mentorship, and involvement in the policy-making process—through which that call can be answered. The chapter then issues a call for new partnerships to tap the full potential of nurses to serve as leaders in the health care system. The final section presents the committee's conclusions regarding the need to transform leadership in the nursing profession.

A NEW STYLE OF LEADERSHIP

Those involved in the health care system—nurses, physicians, patients, and others—play increasingly interdependent roles. Problems arise every day that do not have easy or singular solutions. Leaders who merely give directions and expect them to be followed will not succeed in this environment. What is needed is a style of leadership that involves working with others as full partners in a context of mutual respect and collaboration. This leadership style has been associated with improved patient outcomes, a reduction in medical errors, and less staff turnover (Gardner, 2005; Joint Commission, 2008; Pearson et al., 2007). It may also reduce the amount of workplace bullying and disruptive behavior, which remains a problem in the health care field (Joint Commission, 2008; Olender-Russo, 2009; Rosenstein and O'Daniel, 2008). Yet while the benefits of collaboration among health professionals have repeatedly been documented with respect to improved patient outcomes, reduced lengths of hospital stay, cost savings, increased job satisfaction and retention among nurses, and improved teamwork, interprofessional collaboration frequently is not the norm in the health care field. Changing this culture will not be easy.

The new style of leadership that is needed flows in all directions at all levels. Everyone from the bedside to the boardroom must engage colleagues, subordinates, and executives so that together they can identify and achieve common goals (Bradford and Cohen, 1998). All members of the health care team must share in the collaborative management of their practice. Physicians, nurses, and other health professionals must work together to break down the walls of hierarchal silos and hold each other accountable for improving quality and decreasing preventable adverse events and medication errors. All must display the capacity to adapt to the continually evolving dynamics of the health care system.

Leadership Competencies

Nurses at all levels need strong leadership skills to contribute to patient safety and quality of care. Yet their history as a profession dominated by females can make it easier for policy makers, other health professionals, and the public to view nurses as "functional doers"—those who carry out the instructions of others—rather than "thoughtful strategists"—those who are informed decision makers and whose independent actions are based on education, evidence, and experience. A 2009 Gallup poll of more than 1,500 national opinion leaders,[1] "Nursing Leadership from Bedside to Boardroom: Opinion Leaders' Perceptions," identified nurses as "one of the most trusted sources of health information" (see Box 5-1) (RWJF, 2010a). The Gallup poll also identified nurses as the health professionals that should have greater influence than they currently do in the critical areas of quality of patient care and safety. The leaders surveyed believed that major obstacles prevent nurses from being more influential in health policy decision making. These findings have crucial implications for front-line nurses,

---

[1] Gallup research staff—Richard Blizzard, Christopher Khoury, and Coleen McMurray—conducted telephone surveys with 1,504 individuals, including university faculty, insurance executives, corporate executives, health services leaders, government leaders, and industry thought leaders.

BOX 5-1
Results of Gallup Poll "Nursing Leadership from Bedside to Boardroom: Opinion Leaders' Perceptions"

- Opinion leaders rate doctors and nurses first and second among a list of options for trusted information about health and health care.
- Opinion leaders perceive patients and nurses as having the least amount of influence on health care reform in the next 5–10 years.
- Reducing medical errors, increasing quality of care, and promoting wellness top the list of areas in which large majorities of opinion leaders would like nurses to have more influence.
- Relatively few opinion leaders say nurses currently have a great deal of influence on increasing access to care, including primary care.
- Opinion leaders identified top barriers to nurses' increased influence and leadership as not being perceived as important decision makers or revenue generators compared with doctors, having a focus on acute rather than preventive care, and not having a single voice on national issues.
- Opinion leaders' suggestions for nurses to take on more of a leadership role were making their voices heard and having higher expectations.

SOURCE: RWJF, 2010a.

---

who possess critical knowledge and awareness of the patient, family, and community but do not speak up as often as they should.

To be more effective leaders and full partners, nurses need to possess two critical sets of competencies: a common set that can serve as the foundation for any leadership opportunity and a more specific set tailored to a particular context, time, and place. The former set includes, among others, knowledge of the care delivery system, how to work in teams, how to collaborate effectively within and across disciplines, the basic tenets of ethical care, how to be an effective patient advocate, theories of innovation, and the foundations for quality and safety improvement. These competencies also are recommended by the American Association of Colleges of Nursing as essential for baccalaureate programs (AACN, 2008). Leadership competencies recommended by the National League for Nursing and National League for Nursing Accrediting Commission are being revised to reflect similar principles. More specific competencies might include learning how to be a full partner in a health team in which members from various professions hold each other accountable for improving quality and decreasing preventable adverse events and medication errors. Additionally, nurses who are interested in pursuing entrepreneurial and business development opportunities need competencies in such areas as economics and market forces, regulatory frameworks, and financing policy.

Leadership in a Collaborative Environment

As noted in Chapter 1, a growing body of research has begun to highlight the potential for collaboration among teams of diverse individuals from different professions (Paulus and Nijstad, 2003; Pisano and Verganti, 2008; Singh and Fleming, 2010; Wuchty et al., 2007). Practitioners and organizational leaders alike have declared that collaboration is a key strategy for improving problem solving and achieving innovation in health care. Two nursing researchers who have studied collaboration among health professionals define it as

> a communication process that fosters innovation and advanced problem solving among people who are of different disciplines, organizational ranks, or institutional settings [and who] band together for advanced problem solving [in order to] discern innovative solutions without regard to discipline, rank, or institutional affiliation [and to] enact change based on a higher standard of care or organizational outcomes. (Kinnaman and Bleich, 2004)

Much of what is called collaboration is more likely cooperation or coordination of care. Katzenbach and Smith (1993) argue that truly collaborative teams differ from high-functioning groups that have a defined leader and a set direction, but in which the dynamics of true teamwork are absent. The case study presented in Box 5-2 illustrates just how important it is for health professionals to work in teams to ensure that care is accessible and patient centered.

Leadership at Every Level

Leadership from nurses is needed at every level and across all settings. Although collaboration is generally a laudable goal, there are many times when nurses, for the sake of delivering exceptional patient and family care, must step into an advocate role with a singular voice. At the same time, effective leadership also requires recognition of situations in which it is more important to mediate, collaborate, or follow others who are acting in leadership roles. Nurses must understand that their leadership is as important to providing quality care as is their technical ability to deliver care at the bedside in a safe and effective manner. They must lead in improving work processes on the front lines; creating new integrated practice models; working with others, from organizational policy makers to state legislators, to craft practice policy and legislation that allows nurses to work to their fullest capacity; leading curriculum changes to prepare the nursing workforce to meet community and patient needs; translating and applying research findings into practice and developing functional models of care; and serving on institutional and policy-making boards where critical decisions affecting patients are made.

Leadership in care delivery is particularly important in community and

BOX 5-2
Case Study: Arkansas Aging Initiative

A Statewide Program Uses Interprofessional Teams
to Improve Access to Care for Older Arkansans

Bonnie Sturgeon was an independent 80-year-old in 2005 when shortness of breath began to slow her down. She had been living on her own for decades, driving herself to church and singing in the choir. She went to the Christus St. Michael Health System in Texarkana, Texas, her home town, for a diagnostic workup. There she met Amyleigh Overton-McCoy, PhD, GNP-BC, RN, a geriatrics nurse practitioner with the Arkansas Aging Initiative (AAI).

"When I first went to see Amyleigh, I was there an hour or more," Ms. Sturgeon said. "She asked me every question she could think of, and I wondered how many questions could be asked?" But the intensive interviewing and testing revealed that she had three blocked arteries and had experienced a heart attack. Ms. Sturgeon was scheduled for a triple coronary artery bypass grafting procedure. Five years later, she credits Ms. Overton-McCoy with saving her life. "I've not ever been in her office that she hasn't gone over the past visit, what progress I made, and if I've had any new problems, even the smallest thing."

Patient centeredness, meticulous diagnostics, and wise counsel represent the kind of nursing that might provide a textbook definition of holistic care. This is the kind of care older Arkansans have been receiving since state voters passed the Tobacco Settlement Proceeds Act of 2000, which ordered that state monies from the Tobacco Master Settlement Agreement go toward health care initiatives, including the AAI.

This is not about making somebody live to be 100 or 110. This is about quality of life. You can make the end [of life] as great as the beginning. That's my job.

—Amyleigh Overton-McCoy, PhD, GNP-BC, RN, geriatrics nurse practitioner and education director, Texarkana Regional Center on Aging, Texarkana, Texas

Affiliated with the Donald W. Reynolds Institute on Aging at the University of Arkansas for Medical Sciences (UAMS) in Little Rock, the AAI has two direct service components. First, a team consisting of a geriatrician, an advanced practice registered nurse (APRN), and a social worker provides care at each of eight satellite centers on aging owned and managed by local hospitals (and financially self-supporting through Medicare). The team follows its patients across settings—hospital, clinic, home, and nursing home—as needed. Second, an education component supported by the tobacco settlement funds targets health professionals and students, older adults and their families, and the community at large.

The AAI's director, Claudia J. Beverly, PhD, RN, FAAN, said that these two components are funded separately but go hand in hand in practice. New patients usually see a physician for an initial examination. APRNs are responsible for health promotion and disease prevention—mammograms and flu shots, for example—as well as analyses of current drug regimens. For patients with complex conditions, social workers make referrals and work with families on nursing home placement.

Almost all older Arkansans can now access interprofessional geriatric care within an hour's drive of their home. Patients are quite satisfied with their care and with the team approach (Beverly et al., 2007). Unpublished analyses of the areas around the centers show lower rates of emergency room use and hospitalization and higher rates of health care knowledge among elderly patients.

Physicians at the eight sites report to Dr. Beverly, who is also director of UAMS's Hartford Center of Geriatric Nursing Excellence, which provides some funding to the AAI. She has hired a nurse with a doctorate and a geriatrician to act as associate directors. Developing teamwork has been a priority. "This is such a beautiful case study in how nursing and medicine can work together," she said, "and how, together, we can do good things."

There have been some obstacles: primary care services are dependent upon Medicare funding, and with an annual budget of $2 million to divide among eight sites, additional revenue is needed. There also may not be enough clinicians trained in geriatrics available. And although Dr. Beverly believes that APRNs "should have

their own panel of patients," they see only returning patients at the centers. She said funding has been secured to further evaluate how best to use team members.

The model has continued to evolve from the first center in Northwest Arkansas that Dr. Beverly started as a Robert Wood Johnson Executive Nurse Fellow. That site is developing a program for the training of in-home caregivers, including home health aides and family members. And a new telehealth project will allow patients and clinicians to "see" a specialist electronically. "Economically, this is going to provide a huge benefit to patients," Ms. Overton-McCoy said.

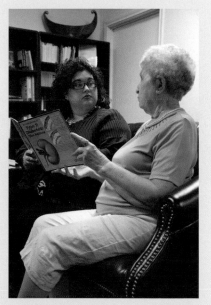

Photomotion Photography/Michelle DeHan

Nurse Amyleigh Overton-McCoy explains to Bonnie Sturgeon how to manage the common health concerns associated with aging.

home settings where nurses work more autonomously with patients and families than they do in the acute care setting. In community and home settings, nurses provide a direct link connecting patients, their caregivers, and other members of the health care team. Other members of the health care team may not have the time, expertise, or first-hand experience with the patient's home environment and circumstances to understand and respond to patient and family needs. For example, a neurologist may not be able to help a caregiver of an Alzheimer's patient understand or curtail excessive spending habits, or a surgeon may not be able to offer advice to a caregiver on ostomy care—roles that nurses are perfectly positioned to assume. Leadership in these situations sometimes requires nurses to be assertive and to have a strong voice in advocating for patients and their families to ensure that their needs are communicated and adequately met.

Box 5-3 describes a nurse who evolved over the course of her career from thinking that being an effective nurse was all about honing her nursing skills and competencies to realize that becoming an agent of change was an equally important part of her job.

A CALL FOR NURSES TO LEAD

Leadership does not occur in a social or political vacuum. As Bennis and Nanus (2003) note, the fast pace of change can be managed only if it is accompanied by leaders who can track the context of the "social architecture" to sustain and implement innovative ideas. Creating innovative care models at the bedside and in the community or taking the opportunity to fill a seat in a policy-making body or boardroom requires nurse leaders to develop ideas; approach management; and courageously make decisions within the political, economic, and social context that will make their solutions real and sustainable. A shift must take place in how nurses view their responsibility to those they care for; they must see themselves as full partners with other health professionals, and practice and education environments must socialize and educate them accordingly.

An important aspect of this socialization is mentoring others along the way. More experienced nurses must take the time to show those who are new and less experienced the most effective ways of being an exceptional nurse at the bedside, in the boardroom, and everywhere between. Technology such as chat rooms, Facebook, and even blogs can be used to support the mentoring role.

A crucial part of working within the social architecture is understanding how leadership and practice produce change over time. The nursing profession's history includes many examples of the effect of nursing leadership on changes in systems and improvements in patient care. In the late 1940s and early 1950s, nurse Elizabeth Carnegie led the fight for the racial integration of nursing in Florida by example and through her extraordinary character and organizational skills. Her efforts to integrate the nursing profession were based in her sense of social justice not just for the profession, but also for the care of African American citizens who had little access to a workforce that was highly skilled or provided adequate access to health care services. Also in Florida, in the late 1950s, Dorothy Smith, the first dean of the new University of Florida College of Nursing, developed nursing practice models that brought nursing faculty into the hospital in a joint nursing service. Students thereby had role models in their learning experiences, and staff nurses had the authority to improve patient care. From this system came the patient kardex and the unit manager system that freed nurses from the constant search for supplies that took them away from the bedside. In the 1980s, nursing research by Neville Strumpf and Lois Evans highlighted the danger of using restraints on frail elders (Evans and Strumpf, 1989; Strumpf and Evans, 1988). Their efforts to translate their findings into practice revolutionized nursing practice in nursing homes, hospitals, and other facilities by focusing nursing care on preventing falls and other injuries related to restraint use, and led to state and federal legislation that resulted in reducing the use of restraints on frail elders.

Nurses also have also led efforts to improve health and access to care through entrepreneurial endeavors. For example, Ruth Lubic founded the first free-standing birth center in the country in 1975 in New York City. In 2000, she opened the Family Health and Birth Center in Washington, DC, which provides care to underserved communities (see Box 2-2 in Chapter 2). Her efforts have improved the care of thousands of women over the years. There are many other examples of nurse entrepreneurs, and a nurse entrepreneur network[2] exists that provides networking, education and training, and coaching for nurses seeking to enter the marketplace and business.

Will Student Nurses Hear the Call?

Leadership skills must be learned and mastered over time. Nonetheless, it is important to obtain a basic grasp of those skills as early as possible—starting in school (see Chapter 4). Nursing educators must give their students the most relevant knowledge and practice opportunities to equip them for their profession, while instilling in them a desire and expectation for new learning in the years to come. Regardless of the basic degree with which a nurse enters the profession, faculty should feel obligated to show students the way to their first or next career placement, as well as to their next degree and continuous learning opportunities.

Moreover, students should not wait for graduation to exercise their potential for leadership. In Georgia, for example, health students came together in 2001 under the banner "Lead or Be Led" to create a student-led, interprofessional nonprofit organization that "seeks to make being active in the health community a professional habit." Named Health Students Taking Action Together (Health-STAT), the group continues to offer workshops in political advocacy, media

---

[2] See http://www.nurse-entrepreneur-network.com/public/main.cfm.

BOX 5-3
Nurse Profile: Connie Hill

*A Nurse Leader Extends Acute Care Nursing
Beyond the Hospital Walls*

It was at a 2002 meeting at Children's Memorial Hospital in Chicago that Connie Hill, MSN, RN, reviewed the chart of a child who had been on a ventilator in her unit for 2 years. She asked her colleagues why the child had not been discharged. "It wasn't because she was not medically stable," Ms. Hill said recently, "but because there was a lack of community resources to support her." Inadequate community services existed for a child with special needs in Chicago, the third-largest city in the nation? "I was dumbfounded," she recalled. "And I said, 'We need to start a consortium. We need to invite policy makers, state agencies, community leaders.' And people just looked at me, like, 'Okay, Connie. How are we going to get that started?'"

As director of 9 West, the 30-bed Allergy/Pulmonary/Transitional Care Unit, Ms. Hill persisted, and in 2004 the Consortium for Children with Complex Medical Needs was formed. The 75-member coalition of parents, clinicians, advocates, and representatives of government agencies and insurance companies meets quarterly, with the goal of "networking, education, and advocacy" on behalf of the city's special-needs children, some of whom may be on ventilators indefi-

nitely. For example, the group identified poor reimbursement of home health care as a serious obstacle, and the hospital established ties to agencies able to tackle the reimbursement issue. Now, some children can go home to receive care.

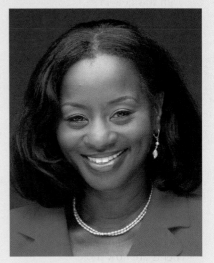

Photo courtesy of Connie Hill

Connie Hill, MSN, RN

Ms. Hill never intended to be a leader. She was working as a staff nurse at the hospital in the mid-1990s when colleagues encouraged

training, networking, and fundraising. Its annual leadership symposium convenes medical, nursing, public health, and other students statewide to learn about health issues facing the state and work together on developing potential solutions (HealthSTAT, 2010). The National Student Nurses Association (NSNA), initiated in 1998, offers an online Leadership University that allows students to enhance

her to apply for a clinical manager position in 9 West. She followed their advice, and in late 2000 when her supervisor failed to return from maternity leave, she proposed a "shared leadership model." After a year or so during which she and two other nurses shared the directorship, Ms. Hill was asked to become sole director (some staff were uncomfortable with the decentralized authority, despite good clinical outcomes). She did so, with a modest goal: "I wanted to provide a venue for all nurses to have a voice."

With this goal in mind, Ms. Hill decided in 2008 that 9 West would be a good fit for Transforming Care at the Bedside (TCAB), a national initiative of The Robert Wood Johnson Foundation with the Institute for Healthcare Improvement. Communication between nurses and rotating medical residents was targeted in the hospital's quest to improve the coordination of care (Quisling, 2009). As Ms. Hill said, "It's disheartening when you receive a patient survey and a family says, 'The doctor said this, but then the nurse told me that.'" A procedure was created for staff nurses to provide orientations to residents, who rotate monthly among units, to foster better team communication. Residents are now more likely to confer with 9 West nurses during rounds, Ms. Hill said, increasing satisfaction among nurses, residents, patients, and families.

As a doctoral student at the University of Wisconsin-Milwaukee College of Nursing, Ms. Hill is examining an often neglected population: teens born with HIV, a majority of whom are African American and Hispanic. Now that many HIV-positive children survive into adulthood, they mature sexually and face the stigma attached to the infection. Ms. Hill's study uses PhotoVoice, which involves putting cameras into the hands of HIV-positive teens and asking them for a visual answer to the question, "Where do you see yourself in five years?" "They're writing their own story" in photographs, she said, a story they can use to raise awareness in others and to remind themselves of their own strengths.

I wanted to make the environment for the child and parents a place where they could feel safe, even though there was a lot of scary stuff going on around them.

—Connie Hill, MSN, RN, director of a 30-bed unit at Children's Memorial Hospital, Chicago

---

Ms. Hill has quite a story herself. As a mother of a grown son, a pediatric nurse who endured many hospitalizations as a child, a researcher whose study is an outgrowth of her advocacy work, and an African American who strives to enhance access to health care for all, she is a woman of both practical ideas and lofty ideals. So when she saw that a child capable of living at home had been in her unit for 2 years, her natural response was to assemble a consortium. Today, that child is doing well at home.

their capacity for leadership through several avenues, such as earning academic credit for participating in the university's leadership activities and discussing leadership issues with faculty. Students work in cooperative relationships with other students from various disciplines, faculty, community organizations, and the public (Janetti, 2003). Box 5-4 profiles two student leaders, one of whom eventu-

BOX 5-4
Nurse Profile: Kenya D. Haney and Billy A. Caceres

Building Diversity in Nursing, One Student at a Time

Despite improvements to the demographic make up of the nursing workforce in recent decades, the workforce remains predominantly white, female, and middle aged. Racial and ethnic minorities make up 34 percent of the U.S. population but only 12 percent of the registered nurse (RN) workforce, and just 7 percent of RNs are men (AACN, 2010). And diversity matters to patients: many studies have shown that a more diverse health care workforce results in greater access to care for minority populations (IOM, 2004). Two nurses, an African American woman and a Hispanic man, both under age 35, illustrate the growing diversity of the profession and the importance of offering various educational paths as an entry into nursing.

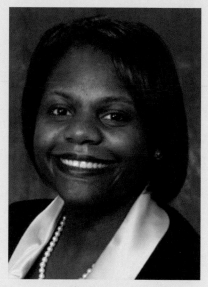

Photo courtesy of Kenya Haney

Kenya D. Haney, RN

Kenya D. Haney, RN, was a married mother of two in 2004 when she was trying to decide between nursing school and law school. She had taken classes toward a bachelor's degree in communications and knew she would need a more flexible program. She chose the associate's degree in nursing program at St. Louis Community College in Missouri: it offered a part-time option and child care at $2 an hour, which her educational grants covered. If the child care had not been available, she would have waited until her children were older, she said, and then "gone back to finish the communications degree and gone on to law school. There's just not a doubt in my mind."

After graduating, Ms. Haney got a job in intensive care; entered the bachelor's of science in nursing (BSN) program for RNs at the University of Missouri, St. Louis; and joined the Breakthrough to Nursing initiative at the National Student Nurses Association (NSNA). The NSNA initiative aims to increase the number of men entering the profession, recruit and retain nurses of diverse ethnic and racial backgrounds, support nursing students with physical disabilities, and increase enrollment of young and nontraditional students. It works toward these goals by making peers available to students in need of support. Ms. Haney became its director in 2008 and NSNA president in 2009. "You know, we're not the answer to everything," she said of Breakthrough to Nursing. "But we're there for support. Maybe we'll just say, 'You can do this. You're not alone, and you really are needed.'"

If we could open up the doors just a little bit wider for foreign nursing students, mothers, nontraditional students, and men, that would make a world of difference to patients.

—Kenya D. Haney, RN, student, University of Missouri, St. Louis, and immediate past president, National Student Nurses Association

Billy A. Caceres, BSN, RN, already had a bachelor's degree in politics and communications and a job in event planning for a New York City nonprofit when he made the decision to pursue a BSN. As an undergraduate at New York University (NYU), he had volunteered to raise awareness of sexual assault and substance abuse on campus and wanted to learn more about health. He applied and was accepted to NYU's College of Nursing in its 15-month accelerated program for students with a bachelor's in another field. Soon he became involved in the Hartford Geriatric Nursing Institute at NYU.

As a nurse, Mr. Caceres has encountered bias at times from patients, especially older women, some of whom feel uncomfortable being cared for by a man. "I don't get offended," he said. "But sometimes I think, What if nobody else was around? What would you do? I'm just trying to provide care for you." He has just begun his first job as a hospital staff nurse, in a New York City orthopedics unit, and hopes one day to merge his interests in geriatrics and health policy, he said.

Both Ms. Haney and Mr. Caceres intend to pursue graduate degrees,

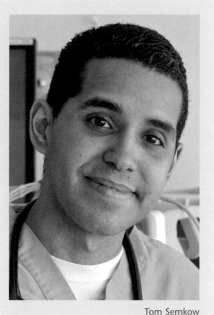

Tom Semkow

Billy A. Caceras, BSN, RN

perhaps even the doctorate. If so, they will be models for a new generation: only 23 percent of students in research-focused doctoral programs in nursing are from minority backgrounds, and only 7 percent are men (AACN, 2010). Regardless, the two have taken significant steps. As Ms. Haney said, "Sometimes it's that initial barrier of getting into nursing school that can hurt so many. But the NSNA is a way to bring us together to see that we have one common goal, and that is to be professional nurses. Basically, it's for the patient."

A lot of nurses get surprised that I have this interest in politics, but I think it's okay to go into nursing as a second career.

—Billy A. Caceres, BSN, RN, staff nurse, New York University Langone Medical Center, New York

ally became NSNA president; both represent as well the growing diversity of the nursing profession, a crucial need if the profession is to rise to the challenge of helping to transform the health care system (see Chapter 4).

Looking to the future, nurse leaders will need the skills and knowledge to understand and anticipate population trends. Formal preparation of student nurses may need to go beyond what has traditionally been considered nursing education. To this end, a growing number of schools offer dual undergraduate degrees in partnership with the university's business or engineering school for nurses interested in starting their own business or developing more useful technology. Graduate programs offering dual degree programs with schools of business, public health, law, design, or communications take this idea one step further to equip students with an interest in administrative, philanthropic, regulatory, or policy-making positions with greater competencies in management, finance, communication, system design, or scope-of-practice regulations from the start of their careers.

Will Front-Line Nurses Hear the Call?

Given their direct and sustained contact with patients, front-line nurses, along with their unit or clinic managers, are uniquely positioned to design new models of care to improve quality, efficiency, and safety. Tapping that potential will require developing a new workplace culture that encourages and supports leaders at the point of care (whether a hospital or the community) and requires all members of a health care team to hold each other accountable for the team's performance; nurses must also be equipped with the communication, conflict resolution, and negotiating skills necessary to succeed in leadership and partnership roles. For example, one new quality and safety strategy requires checklists to be completed before certain procedures, such as inserting a catheter, are begun. Nurses typically are asked to enforce adherence to the checklist. If another nurse or a physician does not wash his/her hands or contaminates a sterile field, nurses must possess the basic leadership skills to remind their colleague of the protocol and stop the procedure, if necessary, until the checklist is followed. And again, nurses must help and mentor each other in their roles as expert clinicians and patient advocates. No one can build the capabilities of an exceptional and effective nurse like another exceptional and effective nurse.

Will Community Nurses Hear the Call?

Nurses working in the community have long understood that to be effective in contributing to improvements in the entire community's health, they must assume the role of social change agent. Among other things, community and public health nurses must promote immunization, good nutrition, and physical activity; detect emergency health threats; and prevent and respond to outbreaks of communicable diseases. In addition, they need to be prepared to assume roles in dealing with public health emergencies, including disaster preparedness, response, and recovery. Recent declines in the numbers of community and public health nurses, however, have made the leadership imperative for these nurses much more challenging.

Community and public health nurses learn to expect the unexpected. For example, a school nurse alerted health authorities to the arrival of the H1N1 influenza virus in New York City in 2009 (RWJF, 2010c). Likewise, an increasing number of nurses are being trained in incident command as part of preparedness for natural disasters and possible terrorist attacks. This entails understanding the roles of and working with community, state, and federal officials to assure the health and safety of the public. For example, when the town of Chehalis, south of Seattle, experienced a 100-year flood in 2007, a public health nurse called the secretary of Washington State's Department of Health, Mary Selecky, to ask how to "deal with and dispose of dead cows, an unforeseen challenge [for] a public health nurse. The nurse knew she needed [to provide] tetanus shots and portable toilets but had not anticipated other, less common, aspects of the emergency" (IOM, 2010).

The profile in Box 5-5 illustrates how nurses lead efforts that provide critical services for communities. The profile also shows how nurses can also become leaders and social change agents in the broader community by serving on the boards of health-related institutions. The importance of this role is discussed in the next section.

Will Chief Nursing Officers Hear the Call?

Although chief nursing officers (CNOs) typically are part of the hierarchical decision-making structure in that they have authority and responsibility for the nursing staff, they need to move up in the reporting structure of their organizations to increase their ability to contribute to key decisions. Not only is this not happening, however, but CNOs appear to be losing ground. A 2002 survey by the American Organization of Nurse Executives (AONE) showed that 55 percent of CNOs reported directly to their institution's CEO, compared with 60 percent in 2000. More CNOs described a direct reporting relationship to the chief operating officer instead. Such changes in reporting structure can limit nurse leaders' involvement in decision making about the most important product of hospitals—patient care. Additionally, the AONE survey showed that most CNOs (70 percent) have seen their responsibilities increase even as they have moved down in the reporting structure (Ballein Search Partners and AONE, 2003). CNOs face growing issues of contending not only with increased responsibilities, but also with budget pressures and difficulties with staffing, retention, and turnover levels during a nursing shortage (Jones et al., 2008).

BOX 5-5
Nurse Profile: Mary Ann Christopher

Cultivating Neighborhood Nursing at the Visiting
Nurse Association of Central Jersey

At the Visiting Nurse Association of Central Jersey (VNACJ), president and chief executive officer Mary Ann Christopher, MSN, RN, FAAN, maintains a $100 million annual budget, a 4,000-patient daily census, and a 1,700-person staff. Services available to residents in 10 central New Jersey counties include home care, primary care, wellness services, mental health care, rehabilitation, homeless services, and hospice and palliative care. Yet despite the size and complexity of the 98-year-old organization, Ms. Christopher's primary objective has remained simple in her 27-year career there. "People need to know that you stand for what you say you stand for," she said. And what the VNACJ stands for is local communities "driving" the services provided. Ms. Christopher has called it Neighborhood Nursing, a collaborative model in which nurses are assigned to specific neighborhoods so they and community members can respond to what they identify as the most pressing health issues.

As an example of the model, she cites a VNACJ nurse who noticed that many residents of a retirement community were exhibiting signs of congestive heart failure. The nurse proposed that the VNACJ set up a

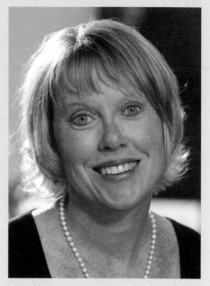

Photo courtesy of Mary Ann Christopher

Mary Ann Christopher, MSN, RN, FAAN

kiosk that would contain a telehealth monitor. The device would permit residents to check their weight, oxygen saturation, and blood pressure levels and automatically transmit the values to a cardiac nurse. If a patient's indicators were outside the desired range, the nurse and patient would converse remotely, in real time, and patients needing a medica-

Nurses also are underrepresented on institution and hospital boards, either their own or others. A biennial survey of hospitals and health systems conducted in 2007 by the Governance Institute found that only 0.8 percent of voting board members were CNOs, compared with 5.1 percent who were vice presidents for medical affairs (Governance Institute, 2007). More recently, a 2009 survey of

tion adjustment would be visited. The VNACJ funded the idea, and outcomes are being monitored.

Ms. Christopher said that the aims of such an initiative are both immediate and long term. In the short run, the VNACJ hopes to reduce rates of emergency room (ER) use and repeated hospitalizations—expensive and inefficient means of managing chronic illness. As for the long-term goal, the VNACJ nurses strive to give individuals as well as entire communities greater control over their health. After the telehealth kiosk was set up, for example, residents began paying attention to one another's weight and blood pressure levels.

Ms. Christopher has secured grants to test a wide range of such ideas. For example, the Mobile Outreach Program has reduced rates of ER use among deinstitutionalized mentally ill and homeless patients; funded in the mid-1980s by The Robert Wood Johnson Foundation and the State of New Jersey, it is now supported by local governments. The Mobile Outreach Program is the VNACJ initiative Ms. Christopher is the most proud of and the one, she said, that may be the most replicable.

In 1998 the Balanced Budget Act resulted in a 15 percent reduction in revenues and left the VNACJ with only $100,000 in reserve. Now, even with $24 million in reserve, Ms. Christopher worries about declines in federal, state, and philanthropic funding, especially in light of the recent increases in un- and underinsured patients being seen as a result of the recession. Still, she said that the agency's focus on providing services the community values, even as those values change, has kept the association fiscally sound.

I make decisions within the context of really understanding the impact of service delivery. I think I can see opportunities quickly, because I'm seeing it more from a nurse's perspective, but also a nurse who grew up on a community-based side [of health care delivery].

—Mary Ann Christopher, MSN, RN, FAAN, president and chief executive officer, Visiting Nurse Association of Central Jersey, Red Bank, New Jersey

---

Not all CEOs of visiting nurse associations are nurses (those in New York City and Boston, for example, are not). Ms. Christopher said she can see why it matters that she is a nurse. First, she knows well what nurses can do. She has cultivated an atmosphere of honoring staff ideas (such as the cardiac monitoring initiative). As a result, the VNACJ has a turnover rate of less than 5 percent for nurses. Second, Ms. Christopher is sought after to serve on governing boards and advisory groups and is the only RN on the board of trustees at the University of Medicine and Dentistry of New Jersey. She believes that her nursing expertise, keen sense of community, and fiscal responsibility give her "legitimacy at any table I'm at...being a guardian for what's best for patients and communities."

community health systems found that nurses made up only 2.3 percent of their boards, compared with 22.6 percent who were physicians (Prybil et al., 2009).[3]

---

[3] It should be noted that, while there are many more physicians than nurses on hospital boards, health care providers still are generally underrepresented.

While most boards focus mainly on finance and business, health care delivery, quality, and responsiveness to the public—areas in which the nature of their work gives nurses particular expertise—also are considered key (Center for Healthcare Governance, 2007). A 2007 survey found that 62 percent of boards included a quality committee (Governance Institute, 2007). A 2006 survey of hospital presidents and CEOs showed the impact of such committees. Those institutions with a quality committee were more likely to adopt various oversight practices; they also experienced lower mortality rates for six common medical conditions measured by the Agency for Healthcare Research and Quality's (AHRQ's) Inpatient Quality Indicators and the State Inpatient Databases (Jiang et al., 2008).

The growing attention of hospital boards to quality and safety issues reflects the increased visibility of these issues in recent years. Several states and the Centers for Medicare and Medicaid Services, for example, are increasing their oversight of specific preventable errors ("never events"), and new payment structures in health care reform may be based on patient outcomes and satisfaction (Hassmiller and Bolton, 2009; IOM, 2000; King, 2009; Wachter, 2009). Given their expertise in quality and safety improvement, nurses are more likely than many other board members to understand the issues involved and often can educate other members about these issues (Mastal et al., 2007). This is one area, then, in which nurse board members can have a significant impact. Recognizing this, the 2009 survey of community health systems mentioned above specifically recommended that community health system boards consider appointing expert nursing leaders as voting board members to strengthen clinical input in deliberations and decision-making processes (Prybil et al., 2009).

More CNOs need to prepare themselves and seek out opportunities to serve on the boards of health-related institutions. If decisions are taking place about patient care and a nurse is not at the decision-making table, important perspectives will be missed. CNOs should also promote leadership activities among their staff, encouraging them to secure important decision-making positions on committees and boards, both internal and external to the organization.

Will Nurse Researchers Hear the Call?

Nurse researchers must develop new models of quality care that are evidence based, patient centered, affordable, and accessible to diverse populations. Developing and imparting the science of nursing is also an important contribution to nurses' ability to deliver high-quality, safe care. Additionally, nurses must serve as advocates and implementers for the program designs they develop. Academic–service partnerships that typically involve nursing schools and nearby, often low-income communities are a first step toward implementation. Given that a nursing school does not exist in every community, however, such partnerships cannot achieve change on the scale needed to transform the health care system. Nurse researchers must become active not only in studying important care delivery questions but also in translating research findings into practice and developing and setting the policy agendas. Their leadership is vital in ensuring that new state- and federal-level policies are based on evidence and will help increase quality and access while decreasing costs and health care disparities. The Affordable Care Act (ACA) provides opportunities for demonstration projects and pilot programs directed at various elements of nursing. If these projects and programs do not adequately track nursing inputs and intended/unintended outcomes, they cannot hope to achieve their potential.

Nurse researchers should seek funding from the National Institute for Nursing Research and other institutes of the National Institutes of Health, as do scientists from other disciplines, to help increase the evidence base for improved models of care. Funding might also be secured from other government entities, such as AHRQ and the Health Resources and Services Administration (HRSA) and local and national foundations, depending on the research topic. To be competitive in these efforts, nurses should hone their analytical skills with training in such areas as statistics and data analysis, econometrics, biometrics, and other qualitative and quantitative research methods that are appropriate to their research topics. Mark Pauly, codirector of the Robert Wood Johnson Foundation's Interdisciplinary Nursing Quality Research Initiative, argues that, for nursing research to achieve parity with other health services research in terms of acceptability, it must be managed by interprofessional teams that include both nurse scholars and scholars from methodological and modeling disciplines. For nurse researchers to achieve parity with other health services researchers, they must develop the skills and initiative to take leadership roles in this research.[4]

Will Nursing Organizations Hear the Call?

The Gallup poll of 1,500 opinion leaders referenced earlier in this chapter also highlighted fragmentation in the leadership of nursing organizations as a challenge. Responding opinion leaders predicted that nurses will have little influence on health care reform over the next 5–10 years (see Figure 5-1). By contrast, they believed that nurses should have more input and impact in areas such as planning, policy development, and management (Figure 5-2) (RWJF, 2010a). No one expects all professional health organizations to coordinate their public agendas, actions, or messaging for every issue. But nursing organizations must continue to collaborate and work hard to develop common messages, including visions and missions, with regard to their ability to offer evidence-based solutions

---

[4] Personal communication, Mark Pauly, Bendheim Professor, Professor of Health Care Management, Professor of Business and Public Policy, Professor of Insurance and Risk Management, and Professor of Economics, Wharton School of the University of Pennsylvania, and Codirector of the Robert Wood Johnson Foundation's Interdisciplinary Nursing Quality Research Initiative, June 25, 2010.

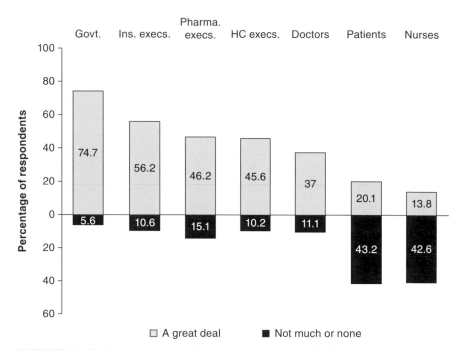

FIGURE 5-1 Opinion leaders' predictions of the amount of influence nurses will have on health care reform.
NOTE: Govt. = Government; Ins. Execs. = Insurance executives; Pharma. execs. = Pharmaceutical executives; HC execs. = Health care executives.
SOURCE: RWJF, 2010b. Reprinted with permission from Frederick Mann, RWJF.

for improvements in patient care. Once common ground has been established, nursing organizations will need to activate their membership and constituents to work together to take action and support shared goals. When policy makers and other key decision makers know that the largest group of health professionals in the country is in agreement on important issues, they listen and often take action. Conversely, when nursing organizations and their members disagree with one another on important issues, decisions are not made, as the decision makers often are unsure of which side to take.

Quality and safety are important areas in which professional nursing organizations have great potential to serve as leaders. The Nursing Alliance for Quality Care (NAQC)[5] is a Robert Wood Johnson Foundation–funded effort with the mission of advancing the quality, safety, and value of patient-centered health care for all individuals, including patients, their families, and the communities where patients live.

---

[5] See http://www.gwumc.edu/healthsci/departments/nursing/naqc/.

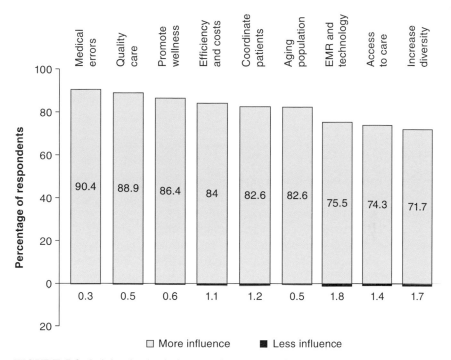

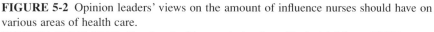

FIGURE 5-2 Opinion leaders' views on the amount of influence nurses should have on various areas of health care.
SOURCE: RWJF, 2010b. Reprinted with permission from Frederick Mann, RWJF.

Based at the George Washington University School of Nursing, the organization stresses the need for nurses to advocate actively for and be accountable to patients for high-quality and safe care. The establishment of the NAQC "is based on the assumption that only with a stronger, more unified 'voice' in nursing policy will dramatic and sustainable achievements in quality and safety be achieved for the American public" (George Washington University Medical Center, 2010).

ANSWERING THE CALL

The call for nurses to assume leadership roles can be answered through leadership programs for nurses; mentorship; and involvement in the policy-making process, including political engagement.

Leadership Programs for Nurses

Leadership is not necessarily innate; many individuals develop into leaders. Sometimes that development comes through experience. For example, nurse leaders at the executive level historically earned their way to their position through their competence, rather than obtaining formal preparation through a business school. However, development as a leader can also be achieved through more formal education and training programs. The wide range of effective leadership programs now available for nurses is illustrated by the examples described below. The challenge is to better utilize these opportunities to develop a greater number of nursing leaders.

Integrated Nurse Leadership Program

The Integrated Nurse Leadership Program (INLP),[6] funded by the Gordon and Betty Moore Foundation, works with hospitals in the San Francisco Bay area that wish to remodel their professional culture and systems of care to improve care while dealing more effectively with continual change. The program develops hospital leaders, offers training and technical assistance, and provides grants to support the program's implementation. INLP has found that the development of stable, effective leadership in nursing-related care is associated with better-than-expected patient care outcomes and improvements in nurse recruitment and retention. The impact of the program will be evaluated to produce models that can be replicated in other parts of the country.

Fellows Program in Management for Nurse Executives at Wharton[7]

When the Johnson & Johnson Company and the Wharton School joined in 1983 to offer a senior nurse executive management fellowship, the program concentrated on helping senior nursing leaders manage their departments by providing them, for example, intense training in accounting (Shea, 2005). The Wharton Fellows program has changed in many ways since then in response to the evolving health care environment, according to a 2005 review (Shea, 2005). For example, the program has strengthened senior nursing executives' ability to argue for quality improvement on the basis of solid evidence, including financial documentation and probabilistic decision making. The program also aims to improve such leadership competencies as systems thinking, negotiation, communications, strategy, analysis, and the development of learning communities. Its offerings will likely undergo yet more changes as hospital chief executive and chief operating officers increasingly come from the ranks of the nursing profession.

---

[6] See http://futurehealth.ucsf.edu/Public/Leadership-Programs/Home.aspx?pid=35.

[7] See http://executiveeducation.wharton.upenn.edu/open-enrollment/health-care-programs/Fellows-Program-Management-Nurse-Executives.cfm.

Robert Wood Johnson Foundation Executive Nurse Fellows Program

The Robert Wood Johnson Foundation Executive Nurse Fellows Program[8] is an advanced leadership program for nurses in senior executive roles who wish to lead improvements in health care from local to national levels. It provides a 3-year in-depth, comprehensive leadership development experience for nurses who are already serving in senior leadership positions. The program is designed to cultivate and expand fellows' capacity to lead teams and organizations. The fellowship program includes curriculum and program activities that provide opportunities for executive coaching and mentoring, team-based and individual leadership projects, professional development that incorporates best practices in leadership, as well as access to online communities and leadership networks. Through the program, fellows master 20 leadership competencies that cover a broad range of knowledge and skills that can be used when "leading self, leading others, leading the organization and leading in health care" (RWJF Executive Nurse Fellows, 2010).

Best on Board

Best on Board[9] is an education, testing, and certification program that helps prepare current and prospective leaders to serve on the governing board of a health care organization. Its CEO, Connie Curran, is a registered nurse (RN) who chaired a hospital nursing department, was the dean of a medical college, and founded her own national management and consulting services firm. A 2010 review cites the growing recognition by blue ribbon panels and management researchers that nurses are an untapped resource for the governing bodies of health care organizations. The authors argue that while nurses have many qualities that make them natural assets to any health care board, they must also "understand the advantages of serving on boards and what it takes to get there" (Curran and Totten, 2010).

Robert Wood Johnson Foundation Health Policy Fellows and Investigator Awards Programs

While not limited to nurses, the Robert Wood Johnson Foundation Health Policy Fellows and Investigator Awards programs[10] offer nurses, other health professionals, and behavioral and social scientists "with an interest in health [the opportunity] to participate in health policy processes at the federal level" (RWJF Scholars, Fellows & Leadership Programs, 2010). Fellows work on Capitol Hill with elected officials and congressional staff. The goal is for fellows to use their academic and practice experience to inform the policy process and to improve

---

[8] See http://www.executivenursefellows.org.

[9] See http://www.bestonboard.org.

[10] See http://www.rwjfleaders.org/programs/robert-wood-johnson-foundation-health-policy-fellow.

the quality of policies enacted. Investigators are funded to complete innovative studies of topics relevant to current and future health policy. Participants in both programs receive intensive training to improve the content and delivery of messages intended to improve health policy and practice. This training is critical, as investigators are often called upon to testify to Congress about the issues they have explored. The health policy fellows bring their more detailed understanding of how policies are formed back to their home organizations. In this way, they are more effective leaders as they strive to bring about policy changes that lead to improvements in patient care.

American Nurses Credentialing Center Magnet Recognition Program

Although not an individual leadership program, the American Nurses Credentialing Center (ANCC) Magnet Recognition Program[11] recognizes health care organizations that advance nursing excellence and leadership. In this regard, achieving Magnet status indicates that the nursing workforce within the institution has attained a number of high standards relating to quality and standards of nursing practice. These standards, as designated by the Magnet process, are called "Forces of Magnetism." According to ANCC, "the full expression of the Forces embodies a professional environment guided by a strong visionary nursing leader who advocates and supports development and excellence in nursing practice. As a natural outcome of this, the program elevates the reputation and standards of the nursing profession" (ANCC, 2010). Some of these Forces include quality of nursing leadership, management style, quality of care, autonomous nursing care, nurses as teachers, interprofessional relationships, and professional development.

Mentorship[12]

Leadership is also fostered through effective mentorship opportunities with leaders in nursing, other health professions, policy, and business. All nurses have a responsibility to mentor those who come after them, whether by helping a new nurse become oriented or by taking on more formal responsibilities as a teacher of nursing students or a preceptor. Nursing organizations (membership associations) also have a responsibility to provide mentoring and leadership guidance, as well as opportunities to share expertise and best practices, for those who join.

Fortunately, a number of nursing associations have organized networks to support their membership and facilitate such opportunities:

---

[11] See http://www.nursecredentialing.org/Magnet/ProgramOverview.aspx.

[12] This section draws on personal communication in 2010 with Susan Gergely, Director of Operations, American Organization of Nurse Executives; Beverly Malone, CEO, National League for Nursing; Robert Rosseter, Chief Communications Officer, American Association of Colleges of Nursing; and Pat Ford Roegner, CEO, American Academy of Nursing.

- The American Association of Colleges of Nursing (AACN) conducts an expertise survey that is used to identify subject matter experts across topic areas within its membership; it also maintains a list of nursing education experts. Names of these experts are shared with members on request. These resources also are used to identify experts to serve on boards, respond to media requests, and serve in other capacities. In addition, AACN offers an annual executive leadership development program and a new deans mentoring program to further promote and foster leadership.

- The National League for Nursing (NLN) has established an Academy of Nurse Educators whose members are available to serve as mentors for NLN members. NLN engages these educators in a variety of mentoring programs, from a National Scholarly Writing Retreat to the Johnson & Johnson mentoring program for new faculty.

- While AONE does not have a formal mentoring program, it has developed online learning communities where members are encouraged to interact, post questions, and learn from each other. These online communities facilitate collaboration; encourage the sharing of knowledge, best practices, and resources; and help members discover solutions to day-to-day challenges in their work.

- The American Academy of Nursing keeps a detailed list of nurse "Edge Runners"[13] that describes the programs nursing leaders have developed and the outcomes of those programs. Edge Runner names and contact information are prominently displayed so that learning and mentoring can take place freely.[14]

- The American Nurses Association just passed a resolution at its 2010 House of Delegates to develop a mentoring program for novice nurses. The program has yet to be developed.

- Over the years, the National Coalition of Ethnic Minority Nurse Associations (NCEMNA) has offered numerous workshops, webinars, and educational materials to develop its members' competencies in leadership, policy, and communications. NCEMNA's highly regarded Scholars program[15] promotes the academic and professional development of ethnic minority investigators, in part through a mentoring program. It serves as a model worth emulating throughout the nursing profession.

---

[13] The Edge Runner program is a component of the American Academy of Nursing's Raise the Voice campaign, funded by the Robert Wood Johnson Foundation. The Edge Runner designation recognizes nurses who have developed innovative, successful models of care and interventions to address problems in the health care delivery system or unmet health needs in a population.

[14] See AAN's Edge Runner Directory, http://www.aannet.org/custom/edgeRunner/index.cfm?page id=3303&showTitle=1.

[15] See http://www.ncemna.org/scholarships.asp.

Involvement in Policy Making

Nurses may articulate what they want to happen in health care to make it more truly patient centered and to improve quality, access, and value. They may even have the evidence to support their conclusions. As with any worthy cause, however, they must engage in the policy-making process to ensure that the changes they believe in are realized. To this end, they must be able to envision themselves as leaders in that process and seek out new partners who share their goals.

The challenge now is to motivate all nurses to pursue leadership roles in the policy-making process. Political engagement is one avenue they can take to that end. As Bethany Hall-Long, a nurse who was elected to the Delaware State House of Representatives in 2002 and is now a state senator, writes, "political actions may be as simple as voting in local school board elections or sharing research findings with state officials, or as complex as running for elected office" (Hall-Long, 2009). For example, engaging school board candidates about the fundamental role of school nurses in the management of chronic conditions among students can make a difference at budget time. And if the goal is broader, perhaps to locate more community health clinics within schools, achieving buy-in from the local school board is absolutely vital. As Hall-Long writes, however, "since nurses do not regularly communicate with their elected officials, the elected officials listen to non-nursing individuals" (Hall-Long, 2009).

Political engagement can be a natural outgrowth of nursing experience. When Marilyn Tavenner first started working in an intensive care unit in Virginia, she thought, "If I were the head nurse or the nurse manager, I would make changes. I would try to influence that unit and that unit's quality and staffing." After she became a nurse manager, she thought, "I wouldn't mind doing this for the entire hospital." After succeeding for several years as a director of nursing, she was encouraged by a group of physicians to apply for the CEO position of her hospital when it became available. Eventually, Timothy Kaine, governor of Virginia from 2006 to 2010, recruited her to be the state's secretary of health and human resources. In February 2010, Ms. Tavenner was named deputy administrator for the federal Centers for Medicare and Medicaid Services. Like many nurses, she had never envisioned working in government. But she realized that she wanted to have an impact on health care and health care reform. She wanted to help the uninsured find resources and access to care. For her, that meant building on relationships and finding opportunities to work in government.[16]

Other notable nurses who have answered the call to serve in government include Sheila Burke, who served as chief of staff to former Senate Majority Leader Robert Dole, has been a member of the Medicare Payment Advisory Commission,

---

[16] This paragraph draws on personal communication with Marilyn Tavenner, principal deputy administrator and chief operating officer, Centers for Medicare and Medicaid Services, May 11, 2010.

and now teaches at Georgetown and Harvard Universities; and Mary Wakefield, who was named administrator of HRSA in 2009 and is the highest-ranking nurse in the Obama Administration. Speaker of the House Nancy Pelosi's office has had back-to-back nurses from The Robert Wood Johnson Foundation Health Policy Fellows Program as staffers since 2007, providing a significant entry point for the development of new health policy leaders. Additionally, in 1989 Senator Daniel Inouye established the Military Nurse Detailee fellowship program. This 1-year fellowship provides an opportunity for a high-ranking military nurse, who holds a minimum of a master's degree, to gain health policy leadership experience in Senator Inouye's office. The fellowship rotates among three branches of service (Army, Navy, and Air Force) annually.[17] During the Clinton Administration, Beverly Malone served as deputy assistant secretary for health in the Department of Health and Human Services (HHS). In 2002, Richard Carmona, who began his education with an associate's degree in nursing from the Bronx Community College in New York, was appointed surgeon general by President George W. Bush. Shirley Chater led the reorganization of the Social Security Administration in the 1990s. Carolyne Davis served as head of the Health Care Finance Administration (predecessor of the Centers for Medicare and Medicaid Services) in the 1980s during the implementation of a new coding system that classifies hospital cases into diagnosis-related groups. From 1979 to 1981, Rhetaugh Dumas was the first nurse, the first woman, and the first African American to serve as a deputy director of the National Institute of Mental Health (Sullivan, 2007). Nurses also have served as regional directors of HHS and as senior advisors on health policy to HHS.

As for elected office, there were three nurse members of the 111th Congress—Eddie Bernice Johnson (D-TX), Lois Capps (D-CA), and Carolyn McCarthy (D-NY)—all of whom had a hand in sponsoring and supporting health care–focused legislation, from AIDS research to gun control. Lois Capps organized and co-chairs the Congressional Nursing Caucus (which also includes members who are not nurses). The group focuses on mobilizing congressional support for health-related issues. Additionally, 105 nurses have served in state legislatures, including Paula Hollinger of Maryland, who sponsored one of the nation's first stem cell research bills. None of these nurses waited to be asked; they pursued their positions, both elected and appointed, because they knew they had the expertise and experience to make changes in health care.

Very little in politics is accomplished without preparation or allies. Health professionals point with pride to multiple aspects of the Prescription for Pennsylvania initiative, a state health care reform initiative that preceded the ACA and is also described in Box 5-6. As is clear from a detailed 2009 review, success was not achieved overnight; smaller legislative and regulatory victories set the stage

---

[17] Personal communication, Corina Barrow, Lieutenant Colonel, Army Nurse Corps, Nurse Corps Detailee, Office of Senator Daniel Inouye (D-HI), August 25, 2010.

BOX 5-6
Case Study: Prescription for Pennsylvania

A Governor's Leadership Improves Access to
Care for Residents of a Rural State

When Pennsylvania Governor Edward Rendell took office in 2003, one-twelfth of the state's 12 million residents had no access to health care, 80 percent of health care expenditures went to treating chronic illnesses, and $3 billion was spent annually on avoidable hospitalizations of chronically ill patients. Pennsylvanians were 11 percent more likely than all other Americans to use the emergency room (ER).

If we look at the workforce and the health care needs of an aging population, we're insane if we don't try to figure out how we can make sure that we have an adequate number of [clinicians] with the skill and knowledge to work together.

—Ann S. Torregrossa, Esq., director, Governor's Office of Health Care Reform for the Commonwealth of Pennsylvania

---

On his first day in office, Governor Rendell established the Office of Health Care Reform to begin to address residents' access to affordable, high-quality health care. In January 2007 he announced a major new blueprint for that reform, Prescription for Pennsylvania (known as Rx for PA, www.rxforpa.com), which would promote access to care for all Pennsylvanians and reduce the state's skyrocketing health care expenses.

In the 3-plus years since, many initiatives have been undertaken, including

- expanding health insurance coverage for the uninsured;
- improving access to electronic health information through the Pennsylvania Health Information Exchange;
- establishing a chronic illness commission, which in 2008 recommended, among other proposals, the patient-centered medical home;
- addressing workforce shortages through the Pennsylvania Center for Health Careers;
- establishing seven "learning collaboratives" that involve about 800 providers and 1 million patients and teach a variety of providers to collaborate on primary care teams; and
- expanding the legal scope of practice for physician assistants, advanced practice registered nurses (APRNs), clinical nurse specialists, certified nurse midwives, and dental hygienists (although legislation is still needed to allow APRNs to prescribe medications independently).

This last strategy has had an impact on access to care, particularly for the uninsured and underinsured. There are now 51 retail clinics that use APRNs in urban, suburban, and rural areas, and they provide care to 60 percent of the state's uninsured, said Ann S. Torregrossa, Esq., who in 2005 was named deputy director and in 2009 director of the Office of Health Care Reform. Ms. Torregrossa said that of 300,000 visits to such clinics, about half would have been ER visits. Retail clinics have been shown to reduce costs and improve access to care (Mehrotra et al., 2009).

Other outcome data after the first year of Rx for PA show an increase in the number of people with diabetes receiving eye and foot examinations and a doubling of the number of children with asthma who have a plan in place for controlling exacerbations (Pennsylvania Governor's Office, 2009). There are about 250 nurse-managed health centers nationwide and 27 in Pennsylvania; many are affiliated with schools of nursing and provide care at a 10 percent lower cost than other models—including a 15 percent reduction in ER use and a 25 percent reduction in prescription drug costs (according to unpublished data from the National Nursing Centers Consortium [NNCC]).

Tine Hansen-Turton, MGA, JD, CEO of the NNCC and vice president of the Public Health Management Corporation, a nonprofit institute, said that nurses involved in Rx for PA have a great deal to teach clinicians and leaders in other states as they grapple with health care reform (Hansen-Turton et al., 2009). The nurse-managed health centers in particular offer a preventive care model that improves access to care. And Pennsylvanians have given high marks to the care they have received from APRNs, Ms. Hansen-Turton said, adding, "It's all about access."

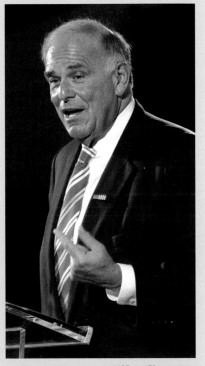

USEventPhotos.com

Governor Edward Rendell speaks about the important role of nurses in improving access to health care in Pennsylvania.

starting in the late 1990s. Even some apparent legislative failures built the foundation for future successes because they caused nurses to spend more time meeting face to face with physicians who had organized opposition to various measures. As a result, nursing leaders developed a better sense of where they could achieve compromises with their opponents. They also found a new ally in the Chamber of Commerce to counter opposition from some sections of organized medicine (Hansen-Turton et al., 2009).

Hansen-Turton and colleagues draw three major lessons from this experience. First, nurses must build strong alliances within their own professional community, an important lesson alluded to earlier in this chapter. Pennsylvania's nurses were able to speak with a unified voice because they first worked out among themselves which issues mattered most to them. Second, nurses must build relationships with key policy makers. Pennsylvania's nurses developed strong relationships with several legislators from both major political parties and earned the support of two successive sitting governors: Thomas Ridge (Republican) and Edward Rendell (Democrat). Third, nurses must find allies outside the nursing profession, particularly in business and other influential communities. Pennsylvania's nurses gained a strong ally in the Chamber of Commerce when they were able to demonstrate how expanding regulations to allow nurses to do all they were educated and demonstrably capable of doing would help lower health care costs (Hansen-Turton et al., 2009).

Perhaps the most important lesson to draw from the Pennsylvania experience lies in the way the campaign was framed. The focus of attention was on achieving quality care and cost reductions. A closer examination of the issues showed that achieving those goals required, among other things, expanding the roles and responsibilities of nurses. What drew the greatest amount of political support for the Prescription for Pennsylvania campaign was the shared goal of getting more value out of the health care system—quality care at a sustainable price. The fact that the campaign also expanded nursing practice was secondary. Those expansions are likely to continue as long as the emphasis is on quality care and cost reduction. Similarly, the committee believes that the goal in any transformation of the health care system should be achieving innovative, patient-centered, high-value care. If all stakeholders—from legislators, to regulators, to hospital executives, to insurance companies—act from a patient-centered point of reference, they will see that many of the solutions they are seeking require a transformation of the nursing profession.

A CALL FOR NEW PARTNERSHIPS

Having enough nurses and having nurses with the right skills and competencies to care for the population is an important societal issue. Having allies from outside the profession is important to achieving this goal. More nurses need to reach out to new partners in arenas ranging from business, government, and philanthropy to state and national medical associations to consumer groups. Additionally, nurses need to fortify alliances that are made through personal connections and relationships. Just as important, society needs to understand its stake in ensuring that nurses are effective full partners and leaders in the quest to deliver quality, high-value care that is accessible to diverse populations. The full potential of the nursing profession in care, leadership, and research must be tapped to deal with the wide range of health care challenges the nation will face in the coming years.

Eventually, to transform the way health care is delivered in the United States, nurses will have to move not just out of the hospital, but also out of health care organizations entirely. For example, nurses are underrepresented on the boards of private nonprofit and philanthropic organizations, which do not provide health care services but often have a large impact on health care decisions. The Commonwealth Fund and the Kaiser Family Foundation, for instance, have no nurses on their boards, although they do have physicians. Without nurses, vital ground-level perspectives on quality improvement, care coordination, and health promotion are likely missing. On the other hand, AARP provides a positive example. At least two nurses at AARP have served in the top leadership and governance roles (president and chair) in the past 3 years. Nurses serve on the health and long-term services policy committee, and the senior vice president of the Public Policy Institute is also a nurse. AARP's commitment to nursing is clear through its sponsorship, along with the Robert Wood Johnson Foundation, of the Center to Champion Nursing.

CONCLUSION

Enactment of the ACA will provide unprecedented opportunities for change in the U.S. health care system for the foreseeable future. Strong leadership on the part of nurses, physicians, and others will be required to devise and implement the changes necessary to increase quality, access, and value and deliver patient-centered care. If these efforts are to be successful, all nurses, from students, to bedside and community nurses, to CNOs and members of nursing organizations, to researchers, must develop leadership competencies and serve as full partners with physicians and other health professionals in efforts to improve the health care system and the delivery of care. Nurses must exercise these competencies in a collaborative environment in all settings, including hospitals, communities, schools, boards, and political and business arenas. In doing so, they must not only mentor others along the way, but develop partnerships and gain allies both within and beyond the health care environment.

REFERENCES

AACN (American Association of Colleges of Nursing). 2008. *The essentials of baccalaureate education for professional nursing practice.* Washington, DC: AACN. Available from http://www.aacn.nche.edu/education/pdf/BaccEssentials08.pdf.

AACN. 2010. *Enhancing diversity in the nursing workforce: Fact sheet updated March 2010.* http://www.aacn.nche.edu/Media/FactSheets/diversity.htm (accessed July 1, 2010).

ANCC (American Nurses Credentialing Center). 2010. *Program overview.* http://www.nursecredentialing.org/Magnet/ProgramOverview.aspx (accessed August 25, 2010).

Ballein Search Partners and AONE (American Organization of Nurse Executives). 2003. *Why senior nursing officers matter: A national survey of nursing executives.* Oak Brook, IL: Ballein Search Partners.

Bennis, W., and B. Nanus. 2003. *Leaders: Strategies for taking charge.* New York: HarperCollins.

Beverly, C. J., R. E. McAtee, R. Chernoff, G. V. Davis, S. K. Jones, and D. A. Lipschitz. 2007. The Arkansas aging initiative: An innovative approach for addressing the health of older rural Arkansans. *Gerontologist* 47(2):235-243.

Bradford, D. L., and A. R. Cohen. 1998. *Power up: Transforming organizations through shared leadership.* Hoboken, NJ: John Wiley & Sons, Inc.

Center for Healthcare Governance. 2007. *A seat at the power table: The physician's role on the hospital board.* Chicago, IL: Center for Healthcare Governance.

Curran, C. R., and M. K. Totten. 2010. Expanding the role of nursing in health care governance. *Nursing Economic$* 28(1):44-46.

Evans, L. K., and N. E. Strumpf. 1989. Tying down the elderly. A review of the literature on physical restraint. *Journal of the American Geriatrics Society* 37(1):65-74.

Gardner, D. B. 2005. Ten lessons in collaboration. *OJIN: Online Journal of Issues in Nursing* 10(1):2.

George Washington University Medical Center. 2010. *NAQC: Nursing alliance for quality care.* http://www.gwumc.edu/healthsci/departments/nursing/naqc/ (accessed August 25, 2010).

Governance Institute. 2007. *Boards x 4: Governance structures and practices.* San Diego, CA: Governance Institute.

Hall-Long, B. 2009. Nursing and public policy: A tool for excellence in education, practice, and research. *Nursing Outlook* 57(2):78-83.

Hansen-Turton, T., A. Ritter, and B. Valdez. 2009. Developing alliances: How advanced practice nurses became part of the prescription for Pennsylvania. *Policy, Politics, & Nursing Practice* 10(1):7-15.

Hassmiller, S. B., and L. B. Bolton (eds.). 2009. Transforming care at the bedside: Paving the way for change. *American Journal of Nursing* 109(11):3-80.

HealthSTAT. 2010. *About us.* http://www.healthstatgeorgia.org/?q=content/about (accessed June 29, 2010).

IOM (Institute of Medicine). 2000. *To err is human: Building a safer health system.* Washington, DC: National Academy Press.

IOM. 2004. *In the nation's compelling interest: Ensuring diversity in the health care workforce.* Washington, DC: The National Academies Press.

IOM. 2010. *A summary of the December 2009 Forum on the Future of Nursing: Care in the community.* Washington, DC: The National Academies Press.

Janetti, A. 2003. NSNA leadership university: A practicum in shared governance. *DEAN'S Notes* 25(1).

Jiang, H. J., C. Lockee, K. Bass, and I. Fraser. 2008. Board engagement in quality: Findings of a survey of hospital and system leaders. *Journal of Healthcare Management* 53(2):121-134; discussion 135.

Joint Commission. 2008. Behaviors that undermine a culture of safety. *Sentinel Event Alert* (40).

Jones, C. B., D. S. Havens, and P. A. Thompson. 2008. Chief nursing officer retention and turnover: A crisis brewing? Results of a national survey. *Journal of Healthcare Management* 53(2):89-105; discussion 105-106.

Katzenbach, J. R., and D. K. Smith. 1993. *The wisdom of teams: Creating the high-performance organization.* Boston, MA: Harvard Business School Press.

King, S. 2009. Channeling grief into action: Creating a culture of safety conference call, February 25, 2009, Hosted by Institute for Healthcare Improvement.

Kinnaman, M. L., and M. R. Bleich. 2004. Collaboration: Aligning resources to create and sustain partnerships. *Journal of Professional Nursing* 20(5):310-322.

Mastal, M. F., M. Joshi, and K. Schulke. 2007. Nursing leadership: Championing quality and patient safety in the boardroom. *Nursing Economic$* 25(6):323-330.

Mehrotra, A., H. Liu, J. L. Adams, M. C. Wang, J. R. Lave, N. M. Thygeson, L. I. Solberg, and E. A. McGlynn. 2009. Comparing costs and quality of care at retail clinics with that of other medical settings for 3 common illnesses. *Annals of Internal Medicine* 151(5):321-328.

Olender-Russo, L. 2009. Creating a culture of regard: An antidote for workplace bullying. *Creative Nursing* 15(2):75-81.

Paulus, P., and B. Nijstad, eds. 2003. *Group creativity: Innovation through collaboration.* New York: Oxford University Press.

Pearson, A., H. Laschinger, K. Porritt, Z. Jordan, D. Tucker, and L. Long. 2007. Comprehensive systematic review of evidence on developing and sustaining nursing leadership that fosters a healthy work environment in healthcare. *International Journal of Evidence-Based Healthcare* 5:208-253.

Pennsylvania Governor's Office. 2009. *Governor Rendell thanks "pioneers" for making Pennsylvania the national leader on chronic care management and creating patient-centered medical homes.* http://www.portal.state.pa.us/portal/server.pt?open=512&objID=3053&PageID=431159&mode=2&contentid=http://pubcontent.state.pa.us/publishedcontent/publish/global/news_releases/governor_s_office/news_releases/governor_rendell_thanks__pioneers__for_making_pennsylvania_the_national_leader_on_chronic_care_management_and_creating_patient_centered_medical_homes.html (accessed July 1, 2010).

Pisano, G. P., and R. Verganti. 2008. Which kind of collaboration is right for you? *Harvard Business Review* 86(12):78-86.

Prybil, L., S. Levey, R. Peterson, D. Heinrich, P. Brezinski, G. Zamba, A. Amendola, J. Price, and W. Roach. 2009. *Governance in high-performing community health systems: A report on trustee and CEO views.* Chicago, IL: Grant Thornton LLP.

Quisling, K. E. 2009. Resident orientation: Nurses create a program to improve care coordination. *American Journal of Nursing* 109(11 Suppl):26-28.

Rosenstein, A. H., and M. O'Daniel. 2008. A survey of the impact of disruptive behaviors and communication defects on patient safety. *Joint Commission Journal on Quality and Patient Safety* 34(8):464-471.

RWJF (Robert Wood Johnson Foundation). 2010a. *Nursing leadership from bedside to boardroom: Opinion leaders' perceptions.* http://www.rwjf.org/pr/product.jsp?id=54350 (accessed May 14, 2010).

RWJF. 2010b. *Nursing leadership from bedside to boardroom: Opinion leaders' views.* http://www.rwjf.org/pr/product.jsp?id=54491 (accessed August 25, 2010).

RWJF. 2010c. Unlocking the potential of school nursing: Keeping children healthy, in school, and ready to learn. *Charting Nursing's Future* July(14):1-8.

RWJF Executive Nurse Fellows. 2010. *Overview.* http://www.executivenursefellows.org/index.php?option=com_content&view=article&id=1&Itemid=34 (accessed September 28, 2010).

RWJF Scholars, Fellows & Leadership Programs. 2010. *Robert Wood Johnson Foundation Health Policy Fellows.* http://www.rwjfleaders.org/programs/robert-wood-johnson-foundation-health-policy-fellow (accessed September 28, 2010).

Shea, G. 2005. Developing the strategic voice of senior nurse executives. *Nursing Administration Quarterly* 29(2):133-136.

Singh, J., and L. Fleming. 2010. Lone inventors as sources of breakthroughs: Myth or reality? *Management Science* 56(1):41-56.

Strumpf, N. E., and L. K. Evans. 1988. Physical restraint of the hospitalized elderly: Perceptions of patients and nurses. *Nursing Research* 37(3):132-137.

Sullivan, P. 2007. Rhetaugh Dumas, 78; nurse rose to become NIMH deputy director. *The Washington Post*, July 27.

Wachter, R. M. 2009. Patient safety at ten: Unmistakable progress, troubling gaps. *Health Affairs* 29(1):165-173.

Wuchty, S., B. Jones, and B. Uzzi. 2007. The increasing dominance of teams in production of knowledge. *Science* 316(5827):1036-1039.

6

Meeting the Need for Better Data
on the Health Care Workforce

Key Message #4: Effective workforce planning and policy making require better data collection and an improved information infrastructure.

Planning for fundamental, wide-ranging changes in the preparation and deployment of the nursing workforce will require comprehensive data on the numbers and types of professionals currently available and required to meet future needs. Such data are needed across the health professions if a fundamental transformation of the health care system is to be achieved. Major gaps exist in currently available workforce data. Filling these gaps should be a priority for the National Health Workforce Commission and other structures and resources authorized under the Affordable Care Act.

Chapters 3 through 5 have argued for the need to transform the nursing profession to achieve the vision of a reformed health care system set forth in Chapter 1. Achieving this vision, however, will also require a balance of skills and perspectives among physicians, nurses, and other health professionals. Yet data are lacking on the numbers and types of health professionals currently employed, where they are employed, and in what roles. Understanding of the impact of bundled payments, medical homes, accountable care organizations, health information technology, comparative effectiveness, patient engagement, and safety, as well as the growing diversification of the American population, will not be complete without information on and analysis of the contributions of the various types of health professionals that will be needed. For cost-effectiveness comparisons, for example, different team configurations, continuing education and on-the-job training programs, incentives, and workflow arrangements—all of which affect the efficient use of the health care workforce—must be evaluated. Having these data is a vital first step in the development of accurate models for projecting workforce capacity. Those projections in turn are needed to inform the transformation of nursing practice and education argued for in Chapters 3 and 4, respectively.

Awareness of impending shortages of nurses, primary care physicians, geriatricians, and dentists and in many of the allied health professions has led to a growing consensus among policy makers that strengthening the health care workforce in the United States is an urgent need. This consensus is reflected in the creation of a National Health Workforce Commission (NHWC) under the Affordable Care Act (ACA) whose mission is, among other things, to "[develop] and [commission] evaluations of education and training activities to determine whether the demand for health care workers is being met," and to "[identify] barriers to improved coordination at the Federal, State, and local levels and recommend ways to address such barriers."[1] The ACA also authorizes a National Center for Workforce Analysis, as well as state and regional workforce centers, and provides funding for workforce data collection and studies. The committee believes these initiatives will prove most successful if they analyze workforce needs across the professions—as the Department of Veterans Affairs did in the 1990s (see Chapter 3)—rather than focusing on one profession at a time. Furthermore, national trend data are not granular enough by themselves to permit accurate projections of regional needs.

This chapter addresses key message #4 set forth in Chapter 1: Effective workforce planning and policy making require better data collection and an improved information infrastructure. The chapter first provides a closer look at what is known about the workforce in two areas of urgent need: primary care providers and nurses. It then examines gaps in currently available workforce data. The third section describes the experience of one regional workforce plan in Texas that aims to maintain the right numbers and types of nurses to meet its needs. The final section presents the committee's conclusions about the need for better data on the health care workforce.

---

[1] *Patient Protection and Affordable Care Act*, HR 3590 § 5101, 111th Congress.

CURRENT ESTIMATES OF PRIMARY CARE PROVIDERS AND NURSES

Primary Care Projections

The United States has nearly 400,000 primary care providers (Bodenheimer and Pham, 2010). As noted in Chapter 3, physicians account for 287,000 of these providers, nurse practitioners for 83,000, and physician assistants for 23,000 (HRSA, 2008; Steinwald, 2008). While the numbers of nurse practitioners and physician assistants are steadily increasing, the number of medical students and residents entering primary care has declined in recent years (Naylor and Kurtzman, 2010). In fact, a 2008 survey of medical students found only 2 percent planned careers in general internal medicine, a common entry point into primary care (Hauer et al., 2008).

There is a great deal of geographic variation in where primary care providers work. About 65 million Americans live in areas that are officially identified as primary care shortage areas according to the Health Resources and Services Administration (HRSA) (Rieselbach et al., 2010). For example, while one in five U.S. residents live in rural areas, only one in ten physicians practice in those areas (Bodenheimer and Pham, 2010). A 2006 survey of all 846 federally funded community health centers (CHCs) by Rosenblatt and colleagues (2006) found that 46 percent of direct care providers in rural CHCs were nonphysician clinicians, including nurse practitioners, nurse midwives, and physician assistants; in urban clinics, the figure was 38.9 percent. The contingent of physicians was heavily dependent on international medical graduates and loan forgiveness programs. Even so, the vacancies for physicians totaled 428 full-time equivalents (FTEs), while those for nurses totaled 376 FTEs (Rosenblatt et al., 2006). Expansion of programs that encourage health care providers to practice primary care, especially those from underrepresented and culturally diverse backgrounds, will be needed to keep pace with the demand for community-based care. For further discussion of variation in the geographic distribution of primary care providers, see the section on expanding access to primary care in Chapter 3.

In 2008, the Government Accountability Office determined that there were few projections of the future need for primary care providers, and those that existed were substantially limited (Steinwald, 2008). Arguably, it is simpler to project the future supply of health professionals than to project future demand for their services. It is difficult to predict, for example, the pattern of increased demand for primary care after full implementation of the ACA adds 32 million newly insured people to the health care system. Will there be a short, marked spike in demand, or will the surge be of longer duration that leaves more time to adapt? Given that there are more than 6,000 health professions primary care shortage areas nationwide (HRSA, 2010), the question remains of whether growing demand for primary care can best be met by an increased number of providers or by better distribution of existing providers.

Nursing Workforce Projections

Trend data consistently point to a substantial shortfall in the numbers of nurses in the near future. HRSA has calculated a shortfall of as many as 1 million FTEs by 2020 (HRSA, 2004). However, that projection is almost certainly too high because it depends on extrapolating today's unsustainable growth rates for health care to the future. A more conservative estimate from 2009 suggests a shortage of 260,000 registered nurses (RNs) by 2025; by comparison, the last nursing shortage peaked in 2001 with a vacancy rate of 126,000 FTEs (Buerhaus et al., 2009). Yet this more conservative projection is almost certainly too low because the new law is "highly likely to increase demand for health care services and hence for nurses" (RWJF, 2010). Figure 6-1 shows a forecast of supply and demand for FTE RNs, 2009–2030. For a more detailed examination of the projected nursing shortage based on the numbers and composition of the workforce,

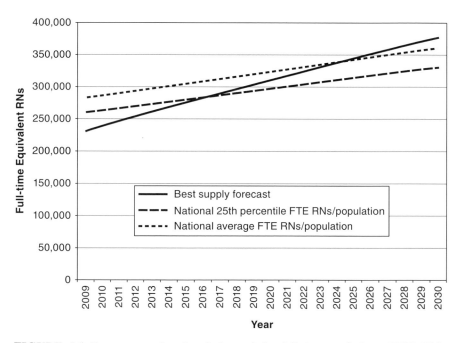

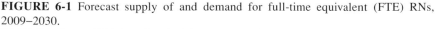

FIGURE 6-1 Forecast supply of and demand for full-time equivalent (FTE) RNs, 2009–2030.
SOURCE: Spetz, 2009. Reprinted with permission from Joanne Spetz. Copyright 2009 by the author.

the effects of health reform on the demand for RNs, and the degree to which the RN workforce measures up to this anticipated demand, see Appendix F (on CD-ROM).

The urgency of the situation is masked by current economic conditions. Nursing shortages have historically eased somewhat during difficult economic times, and the past few years of financial turmoil have been no exception (Buerhaus et al., 2009). Nursing is seen as a stable profession—a rare point of security in an unsettled economy. A closer look at the data, however, shows that during the past two recessions, more than three-quarters of the increase in the employment of RNs is accounted for by women and men over age 50, and there are currently more than 900,000 nurses over age 50 in the workforce (BLS, 2009). Meanwhile, the trend from 2001 to 2008 among middle-aged RNs was actually negative, with 24,000 fewer nurses aged 35 to 49. In a hopeful sign for the future, the number of nurses under age 35 increased by 74,000. In terms of absolute numbers, however, the cohorts of younger nurses are still vastly outnumbered by their older Baby Boom colleagues. In other words, the past practice of dependence on a steady supply of older nurses to fill the gaps in the health care system will eventually fail as a strategy (Buerhaus et al., 2009).

Additionally, a 2008 review by Aiken and Cheung (2008) explains in detail why international migration will no longer be as effective in plugging gaps in the nursing workforce of the United States as it has in the past. Since 1990, recurring shortages have been addressed by a marked increase in the recruitment of nurses from other countries, and the United States is now the major importer of RNs in the world. Figure 6-2 compares trends in new licenses between U.S.- and foreign-educated RNs from 2002 to 2008. Although exact figures are difficult to come by, foreign recruitment has resulted in the addition of tens of thousands of RNs each year. However, the numbers are insufficient to meet the projected demand for hundreds of thousands of nurses in the coming years. U.S. immigration policy would have to substantially favor nursing over all other professional categories, and the migration would exacerbate the current global nursing shortage to politically untenable levels (Aiken and Cheung, 2008).

GAPS IN CURRENT WORKFORCE DATA

As the committee considered how best to inform health care workforce policy and development, it realized it could not answer several basic questions about the workforce numbers and composition that will be needed by 2025. How many primary care providers does the nation require to deliver on its promise of more accessible, quality health care? What are the various proportions of physicians, nurses, physician assistants, and other providers that can be used to meet that need? What is the current educational capacity to meet the need, and how quickly can it be ramped up? Yet the Robert Wood Johnson Foundation Nursing Research Network, when consulted by the committee, suggested that these pro-

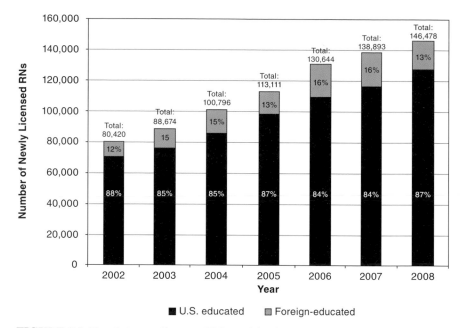

FIGURE 6-2 Trends in new licenses, U.S.- and foreign-educated RNs, 2002–2008.
SOURCE: NCSBN, 2010.

jections could be reliably generated within 5 years if better national and regional data were collected to support workforce prediction models.[2]

Research on the health care workforce to inform policy deliberations is fragmented and dominated by historical debates over what numbers of a particular health profession are needed and the extent (if at all) to which government should be involved in influencing the supply of and demand for health professionals. The methods used to develop projection models are notoriously deficient and focus on single professions, typically assuming the continuation of current practice and utilization patterns. Projection models do not allow policy makers to test and evaluate the impact of different policy scenarios on supply and demand estimates; whether and how health outcomes are associated with various health professions;

---

[2] Personal communication with David Auerbach, Analyst, Health and Human Resource Division, Congressional Budget Office; Peter Buerhaus, Valere Potter Professor of Nursing, and Director, Center for Interdisciplinary Health Workforce Studies, Institute for Medicine and Public Health, Vanderbilt University Medical Center; Tim Dall, Vice President, The Lewin Group; Jean Moore, Director, School of Public Health, University at Albany State University of New York; Edward Salsberg, Director, Center for Workforce Studies, Association of American Medical College; Sue Skillman, Deputy Director, Rural Health Research Center and WWAMI Rural Health Research Center, University of Washington; and Joanne Spetz, Professor, Community Health Systems, University of California, San Francisco, April 15, 2010.

and whether interprofessional team–based care is more efficient, lowers costs, and leads to safer care and improved patient outcomes.

In a paper prepared for the committee, Julie Sochalski and Jonathan Weiner emphasize the importance of collecting data that allow for flexible workforce projections. Meeting the need for adequate numbers of RNs "to support health care delivery reform will require a wholesale paradigm shift in the framework and context used to prepare and deploy the RN workforce and to forecast future requirements" (Sochalski and Weiner, 2010).

The Robert Wood Johnson Foundation Nursing Research Network assessed for the committee the quantity and quality of workforce data across health professions and suggested three key areas of need:

- **Core data sets on health care workforce supply and demand—** Researchers should develop and routinely update core data sets that facilitate analysis of the supply, demand, and distribution of the health care workforce across health professions. To this end, technical assistance and partnerships with licensure boards, educational organizations, and professional associations at the national, state, and local levels will be necessary.
- **Surveillance of health care workforce market conditions—**Researchers should develop a workforce surplus/shortage surveillance system that provides regular and frequent data (e.g., every 6–12 months) on key workforce indicators. This system would employ surveillance methods similar to those of other economic monitoring systems designed to track trends and provide early warning of changes in the marketplace. The development of such a system will require partnerships with public and private employers and organizations.
- **Health care workforce effectiveness research—**Researchers should develop data and support research to evaluate the impact of new models of care delivery on the health care workforce and the impact of workforce configurations on health care costs, quality, and access. This effort should include coordination with other federal agencies to ensure that key data elements are incorporated into federal surveys, claims data, and clinical data. Research should include evaluation of strategies for increasing the efficient education, preparation, and distribution of the health care workforce. Finally, workforce research needs to be included in federal pilot and demonstration projects involving payment innovation, introduction of new technologies, team-based care models, and other advances.

A major barrier to more strategic health care workforce planning efforts is insufficient basic data on the activities performed by health professionals. While claims data can yield information on the services provided by physicians and some allied health professionals, the efforts of other health professionals—including nurses—is invisible in most federal data sets.

As discussed above, the ACA authorizes the NHWC. It also authorizes a National Center for Workforce Analysis, as well as state and regional workforce centers, and provides funding for workforce data collection and studies. A priority for these new structures and resources should be systematic monitoring of health care workforce shortages and surpluses, review of the data and methods needed to predict future workforce needs, and coordination of the collection of data relating to the health care workforce in federal surveys and in the private sector. These three functions must be actively assumed by the federal government to build the necessary capacity for workforce planning in the United States. The NHWC has the potential to build a robust workforce data infrastructure and a high-level analytic capacity.

HRSA's Bureau of Primary Care and Bureau of Health Professions conduct some monitoring—primarily for nurses, primary care clinicians, mental health professionals, dentists, and pharmacists—for purposes of designating health professional shortage areas/facilities and medically underserved areas/populations and informing funding decisions to support clinician training. Thus, HRSA is well positioned to assume leadership in directing resources needed to build a data infrastructure to support health care workforce research.

One currently available resource for examining the role of providers in primary care is the National Provider Indicator (NPI). While the NPI is a mechanism for tracking billing services, this data source at the Centers for Medicare and Medicaid Services (CMS) could be thought of as an opportunity to collect workforce data and conduct research on those nurses who bill for services, primarily nurse practitioners. The committee believes the NPI presents a unique opportunity to track and measure nurse practitioners with regard to their practice, such as where they are located, how many are billing patients, what kinds of patients they are seeing, and what services they are providing. These data would be a significant contribution to the supply data currently being collected, adding to the knowledge base about practice partnerships, utilization of services, and primary care shortages. The committee encourages CMS to make these data available in a useful way to workforce researchers and others who might contribute to this knowledge base.

The NHWC needs to develop predictions for a range of assumptions about future delivery systems and patterns, including the future workforce supply across the professions (see Figure 6-3 for factors to consider) and the demand for services that can be provided by more than one profession or specialty (see Figure 6-4 for factors to consider). The following example illustrates the complexity of developing workforce projections and the depth of the data needs with respect to a single profession, as well as the innovative solutions the Gulf Coast region of Texas found for meeting its nursing needs. The committee commends this example to the NHWC while encouraging it to extend this innovation by looking at workforce needs across professions.

Supply = (Current + New − Exiting) × Efficiency

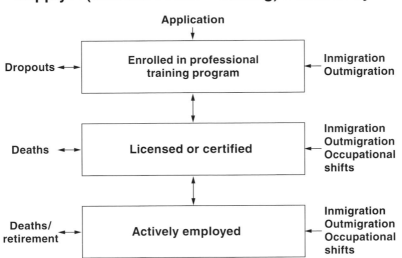

FIGURE 6-3 Factors to consider when assessing the health care workforce supply. SOURCE: HRSA, 2000. Adapted from Figure 3, page 84. Reprinted with permission from Jean Moore, Center for Health Workforce Studies, University of Albany.

Demand = Population × Health × Utilization Rates

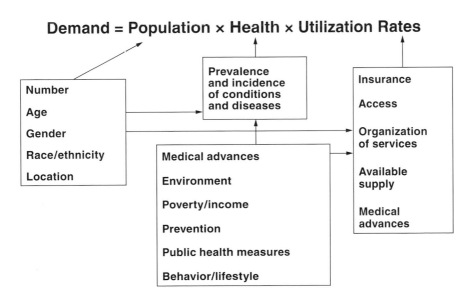

FIGURE 6-4 Factors to consider when assessing health care workforce demand. SOURCE: Salsberg, 2009.

GULF COAST HEALTH SERVICES STEERING COMMITTEE

In the 1990s, a group of CEOs of Houston-area businesses and philanthropic groups formed the Gulf Coast Health Services Steering Committee (GCHSSC)[3] to address a local nursing shortage. This partnership brings together executives from area hospitals, health care systems, and academic institutions. The group was determined to work together to develop regional solutions to workforce challenges that affected the 13 counties of the greater Houston area. One of the four initial areas of focus for the GCHSSC was building educational capacity to accommodate more nursing students. The other three focus areas addressed legislation and regulations, advancing health careers, and improving the work environment where nurses practice. Building educational capacity remains a central focus of the GCHSSC to this day. Thanks to its efforts, more than $30 million was infused into Houston area nursing schools from 2001 to 2008.[4]

Use of Data

One of the first things the GCHSSC's educational capacity work group decided to do was to start tracking the numbers of enrollments, graduates, and qualified applicants who are turned away from nursing schools in the greater Houston area. The GCHSSC quickly concluded that nursing schools were graduating the bulk of their students at the wrong time. Nearly all students graduated in May and took their licensing exam shortly thereafter. Yet this is the time that hospitals—still the major employers of nurses in the Houston area—have their lowest number of inpatient admissions; the highest number of inpatient admissions typically occurs in January and February. The GCHSSC therefore approached the nursing schools about implementing rolling admissions so that entry-level nurses would graduate in the fall, winter, and spring. Results thus far are promising. The GCHSSC projects that the spring surge in graduates will nearly disappear in the next 2 years.

Increased Student Enrollment

The various initiatives undertaken by the GCHSSC have resulted in a 73 percent increase in student enrollment in Houston prelicensure nursing programs, from 2,211 in fall 1998 to 3,829 in fall 2008. Several schools are opening branch campuses and offering online programs to further increase the pool of eligible students. With an eye toward increasing both the numbers and diversity of the nursing student body, the University of Houston has launched a nursing program in Victoria, Texas, a city located about 120 miles outside of Houston. Victoria has a population of 60,000, approximately 45 percent of which is Hispanic (U.S.

---

[3] See http://www.gchssc.com/.

[4] This section draws on personal communication in March 2010 with Mary Koch, Health Services Liason, Workforce Solutions/Houston-Galveston Area Council; and Michael Jhin, who was CEO of St. Luke's Episcopal Hospital at the time the GCHSSC launched.

Census Bureau, 2010). Meanwhile, the University of Texas at Austin has developed an online nursing program that partners with health care institutions and enrolls students from across the state. The GCHSSC is identifying which institutions from the Gulf Coast area have joined with this online program so they can participate in developing a workforce plan for the region.

Faculty Shortage

The GCHSSC is addressing the local nursing faculty shortage in several ways. Nursing schools in three major area universities—the University of Texas Health Science Center at Houston, the University of Texas Medical Branch at Galveston, and the Houston campus of Texas Woman's University—have launched accelerated master's of science in nursing (MSN) programs. In tracking the employment of these MSN graduates, however, the GCHSSC has concluded that most will be working in hospitals and not taking teaching positions. It is easy to understand why. Local hospitals pay RNs with an MSN degree 40 to 60 percent higher salaries than MSN-credentialed professors receive. The GCHSSC is working to address this problem.

Meanwhile, the George Foundation, a local philanthropic organization, is helping the University of Texas School of Nursing at Houston launch an accelerated PhD nursing program. Starting in fall 2010, a cohort of 10 MSN-prepared nurses will begin the program with the aim of completing their degree in 3 years. All students will receive an annual stipend of $60,000, allowing them to attend full time. In return, the new PhDs must teach for at least 3 years at the University of Texas School of Nursing at Houston or in any other nursing education program in the Gulf Coast region. This program is similar to programs in New Jersey and California that are funded by the Robert Wood Johnson Foundation and the Gordon and Betty Moore Foundation, respectively.[5]

CONCLUSION

Taking into account the need to transform the way health care is delivered in the United States and the observations and goals outlined in Chapters 3 through 5, policy makers must have reliable, sufficiently granular data on workforce supply and demand, both present and future, across the health professions. In the context of this report, such data are essential for determining what changes are needed in nursing practice and education to advance the vision for health care set forth in Chapter 1. Major gaps exist in currently available data on the health care workforce. A priority for the NHWC and other structures and resources authorized under the ACA should be systematic monitoring of the supply of health care workers, review of the data and methods needed to develop accurate predictions of future workforce needs, and coordination of the collection of data on the health

---

[5] See http://www.njni.org/?county=42 and http://www.moore.org/nursing.aspx.

care workforce. The building of an infrastructure for the collection and analysis of workforce data is a crucial need if the overarching goal of a transformed health care system is to be realized.

REFERENCES

Aiken, L., and R. Cheung. 2008. *Nurse workforce challenges in the United States: Implications for policy.* OECD Health Working Paper No. 35. Available from http://www.oecd.org/dataoecd/34/9/41431864.pdf.

BLS (Bureau of Labor Statistics). 2009. *Employment projections: Replacement needs.* http://www.bls.gov/emp/ep_table_110.htm (accessed September 10, 2010).

Bodenheimer, T., and H. H. Pham. 2010. Primary care: Current problems and proposed solutions. *Health Affairs* 29(5):799-805.

Buerhaus, P. I., D. I. Auerbach, and D. O. Staiger. 2009. The recent surge in nurse employment: Causes and implications. *Health Affairs* 28(4):w657-668.

Hauer, K. E., S. J. Durning, W. N. Kernan, M. J. Fagan, M. Mintz, P. S. O'Sullivan, M. Battistone, T. DeFer, M. Elnicki, H. Harrell, S. Reddy, C. K. Boscardin, and M. D. Schwartz. 2008. Factors associated with medical students' career choices regarding internal medicine. *JAMA* 300(10):1154-1164.

HRSA (Health Resources and Services Administration). 2000. *HRSA state health workforce data resource guide.* Rockville, MD: HRSA.

HRSA. 2004. *What is behind HRSA's projected supply, demand, and shortage of registered nurses?* Rockville, MD: HRSA.

HRSA. 2008. *The physician workforce.* Rockville, MD: HRSA.

HRSA. 2010. *Shortage designation: HPSAs, MUAs & MUPs.* http://bhpr.hrsa.gov/shortage/ (accessed September 10, 2010).

Naylor, M. D., and E. T. Kurtzman. 2010. The role of nurse practitioners in reinventing primary care. *Health Affairs* 29(5):893-899.

NCSBN (National Council of State Boards of Nursing). 2010. *Nurse licensure and NCLEX examination statistics.* https://www.ncsbn.org/1236.htm (accessed August 20, 2010).

Rieselbach, R. E., B. J. Crouse, and J. G. Frohna. 2010. Teaching primary care in community health centers: Addressing the workforce crisis for the underserved. *Annals of Internal Medicine* 152:118-122.

Rosenblatt, R. A., C. H. Andrilla, T. Curtin, and L. G. Hart. 2006. Shortages of medical personnel at community health centers: Implications for planned expansion. *JAMA* 295(9):1042-1049.

RWJF (Robert Wood Johnson Foundation). 2010. Expanding America's capacity to educate nurses: Diverse, state-level partnerships are creating promising models and results. *Charting Nursing's Future* April (13):1-8.

Salsberg, E. 2009. *State of the national physician workforce.* Paper presented at Annual Meeting of the Association of American Medical Colleges, Boston, MA.

Sochalski, J., and J. Weiner. 2010 (unpublished). *Health care system reform and the nursing workforce: Matching nursing practice and skills to future needs, not past demands.* University of Pennsylvania School of Nursing.

Spetz, J. 2009. *Forecasts of the registered nurse workforce in California.* San Francisco, CA: UCSF.

Steinwald, B. 2008. *Primary care professionals: Recent supply trends, projections, and valuation of services.* Washington, DC: GAO.

U.S. Census Bureau. 2010. *Fact sheet: Victoria city, Texas.* http://factfinder.census.gov/servlet/ACSSAFFFacts?_event=&geo_id=16000US4875428&_geoContext=01000US%7C04000US48%7C16000US4875428&_street=&_county=Victoria&_cityTown=Victoria&_state=04000US48&_zip=&_lang=en&_sse=on&ActiveGeoDiv=&_useEV=&pctxt=fph&pgsl=160&_submenuId=factsheet_1&ds_name=ACS_2008_3YR_SAFF&_ci_nbr=null&qr_name=null&reg=null%3Anull&_keyword=&_industry= (accessed September 28, 2010).

Part III

A Blueprint for Action

7

Recommendations and Research Priorities

Reflecting the charge to the committee, the purpose of this report is to consider reconceptualized roles for nurses, ways in which nursing education system can be designed to educate nurses who can meet evolving health care demands, the role of nurses in creating innovative solutions for health care delivery, and ways to attract and retain well-prepared nurses in a variety of settings. The report comes at a time of opportunity in health care resulting from the passage of the Affordable Care Act (ACA), which will provide access to care for an additional 32 million Americans. In the preceding chapters, the committee has described both barriers and opportunities in nursing practice, education, and leadership. It has also discussed the workforce data needed to guide policy and workforce planning with respect to the numbers, types, and mix of professionals that will be required in an evolving health care environment.

The primary objective of the committee in fulfilling its charge was to define a blueprint for action that includes recommendations for changes in public and institutional policies at the national, state, and local levels. This concluding chapter presents the results of that effort. The committee's recommendations are focused on maximizing the full potential and vital role of nurses in designing and implementing a more effective and efficient health care system, as envisioned by the committee in Chapter 1. The changes recommended by the committee are intended to advance the nursing profession in ways that will ensure that nurses are educated and prepared to meet the current and future demands of the health care system and those it serves.

This chapter first provides some context for the development of the committee's recommendations. It details what the committee considered to be its scope and focus, the nature of the evidence that supports its recommendations, cost considerations associated with the recommendations, and how the recommendations might be implemented. The chapter then presents recommendations for nursing practice, education, and leadership, as well as improved collection and analysis of interprofessional health care workforce data, that resulted from the committee's review of the evidence.

CONSIDERATIONS THAT INFORMED THE COMMITTEE'S RECOMMENDATIONS

As discussed throughout this report, the challenges facing the health care system and the nursing profession are complex and numerous. Challenges to nursing practice include regulatory barriers, professional resistance to expanded scopes of practice, health system fragmentation, insurance company policies, high turnover among nurses, and a lack of diversity in the nursing workforce. With regard to nursing education, there is a need for greater numbers, better preparation, and more diversity in the student body and faculty, the workforce, and the cadre of researchers. Also needed are new and relevant competencies, lifelong learning, and interprofessional education. Challenges with regard to nursing leadership include the need for leadership competencies among nurses, collaborative environments in which nurses can learn and practice, and engagement of nurses at all levels—from students to front-line nurses to nursing executives and researchers—in leadership roles. Finally, comprehensive, sufficiently granular workforce data are needed to ascertain the necessary balance of skills among nurses, physicians, and other health professionals for a transformed health care system and practice environment.

Solutions to some of these challenges are well within the purview of the nursing profession, while solutions to others are not. A number of constraints affect the profession and the health care system more broadly. While legal and regulatory constraints affect scopes of practice for advanced practice registered nurses, the major cross-cutting constraints originate in limitations of available resources—both financial and human. These constraints are not new, nor are they unique to the nursing profession. The current economic landscape has magnified some of the challenges associated with these constraints while also reinforcing the need for change. To overcome these challenges, the nursing workforce needs to be well educated, team oriented, adaptable, and able to apply competencies such as those highlighted throughout this report, especially those relevant to leadership.

The nursing workforce may never have the optimum numbers to meet the needs of patients, nursing students, and the health care system. To maximize the available resources in care environments, providers need to work effectively and efficiently with a team approach. Teams need to include patients and their families, as well as a variety of health professionals, including nurses, physicians, pharmacists, physical and occupational therapists, medical assistants, and social workers, among others. Care teams need to make the best use of each member's education, skill, and expertise, and health professionals need to practice to the full extent of their license and education. Just as physicians delegate to registered nurses, then, registered nurses should delegate to front-line caregivers such as nursing assistants and community health workers. Moreover, technology needs to facilitate seamless care that is centered on the patient, rather than taking time away from patient care. In terms of education, efforts must be made to expand the number of nurses who are qualified to serve as faculty. Meanwhile, curricula need to be evaluated, and streamlined and technologies such as high-fidelity simulation and online education need to be utilized to maximize available faculty. Academic–practice partnerships should also be used to make efficient use of resources and expand clinical education sites.

In conducting its work and evaluating the challenges that face the nursing profession, the committee took into account a number of considerations that informed its recommendations and the content of this report. The committee carefully considered the scope and focus of the report in light of its charge (see Box P-1 in the preface to the report), the evidence that was available, costs associated with its recommendations, and implementation issues. Overall, the committee's recommendations are geared toward advancing the nursing profession as a whole, and are focused on actions required to best meet long-term future needs rather than needs in the short term.

Scope and Focus of the Report

Many of the topics covered in this report could have been the focus of the entire report. As indicated in Chapter 4, for example, the report could have focused entirely on nursing education. Given the nature of the committee's charge and the time allotted for the study, however, the committee had to cover each topic at a high level and formulate relatively broad recommendations. This report could not be an exhaustive compendium of the challenges faced by the nursing workforce, nor was it meant to serve as a step-by-step guide detailing solutions to all of those challenges.

Accordingly, the committee limited its recommendations to those it believed had the potential for greatest impact and could be accomplished within the next decade. Taken together, the recommendations are meant to provide a strong foundation for the development of a nursing workforce whose members are well educated and well prepared to practice to the full extent of their education, to meet the current and future health needs of patients, and to act as full partners in leading change and advancing health. Implementation of these recommendations will take time, resources, and a significant commitment from nurses and other health professionals; nurse educators; researchers; policy makers and government leaders at the federal, state, and local levels; foundations; and other key stakeholders.

An emphasis of the committee's deliberations and this report is nurses' role in advancing care in the community, with a particular focus on primary care. While the majority of nurses currently practice in acute care settings, and much of nursing education is directed toward those settings, the committee sees primary care and prevention as central drivers in a transformed health care system, and therefore chose to focus on opportunities for nurses across community settings. The committee believes nurses have the potential to play a vital role in improving the quality, accessibility, and value of health care, and ultimately health in the community, beyond their critical contributions to acute care. The current landscape also directed the committee's focus on primary care; concern over an adequate supply of primary care providers has been expressed and demand for primary care is expected to grow as millions more Americans gain insurance coverage through implementation of the ACA (see Chapters 1 and 2). Additionally, many provisions of the ACA focus on improving access to primary care, offering further opportunities for nurses to play a role in transforming the health care system and improving patient care.

The committee recognizes that improved primary care is not a panacea and that acute care services will always be needed. However, the committee sees primary care in community settings as an opportunity to improve health by reaching people where they live, work, and play. Nurses serving in primary care roles could expand access to care, educate people about health risks, promote healthy lifestyles and behaviors to prevent disease, manage chronic diseases, and coordinate care.

The committee also focused on advanced practice registered nurses in its discussion of some topics, most notably scope of practice. Recognizing the importance of primary care as discussed above, the committee viewed the potential contributions of these nurses to meeting the great need for primary care services if they could practice uniformly to the full extent of their education and training.

Available Evidence

The charge to the committee called for the formulation of a set of bold national-level recommendations—a considerable task. To develop its recommendations, the committee examined the available published evidence, drew on committee members' expert judgment and experience, consulted experts engaged in the Robert Wood Johnson Foundation Nursing Research Network, and commissioned the papers that appear in Appendixes F through J on the CD-ROM in the back of this report. The committee also called on foremost experts in nursing, nursing research, and health policy to provide input, perspective, and expertise during its public workshops and forums (described in Appendix C).

In addition to the peer-reviewed literature and newly commissioned research, the committee considered anecdotal evidence and self-evaluations for emerging models of care being implemented across the country. Evidence to support the diffusion of a variety of promising innovative models informed the committee's deliberations and recommendations. Many of these innovations are highlighted as case studies throughout the report, and others are discussed in the appendixes. These case studies offer real-life examples of successful innovations that were developed by nurses or feature nurses in a leadership role, and are meant to complement the peer-reviewed evidence presented in the text. The committee believes these case studies contribute to the evidence base on how nurses can serve in reconceptualized roles to directly affect the quality, accessibility, and value of care. Cumulatively, the case studies and nurse profiles demonstrate what is possible and what the future of nursing could look like under ideal circumstances in which nurses would be highly educated and well prepared by an education system that would promote seamless academic progression, in which nurses would be practicing to the full extent of their education and training, and in which they would be acting as full partners in efforts to redesign the health care system.

The committee drew on a wealth of sources of evidence to support its recommendations. The recommendations presented are based on the best evidence available. There is a need, however, to continue building the evidence base in a variety of areas. The committee identified several research priorities to build upon its recommendations. For example, data are lacking on the work of nurses and the nursing workforce in general, primarily because of a dearth of large and well-designed studies explicitly exploring these issues. Accordingly, the committee calls for research in a number of areas that would yield evidence related to the future of nursing to address some of the shortcomings in the data it encountered. Boxes 7-1 through 7-3 list research questions that are directly connected to the recommendations and the discussion in Chapters 3 through 5. The committee believes that answers to these research questions are needed to help advance the profession.

Costs Associated with the Recommendations

The current state of the U.S. economy and its effects on federal, state, and local budgets pose significant challenges to transforming the health care system. These fiscal challenges also will heavily influence the implementation of the committee's recommendations. While providing cost estimates for each recommendation was beyond the scope of this study, the committee does not deny that there will be costs—in some cases sizable—associated with implementing its recommendations. These costs must be carefully weighed against the potential for long-term benefit. Expanding the roles and capacity of the nursing profession will require significant up-front financial resources, but this investment, in the committee's view, will help secure a strong foundation for a future health care system that can provide high-quality, accessible, patient-centered care. Based on its expert opinion and the available evidence, the committee believes that, despite the fiscal challenges, implementation of its recommendations is necessary

---

BOX 7-1
Research Priorities for Transforming Nursing Practice

Scope of Practice

- Comparison of costs, quality outcomes, and access associated with a range of primary care delivery models.
- Examination of the impact of expanding the range of providers allowed to certify patients for home health services and for admission to hospice or a skilled nursing facility.
- Examination of the impact of expanding the range of providers allowed to perform initial hospital admitting assessments.
- Capture of intended and unintended consequences of alternative reimbursement mechanisms for advanced practice registered nurses (APRNs), physicians, and other providers of primary care.
- Exploration of the impact of alternative payment reform policies on the organization and effectiveness of care teams and on the role played by registered nurses (RNs), physician assistants, and APRNs on care teams.
- Capture of the impact of health insurance exchanges on the role of APRNs in the provision of primary care in the United States.

Residencies

- Identification of the key features of residencies that result in nurses acquiring confidence and competency at a reasonable cost.
- Analysis of the possible unintended consequences of reallocating federal, state, and/or facility budgets to support residencies and other nurse training opportunities.

---

to increase the quality, accessibility, and value of care through the contributions of nurses.

Implementation of the Recommendations

Each of the recommendations presented in this report is supported by a level of evidence necessary to warrant its implementation. This does not mean, however, that the evidence currently available to support the committee's recommendations is sufficient to guide or motivate their implementation. The research priorities presented in Boxes 7-1 through 7-3 constitute key evidence gaps that need to be filled to convince key stakeholders that each recommendation is fundamental to the transformation of care delivered by nurses. For example, to be convinced to purchase equipment necessary to expand the number of nurses that can be educated using expensive new teaching technologies, such as high-fidelity

Teamwork

- Identification of the main barriers to collaboration between nurses and other health care staff in a range of settings.
- Identification and testing of new or existing models of care teams that have the potential to add value to the health care system if widely implemented.
- Identification and testing of educational innovations that have the potential to increase health care professionals' ability to serve as productive, collaborative care team members.

Technology

- Identification and testing of new and existing technologies intended to support nurses' decision making and care delivery.
- Capture of the costs and benefits of a range of care technologies intended to support nurses' decision making and care delivery.
- Identification of the contributions of various health professionals to the design and development, purchase, implementation, and evaluation of devices and information technology products.
- Development of a measure of "meaningful use" of information technology by nurses.

Value

- Capture of the impact of changes made to the system of care delivery on costs and quality over the next 5–10 years.
- Capture of the costs of implementing the recommendations in this report.
- Capture of the impact of implementing the recommendations in this report on the cost and quality of health care provided in the United States.
- Analysis of the intended and unintended effects of increasing payment for primary care provided by physicians and other providers.

simulation, distance learning, and online education modalities, decision makers in nursing schools will likely need evidence for the impact of these technologies on increasing the capacity of the nursing education system, as well as assurance that these technologies are an effective way to educate students. Likewise, before agreeing to reorganize care and training in a way that supports nursing residencies, hospitals will likely want to understand the true costs of such programs, as well as the key ingredients for their success. And before state political leaders can be persuaded to enact legislation to expand and standardize the scope of practice for advanced practice registered nurses, they will need messages to convey to their constituents about what these changes will mean for acquiring timely access to high-quality primary care services.

The committee urges the health services research community to embark on research agendas that can produce the evidence needed to guide the implementation of its recommendations. At the same time, the committee recognizes, from

---

BOX 7-2
Research Priorities for Transforming Nursing Education

- Identification of the combination of salary, benefits, and job attributes that results in the most highly qualified nurses being recruited and retained in faculty positions.
- Analysis of how alternative nurse faculty/student ratios affect instruction and the acquisition of knowledge.
- Capture of how optimal nurse faculty/student ratios vary with the implementation of new or existing teaching technologies, including distance learning.
- Identification of the features of online, simulation, and telehealth nursing education that most cost-effectively expand nursing education capacity.
- Capture of the experience in nursing schools that include new curriculum related to expanded clinical settings, evidence-based practice, and interprofessional and patient-centered care.
- Identification and evaluation of new and existing models of nursing education implemented to ensure that nurses acquire fundamental competencies needed to lead and engage in continuous quality improvement initiatives.
- Identification or development of an assessment tool to ensure that nurses have acquired the full range of competence required to practice nursing in undergraduate, postgraduate, and continuing education.
- Analysis of the impact of a range of strategies for increasing the number of nurses with a doctorate on the supply of nurse faculty, scientists, and researchers.
- Identification of the staff and environmental characteristics that best support the success of diverse nurses working to acquire doctoral degrees.
- Identification and testing of new and existing models of education to support nurses' engagement in team-based, patient-centered care to diverse populations, across the lifespan, in a range of settings.
- Development of workforce demand models that can predict regional faculty shortages.

---

the work of Mary Naylor and colleagues (2009), that a strong evidence base, even if supported by the results of multiple randomized clinical trials funded by the National Institutes of Health, will not be sufficient to propel a new model, policy, or practice to a position of widespread acceptance and implementation. "Health care is rich in evidence-based innovations, yet even when such innovations are implemented successfully in one location, they often disseminate slowly—if at all. Diffusion of innovations is a major challenge in all industries including health care" (Berwick, 2003).

Experience with the Transitional Care Model (TCM), described in Chapter 2, illustrates this point. In this case, barriers intrinsic to the way care is currently organized, regulated, reimbursed, and delivered have delayed the ability of a cost-effective, quality-enhancing model to improve the lives of the chronically

---

BOX 7-3
Research Priorities for Transforming Nursing Leadership

- Identification of the personal and professional characteristics most critical to leadership of health care organizations, such as accountable care organizations, health care homes, medical homes, and clinics.
- Identification of the skills and knowledge most critical to leaders of health care organizations, such as accountable care organizations, health care homes, medical homes, and clinics.
- Identification of the personal and professional characteristics most important to leaders of quality improvement initiatives in hospitals and other settings.
- Identification of the characteristics of mentors that have been (or could be) most successful in recruiting and training diverse nurses and nurse faculty.
- Identification of the influence of nursing on important health care decisions at all levels.
- Identification of the unique contributions of nurses to health care committees or boards.

---

ill. Learning from barriers to diffuse evidence-based health care interventions within health systems, Naylor and colleagues identified several ingredients crucial to successful diffusion. First, the model or innovation should be a good fit in response to a critical need, either within an organization or nationwide. Second, without strong champions, especially those with decision-making power, there is very little chance of widespread adoption. The researchers learned the hard way the cost of failure to engage all stakeholders in a project—early, continually, and throughout. Engagement with the media is especially important. An understanding of the landscape is necessary as well and should guide efforts to market the innovation to others. Milestones and measures of success are important to all team members and throughout the entire diffusion process. Finally, flexibility, or the willingness to adapt the model or innovation to meet environmental or organizational demands, increases the probability of success (Naylor et al., 2009).

Planning for the implementation of the committee's recommendations is beyond the scope of this report. However, the committee urges health care providers, organizations, and policy makers to carry out the eight recommendations presented below to enable nurses to lead in the transformation of the health care system and advance the health of patients and communities throughout the nation.

CONCLUSION

The committee believes the implementation of its recommendations will help establish the needed groundwork in the nursing profession to further the work of nurses in innovating and improving patient care. The committee sees its recommendations as the building blocks required to expand innovative models of care, as well as to improve the quality, accessibility, and value of care, through nursing. The committee emphasizes that the synergistic implementation of all of its recommendations as a whole will be necessary to truly transform the nursing profession into one that is capable of leading change to advance the nation's health.

RECOMMENDATIONS

Recommendation 1: Remove scope-of-practice barriers. *Advanced practice registered nurses should be able to practice to the full extent of their education and training. To achieve this goal, the committee recommends the following actions.*

For the Congress:

- Expand the Medicare program to include coverage of advanced practice registered nurse services that are within the scope of practice under applicable state law, just as physician services are now covered.
- Amend the Medicare program to authorize advanced practice registered nurses to perform admission assessments, as well as certification of patients for home health care services and for admission to hospice and skilled nursing facilities.
- Extend the increase in Medicaid reimbursement rates for primary care physicians included in the ACA to advanced practice registered nurses providing similar primary care services.
- Limit federal funding for nursing education programs to only those programs in states that have adopted the National Council of State Boards of Nursing Model Nursing Practice Act and Model Nursing Administrative Rules (Article XVIII, Chapter 18).

For state legislatures:

- Reform scope-of-practice regulations to conform to the National Council of State Boards of Nursing Model Nursing Practice Act and Model Nursing Administrative Rules (Article XVIII, Chapter 18).
- Require third-party payers that participate in fee-for-service payment arrangements to provide direct reimbursement to advanced practice registered nurses who are practicing within their scope of practice under state law.

For the Centers for Medicare and Medicaid Services:

- Amend or clarify the requirements for hospital participation in the Medicare program to ensure that advanced practice registered nurses are eligible for clinical privileges, admitting privileges, and membership on medical staff.

For the Office of Personnel Management:

- Require insurers participating in the Federal Employees Health Benefits Program to include coverage of those services of advanced practice registered nurses that are within their scope of practice under applicable state law.

For the Federal Trade Commission and the Antitrust Division of the Department of Justice:

- Review existing and proposed state regulations concerning advanced practice registered nurses to identify those that have anticompetitive effects without contributing to the health and safety of the public. States with unduly restrictive regulations should be urged to amend them to allow advanced practice registered nurses to provide care to patients in all circumstances in which they are qualified to do so.

Recommendation 2: Expand opportunities for nurses to lead and diffuse collaborative improvement efforts. *Private and public funders, health care organizations, nursing education programs, and nursing associations should expand opportunities for nurses to lead and manage collaborative efforts with physicians and other members of the health care team to conduct research and to redesign and improve practice environments and health systems. These entities should also provide opportunities for nurses to diffuse successful practices.*

To this end:

- The Center for Medicare and Medicaid Innovation should support the development and evaluation of models of payment and care delivery that use nurses in an expanded and leadership capacity to improve health outcomes and reduce costs. Performance measures should be developed and implemented expeditiously where best practices are evident to reflect the contributions of nurses and ensure better-quality care.
- Private and public funders should collaborate, and when possible pool funds, to advance research on models of care and innovative solutions,

including technology, that will enable nurses to contribute to improved health and health care.

- Health care organizations should support and help nurses in taking the lead in developing and adopting innovative, patient-centered care models.
- Health care organizations should engage nurses and other front-line staff to work with developers and manufacturers in the design, development, purchase, implementation, and evaluation of medical and health devices and health information technology products.
- Nursing education programs and nursing associations should provide entrepreneurial professional development that will enable nurses to initiate programs and businesses that will contribute to improved health and health care.

Recommendation 3: Implement nurse residency programs. *State boards of nursing, accrediting bodies, the federal government, and health care organizations should take actions to support nurses' completion of a transition-to-practice program (nurse residency) after they have completed a prelicensure or advanced practice degree program or when they are transitioning into new clinical practice areas.*

The following actions should be taken to implement and support nurse residency programs:

- State boards of nursing, in collaboration with accrediting bodies such as the Joint Commission and the Community Health Accreditation Program, should support nurses' completion of a residency program after they have completed a prelicensure or advanced practice degree program or when they are transitioning into new clinical practice areas.
- The Secretary of Health and Human Services should redirect all graduate medical education funding from diploma nursing programs to support the implementation of nurse residency programs in rural and critical access areas.
- Health care organizations, the Health Resources and Services Administration and Centers for Medicare and Medicaid Services, and philanthropic organizations should fund the development and implementation of nurse residency programs across all practice settings.
- Health care organizations that offer nurse residency programs and foundations should evaluate the effectiveness of the residency programs in improving the retention of nurses, expanding competencies, and improving patient outcomes.

Recommendation 4: Increase the proportion of nurses with a baccalaureate degree to 80 percent by 2020. *Academic nurse leaders across all schools of nursing should work together to increase the proportion of nurses with a baccalaureate degree from 50 to 80 percent by 2020. These leaders should partner with education accrediting bodies, private and public funders, and employers to ensure funding, monitor progress, and increase the diversity of students to create a workforce prepared to meet the demands of diverse populations across the lifespan.*

- The Commission on Collegiate Nursing Education, working in collaboration with the National League for Nursing Accrediting Commission, should require all nursing schools to offer defined academic pathways, beyond articulation agreements, that promote seamless access for nurses to higher levels of education.
- Health care organizations should encourage nurses with associate's and diploma degrees to enter baccalaureate nursing programs within 5 years of graduation by offering tuition reimbursement, creating a culture that fosters continuing education, and providing a salary differential and promotion.
- Private and public funders should collaborate, and when possible pool funds, to expand baccalaureate programs to enroll more students by offering scholarships and loan forgiveness, hiring more faculty, expanding clinical instruction through new clinical partnerships, and using technology to augment instruction. These efforts should take into consideration strategies to increase the diversity of the nursing workforce in terms of race/ethnicity, gender, and geographic distribution.
- The U.S. Secretary of Education, other federal agencies including the Health Resources and Services Administration, and state and private funders should expand loans and grants for second-degree nursing students.
- Schools of nursing, in collaboration with other health professional schools, should design and implement early and continuous interprofessional collaboration through joint classroom and clinical training opportunities.
- Academic nurse leaders should partner with health care organizations, leaders from primary and secondary school systems, and other community organizations to recruit and advance diverse nursing students.

Recommendation 5: Double the number of nurses with a doctorate by 2020. *Schools of nursing, with support from private and public funders, academic administrators and university trustees, and accrediting bodies, should double the number of nurses with a doctorate by 2020 to add to the cadre of nurse faculty and researchers, with attention to increasing diversity.*

- The Commission on Collegiate Nursing Education and the National League for Nursing Accrediting Commission should monitor the progress of each accredited nursing school to ensure that at least 10 percent of all baccalaureate graduates matriculate into a master's or doctoral program within 5 years of graduation.
- Private and public funders, including the Health Resources and Services Administration and the Department of Labor, should expand funding for programs offering accelerated graduate degrees for nurses to increase the production of master's and doctoral nurse graduates and to increase the diversity of nurse faculty and researchers.
- Academic administrators and university trustees should create salary and benefit packages that are market competitive to recruit and retain highly qualified academic and clinical nurse faculty.

Recommendation 6: Ensure that nurses engage in lifelong learning. *Accrediting bodies, schools of nursing, health care organizations, and continuing competency educators from multiple health professions should collaborate to ensure that nurses and nursing students and faculty continue their education and engage in lifelong learning to gain the competencies needed to provide care for diverse populations across the lifespan.*

- Faculty should partner with health care organizations to develop and prioritize competencies so curricula can be updated regularly to ensure that graduates at all levels are prepared to meet the current and future health needs of the population.
- The Commission on Collegiate Nursing Education and the National League for Nursing Accrediting Commission should require that all nursing students demonstrate a comprehensive set of clinical performance competencies that encompass the knowledge and skills needed to provide care across settings and the lifespan.
- Academic administrators should require all faculty to participate in continuing professional development and to perform with cutting-edge competence in practice, teaching, and research.
- All health care organizations and schools of nursing should foster a culture of lifelong learning and provide resources for interprofessional continuing competency programs.
- Health care organizations and other organizations that offer continuing competency programs should regularly evaluate their programs for adaptability, flexibility, accessibility, and impact on clinical outcomes and update the programs accordingly.

Recommendation 7: Prepare and enable nurses to lead change to advance health. *Nurses, nursing education programs, and nursing associations should* *prepare the nursing workforce to assume leadership positions across all levels, while public, private, and governmental health care decision makers should ensure that leadership positions are available to and filled by nurses.*

- Nurses should take responsibility for their personal and professional growth by continuing their education and seeking opportunities to develop and exercise their leadership skills.
- Nursing associations should provide leadership development, mentoring programs, and opportunities to lead for all their members.
- Nursing education programs should integrate leadership theory and business practices across the curriculum, including clinical practice.
- Public, private, and governmental health care decision makers at every level should include representation from nursing on boards, on executive management teams, and in other key leadership positions.

Recommendation 8: Build an infrastructure for the collection and analysis of interprofessional health care workforce data. *The National Health Care Workforce Commission, with oversight from the Government Accountability Office and the Health Resources and Services Administration, should lead a collaborative effort to improve research and the collection and analysis of data on health care workforce requirements. The Workforce Commission and the Health Resources and Services Administration should collaborate with state licensing boards, state nursing workforce centers, and the Department of Labor in this effort to ensure that the data are timely and publicly accessible.*

- The Workforce Commission and the Health Resources and Services Administration should coordinate with state licensing boards, including those for nursing, medicine, dentistry, and pharmacy, to develop and promulgate a standardized minimum data set across states and professions that can be used to assess health care workforce needs by demographics, numbers, skill mix, and geographic distribution.
- The Workforce Commission and the Health Resources and Services Administration should set standards for the collection of the minimum data set by state licensing boards; oversee, coordinate, and house the data; and make the data publicly accessible.
- The Workforce Commission and the Health Resources and Services Administration should retain, but bolster, the Health Resources and Services Administration's registered nurse sample survey by increasing the sample size, fielding the survey every other year, expanding the data collected on advanced practice registered nurses, and releasing survey results more quickly.
- The Workforce Commission and the Health Resources and Services Administration should establish a monitoring system that uses the most

current analytic approaches and data from the minimum data set to systematically measure and project nursing workforce requirements by role, skill mix, region, and demographics.

- The Workforce Commission and the Health Resources and Services Administration should coordinate workforce research efforts with the Department of Labor, state and regional educators, employers, and state nursing workforce centers to identify regional health care workforce needs, and establish regional targets and plans for appropriately increasing the supply of health professionals.
- The Government Accountability Office should ensure that the Workforce Commission membership includes adequate nursing expertise.

REFERENCES

Berwick, D. M. 2003. Disseminating innovations in health care. *JAMA* 289(15):1969-1975.

Naylor, M. D., P. H. Feldman, S. Keating, M. J. Koren, E. T. Kurtzman, M. C. Maccoy, and R. Krakauer. 2009. Translating research into practice: Transitional care for older adults. *Journal of Evaluation in Clinical Practice* 15(6):1164-1170.

A

Methods and Information Sources

The Committee on the Robert Wood Johnson Foundation (RWJF) Initiative on the Future of Nursing, at the Institute of Medicine (IOM) was asked to produce a report providing recommendations for an action-oriented blueprint for the future of nursing. The broad scope of this 13-month study included an examination of public and private policies at the national, state, and local levels. The recommendations presented in this report identify vital roles for nurses in designing and implementing a transformed health care system that provides Americans with high-quality care that is accessible, affordable, patient centered, and evidence based. To provide a comprehensive response to its charge, the committee tapped the wide-ranging expertise of its members and reviewed data from a variety of sources, including recent literature; data and reports from the Nursing Research Network, supported by RWJF; public and stakeholder input gathered through a series of technical workshops and public forums; site visits to a variety of health care settings where nurses do their work; and commissioned papers on selected topics.

EXPERTISE

The committee was composed of 18 members with expertise and experience in diverse areas, including nursing, federal and state administration and regulations, hospital and health plan administration, business administration, health information and technology, public health, health services research, health policy, workforce research and policy, and economics. On occasion, the committee identified areas related to its charge that required specialized knowledge and expertise not available within its membership, such as specific areas of law, scope-of-practice regulations, nursing research methods and data analysis, and health policy. In such cases, the committee called upon the foremost experts in those fields to serve as consultants and advisors during its deliberations (see the acknowledgments section of the report for a list of these individuals). In addition, the committee benefited from resources made available through the unique partnership between the IOM and RWJF, which allowed for borrowed-staff agreements that provided the committee with additional expertise from RWJF on nursing, nursing research, and communications. This partnership also facilitated the availability of additional information resources that were provided through AARP's Center for Championing Nursing in America and AcademyHealth.

LITERATURE REVIEW

Over the course of the study, the committee received and reviewed a wide range of literature from a variety of sources that was relevant to all aspects of its charge. Staff monitored key developments related to nursing, including newly published literature and legislative activity on both on the federal and state levels, with input from the Center to Champion Nursing in America, the NRN (described below), and GYMR public relations. Each committee meeting and public forum provided an opportunity for distinguished experts to submit articles and reports relevant to their presentations. Finally, committee members and the public were invited to submit articles and reports that would further support the committee's work. In total, the committee's database of relevant documents included almost 400 articles and reports.

Nursing is a frequently studied profession. Since the 1923 release of the Goldmark Report, funded by the Rockefeller Foundation, hundreds of public and private commissions and task forces have examined many facets of the profession, including its education system, diversity, scope of practice, workforce capacity, and relationship to other health professions and the public (Goldmark, 1923). The primary driver for this interest in the profession is nurses' essential role in caring for the sick and supporting the well. A number of factors affect the implementation of recommendations contained in previous reports, such as the exclusion of nurses from their production; the failure of the profession itself, through a lack of either resources or political will, to act on the recommendations; or the failure to redirect the focus from nurses to what is necessary to improve patient care. Additional factors, such as context, time, and place, also influence the success of a study and the implementation of its recommendations.

Since 1997, the IOM has produced at least 20 reports or workshop summaries related directly or indirectly to the nursing profession. They all share at least four common themes: nurses are a critical factor in health care because they are the closest to and spend the most time with patients; nurses need the skills and knowledge to keep patients safe and help them stay healthy or recover from illness; new models of care should be developed to better utilize nurses' skills and knowledge while improving patient care and decreasing costs; and patients receive better care when nurses and other health professionals work together effectively. The last broad-based study of the nursing profession published by the IOM was *Nursing and Nursing Education: Public Policies and Private Actions* (IOM, 1983). More recently, the IOM published *Keeping Patients Safe: Transforming the Work Environment of Nurses* (IOM, 2004). This report describes strategies for improving nurses' work environments and responding to the overwhelming demands they often face, with the ultimate goal of improving the safety and quality of care.

As the committee was conducting this study, a number of additional reports about nursing and nursing education, in particular, were released. Four months prior to the launch of the study, Prime Minister Gordon Brown charged a commission in England to examine the future of nursing and midwifery. The commission's report, *Front Line Care: The Future of Nursing and Midwifery in England* (Prime Minister's Commission on the Future of Nursing and Midwifery in England, 2010) states that nurses and midwives have great potential to influence health and must renew their pledge to society to deliver high-quality, compassionate care, and that they must be well supported to do so. A report released by the Josiah Macy, Jr. Foundation, *Who Will Provide Primary Care and How Will They Be Trained?* (Cronenwett and Dzau, 2010), likewise suggests that nurses are well positioned to improve health and recommends that any barriers preventing nurse practitioners from serving as primary care providers or leading models of primary care delivery be removed.

Several reports emphasize that continuing education is crucial if nurses, and other health professionals, are to deliver high-quality and safe care throughout their careers. They include *Continuing Education in the Health Professions: Improving Healthcare Through Lifelong Learning* (Hager et al., 2008), another report from the Macy Foundation; the IOM's *Redesigning Continuing Education in the Health Professions* (IOM, 2009); and *Lifelong Learning in Medicine and Nursing* (AACN and AAMC, 2010), which was cosponsored by the American Association of Colleges of Nursing and the Association of American Medical Colleges. A report specifically addressing the initial education of nurses, published by Dr. Patricia Benner and her team at the Carnegie Foundation, *Educating Nurses: A Call for Radical Transformation* (Benner et al., 2009), calls for a more highly educated nursing workforce, recommending that all entry-level registered nurses (RNs) be prepared at the baccalaureate level and that all RNs earn at least a master's degree within 10 years of initial licensure.

RWJF NURSING RESEARCH NETWORK

To increase the amount, relevance, and accessibility of research available to the committee, RWJF launched a parallel project called the Nursing Research Network (NRN) that generated, synthesized, and disseminated a broad range of research findings. These products both anticipated the committee's information needs and were responsive to requests made by committee members throughout the study process. Many of these products informed the committee's discussions of the present and future of nursing.

Lori Melichar served as research director for the NRN initiative. She supervised the NRN and led efforts to prioritize a research agenda that would meet the committee's information needs. The majority of the NRN's research activities were led and conducted by four research managers from across the country who served as consultants to the committee: Linda Aiken, University of Pennsylvania; Peter Buerhaus, Vanderbilt University; Christine Kovner, New York University; and Joanne Spetz, University of California, San Francisco. Additional researchers and experts were engaged to fill gaps as needed. The production and delivery of NRN products, including reports, research briefs, charts, tables, and commentaries, were coordinated by Patricia (Polly) Pittman, of AcademyHealth and subsequently The George Washington University, and her staff.

The NRN began by providing the committee with a foundational set of 20 articles in the following areas of nursing policy: chronic and long-term care, education policy, expansion of access to primary care, foreign-educated nurses, human resource management (including nurse turnover rates), improvement of quality and safety (including workforce environment and staffing issues), prevention and wellness, promotion of health information technology, cost containment, and workforce estimations. To date, the NRN has produced 6 reports, 48 charts and tables, and 13 research briefs. A broad range of topics has been covered, including estimates of supply and demand, scope of practice, faculty shortages, career ladders, payment systems, health information technology, and physician and patient perceptions of nursing care. All of these products will be available to the public through either RWJF's website or peer-reviewed publications.

COMMITTEE MEETINGS

The committee convened for five meetings and participated in several conference calls throughout the study to deliberate on the content of this report and its recommendations. To obtain additional information on specific aspects of the study charge, the committee included in three of its meetings technical workshops that were open to the public and held three public forums on the future of nursing and the role of nurses across various settings. Subject matter experts were invited to these public sessions to present information and recommendations for the committee's consideration, answer the committee's questions, and participate in subsequent discussions.

The three technical workshops were held in conjunction with the committee's July, September, and November 2009 meetings. The purpose of these workshops was to gather information on specified topics. The committee determined the topics and speakers based on its information needs. The first meeting included a review and discussion of the committee's charge with the study's sponsor, RWJF; an overview and description of the current nursing workforce and future workforce needs; and an introduction to the NRN and the resources that would be made available to the committee through the network. The second workshop was intended to provide an overview of the Prime Minister's Commission on the Future of Nursing and Midwifery and the efforts in England to transform the nursing profession; a discussion of possible ways for the nursing profession to fulfill its promise; and a review of ongoing health care reform efforts in the United States. The third workshop looked at nurses' role in addressing disparities; ways to ensure quality, access, and value in health care; and reimbursement and financing of care delivered by nurses. The agendas for these three workshops are provided in Boxes A-1 through A-3 at the end of this appendix.

The three public forums were held in locations across the United States to engage a broader range of stakeholders and the public. The first, held in October 2009 at Cedars-Sinai Medical Center in Los Angeles, focused on quality and safety, technology, and interdisciplinary collaboration in acute care settings. The second, held in December 2009 at the Community College of Philadelphia, featured presentations and discussion of achievements and challenges in care in the community and focused on community health, public health, primary care, and long-term care. The final forum, held in February 2010 at the University of Texas M. D. Anderson Cancer Center, featured discussion of three topics in nursing education: what to teach, how to teach, and where to teach. Summaries of each of these forums were published separately and are available on the CD-ROM in the back of this report. The agendas for these forums are provided in Boxes A-4 through A-6 at the end of this appendix, and highlights from the forums appear in Appendix C.

In preparation for each of the forums and to augment the information gathered from presenters and discussants, the committee solicited written testimony through an online questionnaire (see Boxes A-7 through A-9 at the end of this appendix for the specific questions that were asked). The public and key stakeholders were invited to provide information on innovations, models, barriers, and opportunities for each of the topics covered at the forums, as well as their vision for the future of nursing overall. The committee received more than 200 submissions of testimony during the course of the study; many of the individuals who submitted this testimony also presented it at the forums. Each forum also included an open microphone session for ad hoc testimony and input from participants on a variety of topics relevant to the forum discussions.

SITE VISITS

In conjunction with each forum, small groups of committee members participated in a series of site visits. These visits highlighted a wide range of settings in which nurses work, as well as their various roles. The sites visited included acute care units in Cedars-Sinai Medical Center—ranging from critical care units to the emergency department and surgical units to child and maternal health and obstetrics units; community health settings in Philadelphia—ranging from a school-based health center to public health clinics and nurse-managed health centers; and education settings in Houston, where committee members saw demonstrations of high-fidelity simulation laboratories and participated in discussions of interprofessional education and educating for quality control. Committee members also talked with nurses, other care providers, and administrators about the challenges nurses encounter daily in their work in these varied settings. Observations made during these site visits informed some of the questions committee members asked speakers at the forums and provided real-world perspectives of seasoned professionals.

COMMISSIONED PAPERS

The committee commissioned a series of papers from experts in subject areas relevant to its statement of task. These papers, included as Appendixes E–I on the CD-ROM in the back of this report, were intended to provide in-depth information on five selected topics:

- A paper written by Barbara L. Nichols, Catherine R. Davis, and Donna R. Richardson from CGFNS International reviews the ways in which other countries educate, regulate, and utilize nurses. This paper also addresses the migration and globalization of the nursing workforce and implications for education, service delivery, and health policy in the United States.
- A paper by Barbara J. Safriet describes federal options for maximizing the value of advanced practice registered nurses (APRNs) in providing quality and cost-effective health care. It includes a review of current mechanisms of payment and financing of services and impediments in the regulatory environment for APRNs, and offers an assessment of policy initiatives that could improve the value of APRNs.
- A paper written by Julie Sochalski of the University of Pennsylvania and Jonathan Weiner of The Johns Hopkins University examines the nursing workforce and possible shortages in the context of a reformed health care system. It examines trends and projections for the workforce, drawbacks of current approaches to assessing the workforce, opportunities and challenges of new workforce approaches, and implications for policy.
- One paper was presented as a series of briefs that provides examples of transformative models of nursing across a variety of settings and locales. This paper was compiled and edited by Linda Norlander of the University of California, San Francisco, and features collaborative

briefs written by 27 fellows of the RWJF Executive Nurse Leadership Program. The briefs cover topics in education, acute care, chronic disease management, palliative and end-of-life care, community health, school-based health, and public–private partnerships.

- A collection of seven papers was written by Linda Aiken of the University of Pennsylvania; Donald Berwick of the Institute for Healthcare Improvement; Linda Cronenwett of the University of North Carolina at Chapel Hill; Kathleen Dracup of the University of California, San Francisco; Catherine Gilliss of Duke University; Chris Tanner of Oregon Health and Science University; and Virginia Tilden of the University of Nebraska. This series of papers describes the most important initiatives required to ensure that future nursing education efforts contribute to improving the health of the population, enhancing the patient's experience of care (including quality, access, and reliability), and reducing or controlling the per capita cost of care.

REFERENCES

AACN and AAMC (American Association of Colleges of Nursing and Association of American Medical Colleges). 2010. *Lifelong Learning in Medicine and Nursing: Final Conference Report.* Washington, DC: AACN and AAMC.

Benner, P., M. Sutphen, V. Leonard, and L. Day. 2009. *Educating Nurses: A Call for Radical Transformation.* San Francisco, CA: Jossey-Bass.

Cronenwett, L., and V. Dzau. 2010. *Who Will Provide Primary Care and How Will They Be Trained?* Proceedings of a Conference Sponsored by the Josiah Macy, Jr. Foundation. Edited by B. Culliton and S. Russell. Durham, NC: Josiah Macy, Jr. Foundation.

Goldmark, J. 1923. *Nursing and nursing education in the United States: Report of the committee for the study of nursing education.* New York: Macmillan Company.

Hager, M., S. Russell, and S. Fletcher, eds. 2008. *Continuing Education in the Health Professions: Improving Healthcare through Lifelong Learning.* Proceedings of a Conference Sponsored by the Josiah Macy, Jr. Foundation. New York: Josiah Macy, Jr. Foundation.

IOM (Institute of Medicine). 1983. *Nursing and Nursing Education: Public Policies and Private Actions.* Washington, DC: National Academy Press.

IOM. 2004. *Keeping Patients Safe: Transforming the Work Environment of Nurses.* Washington, DC: The National Academies Press.

IOM. 2009. *Redesigning Continuing Education in the Health Professions.* Washington, DC: The National Academies Press.

Prime Minister's Commission on the Future of Nursing and Midwifery in England. 2010. *Front Line Care: The Future of Nursing and Midwifery in England.* London: Crown.

BOX A-1
Technical Workshop #1

July 14, 2009

National Academy of Sciences
Lecture Room
2100 C Street, NW, Washington, DC 20037

Public Agenda

11:00 AM   **Delivery of Charge to the Committee**
               John Lumpkin, Robert Wood Johnson Foundation

12:00 PM   **Lunch Available**

12:30–1:00 PM **Outlook for the Nursing Workforce in the United States:
               Can Nursing Win the Game?**
               Peter Buerhaus, Vanderbilt University

1:00–2:30 PM   **Robert Wood Johnson Foundation Nursing Research
               Network**
               • Introduction to the Research Network
                   - *Susan Hassmiller, Robert Wood Johnson Foundation*
                   - *Lori Melichar, Robert Wood Johnson Foundation*
               • Panel discussion with members of the Nursing Research
                 Network
                   - *Peter Buerhaus, Vanderbilt University*
                   - *Christine Kovner, New York University*
                   - *Arnold Milstein, Mercer Consulting*
                   - *Mark Pauly, University of Pennsylvania*

2:30 PM   **Open Session Adjourns**

BOX A-2
Technical Workshop #2

September 14, 2009

Kaiser Family Foundation
Barbara Jordan Conference Center
1330 G Street, NW, Washington, DC

Public Agenda

9:00–10:00 AM	**Overview of the Prime Minister's Commission on the Future of Nursing and Midwifery** *Ann Keen, Chair, and Parliamentary Under Secretary for Health Services* *Anne Marie Rafferty, Commissioner (via videoconference)* *Jane Salvage, Joint Lead, Support Office*
10:00–11:30 AM	**Fulfilling the Potential of the Nursing Workforce** *Ann Hendrich, Ascension Health* *Mary Naylor, University of Pennsylvania* *Ed O'Neil, University of California, San Francisco (via videoconference)*
11:30–11:45 AM	**Break**
11:45 AM–1:00 PM	**Overview of the Status of Health Care Reform** *Chris Jennings, Jennings Policy Strategies, Inc.* *Dean Rosen, Mehlman Vogel Castagnetti, Inc.* *Peter Reinecke, Reinecke Strategic Solutions, Inc.*

BOX A-3
Technical Workshop #3

November 2, 2009

National Academy of Sciences
Lecture Room
2100 C Street, NW, Washington, DC

Public Agenda

8:00–9:00 AM   **The Role of Nurses in Addressing Health Disparities**
Linda Burnes Bolton, Facilitator
David R. Williams, Harvard University
Nilda Peragallo, University of Miami School of Nursing
Antonia M. Villarruel, University of Michigan School of Nursing
Alicia Georges, Lehman College Department of Nursing

9:00–10:30 AM   **Reimbursement and Financing for Nursing Care**
David Goodman and Jennie Chin Hansen, Facilitators
Mark McClellan, Brookings Institute
Gail Wilensky, Project HOPE
Ellen Kurtzman, The George Washington University
Meredith Rosenthal, Harvard University

10:30–10:45 AM   **Break**

10:45–11:45 AM   **Quality, Access, and Value: Nursing Roles for the 21st Century**
Donna Shalala, Facilitator
- Prevention/Wellness
  Susan Cooper, Tennessee Department of Health
- Chronic Disease Management
  Mary Mundinger, Dean and Professor in Health Policy, Columbia University School of Nursing
- End-of-Life Care
  Judy Lentz, CEO, Hospice and Palliative Nurses Association

11:45 AM   **Adjourn**

BOX A-4
Forum on the Future of Nursing: Acute Care

October 19, 2009

Harvey Morse Auditorium
Cedars-Sinai Medical Center
8700 Beverly Boulevard, Los Angeles, CA 90048

Public Agenda

12:30 PM   **Welcome and Introductions**
Linda Burnes Bolton, Cedars-Sinai Medical Center
Tom Priselac, Cedars-Sinai Medical Center

1:00 PM   **Acute Care: Current and Future State**
Marilyn Chow, Kaiser Permanente

1:30 PM   **Panel on Quality and Safety**
Maureen Bisognano, Institute for Healthcare Improvement
Tami Minnier, University of Pittsburgh Medical Center
Reactor Panel
Bernice Coleman, Cedars-Sinai Medical Center
Nancy Chiang, California Student Nurses Association
Kurt Swartout, Kaiser Permanente
Joseph Guglielmo, University of California, San Francisco
Julia Hallisy, The Empowered Patient Coalition

Committee Q&A and Discussion

2:15 PM   **Break**

2:30 PM   **Panel on Technology**
Steve DeMello, Public Health Institute
Pam Cipriano, University of Virginia Health System

Reactor Panel

Committee Q&A and Discussion

3:15 PM   **Panel on Interdisciplinary Collaboration**
Alan Rosenstein, VHA West Coast
Pamela Mitchell, University of Washington

Reactor Panel

Committee Q&A and Discussion

4:00 PM   **Presentation of Testimony**
[A limited number of preselected individuals will be given the
opportunity to present testimony.]

5:25 PM   **Closing Remarks**
Josef Reum, The George Washington University

5:30 PM   **Adjourn**

BOX A-5
Forum on the Future of Nursing: Care in the Community

December 3, 2009

Community College of Philadelphia
Great Hall (S2.19), Winnet Student Life Building
1700 Spring Garden, Philadelphia, PA 19130

Public Agenda

12:30 PM   **Welcome and Introductions**
              Donna E. Shalala, University of Miami
              Josef Reum, The George Washington University

12:45 PM   **Notes on Prescription for Pennsylvania**
              Governor Ed Rendell

1:15 PM   **Committee Q&A and Discussion**

1:30 PM   **Keynote Presentation**
              Mary Selecky, Washington State Department of Health

2:00 PM   **Panel on Community and Public Health**
              Carol Raphael, Visiting Nurse Service of New York
              Eileen Sullivan-Marx, University of Pennsylvania School of Nursing

              Committee Q&A and Discussion

              Preselected Testimony

3:00 PM	**Break**
3:15 PM	**Panel on Primary Care** *Tine Hansen-Turton, National Nursing Centers Consortium* *Sandra Haldane, Indian Health Service* **Committee Q&A and Discussion** **Preselected Testimony**
4:15 PM	**Panel on Chronic and Long-Term Services and Supports** *Claudia Beverly, University of Arkansas for Medical Sciences* *School of Nursing* *Lynda Hedstrom, Ovations-Evercare by UnitedHealthcare®* *Medicare Solutions* **Committee Q&A and Discussion** **Preselected Testimony**
5:10 PM	**Open Microphone Listening Session: Visions for the** **Future of Nursing**
5:30 PM	**Closing Remarks** *Josef Reum, The George Washington University*
5:35 PM	**Adjourn**

BOX A-6
Forum on the Future of Nursing: Education

February 22, 2010

University of Texas, MD Anderson Cancer Center
Cancer Prevention Building (CPB), 8th floor
1155 Pressler Street, Houston, TX 77030

Public Agenda

8:00 AM   **Welcomes and Introductions**
Donna E. Shalala, University of Miami
John Lumpkin, The Robert Wood Johnson Foundation
John Mendelsohn, University of Texas, MD Anderson
Cancer Center

8:15 AM   **What We Should Teach: Arm Chair Discussion #1**
Michael Bleich, Oregon Health and Science University,
Moderator
Linda Cronenwett, University of North Carolina at Chapel
Hill, School of Nursing
M. Elaine Tagliareni, National League for Nursing, formerly
Community College of Philadelphia
Terry Fulmer, College of Nursing, New York University
Marla Salmon, University of Washington School of Nursing

9:15 AM   **Preselected Testimony**
Donna E. Shalala, Facilitator

9:30 AM   **How We Should Teach: Arm Chair Discussion #2**
Linda Burnes Bolton, Cedars-Sinai Medical Center,
Moderator
Pamela Jeffries, The Johns Hopkins University
Divina Grossman, Florida International University
John Rock, Florida International University
Bob Mendenhall, Western Governors University
Cathleen Krsek, University HealthSystem Consortium, UHC/
AACN Nurse Residency Program™

10:30 AM	**Preselected Testimony**
	Donna E. Shalala, Facilitator
10:45 AM	**Break**
11:00 AM	**Where We Should Teach: Arm Chair Discussion #3**
	Jennie Chin Hansen, AARP, Moderator
	Rose Yuhos, AHEC of Southern Nevada
	Cathy Rick, Department of Veterans Affairs Nursing Academy
	Christine Tanner, Oregon Health and Science University
	Willis N. Holcombe, The Florida College System
12:00 PM	**Preselected Testimony**
	Donna E. Shalala, Facilitator
12:15 PM	**Open Microphone Listening Session: Visions for the Future of Nursing**
	Donna E. Shalala, Facilitator
12:35 PM	**Closing Remarks**
	Donna E. Shalala
12:40 PM	**Adjourn**

BOX A-7
Testimony Questions for the Forum on
the Future of Nursing: Acute Care

Question 1: Quality and Safety
Please describe any or all of the following:
- innovative models in which nurses have been used to improve quality and/or safety in acute care settings
- barriers that acute care nurses face in maximizing quality and safety
- how nurses could be further engaged or effectively used to improve acute care quality and safety

Question 2: Technology
Please describe any or all of the following:
- how innovative technologies have been used in acute care settings to improve nurse-led patient care (include information on the measurement of the improvements)
- barriers to the adoption and use of innovative technology in acute care settings
- opportunities in acute care settings for further improvements in the delivery of care through the use of technology

Question 3: Interdisciplinary Collaboration

Please describe any or all of the following:

- innovations in acute care settings that have successfully advanced inter-disciplinary collaboration or have been used to resolve limitations related to scope of practice
- limitations to interdisciplinary collaboration in acute care settings
- how interdisciplinary collaboration could be advanced to improve delivery of acute care and what the role of nurses should be in advancing this collaboration

Question 4: Additional Comments

If you have additional thoughts about nursing in acute care settings or if you would like to share information on innovations or models of care that does not fit within the categories listed above, please use the space provided below.

Question 5: Presentation of Testimony

If you are interested in presenting your testimony in person at the forum on October 19th in Los Angeles, please check the box below. (Please note that there are only a limited number of 2-minute slots available, and there is no funding available to cover travel expenses to the forum.)

BOX A-8
Testimony Questions for the Forum on the
Future of Nursing: Care in the Community

Question 1a: Community Health

Please describe any or all of the following:
- innovative models or initiatives in community health settings in which nurses have played a major role in the design, implementation, or evaluation (include information on improvement measures and outcomes)
- barriers in community health settings that nurses face in providing services or improving community health
- suggestions for how nurses could be further engaged or effectively used to improve care provided at the community level

Question 1b: Presentation of Testimony on Community Health

If you are interested in presenting your testimony on *community health* in person at the forum on December 3 in Philadelphia, please check the box below. (Please note that there are only a limited number of 2-minute slots available, and there is no funding available to cover travel expenses to the forum.)

Question 2a: Public Health

Please describe any or all of the following:
- innovative models or initiatives in public health in which nurses have played a major role in the design, implementation, or evaluation (include information on improvement measures and outcomes)
- barriers in public health that nurses face in providing services or improving the health of the public
- suggestions for how nurses could be further engaged or effectively used to improve public health

Question 2b: Presentation of Testimony on Public Health

If you are interested in presenting your testimony on *public health* in person at the forum on December 3 in Philadelphia, please check the box below. (Please note that there are only a limited number of 2-minute slots available, and there is no funding available to cover travel expenses to the forum.)

Question 3a: Primary Care

Please describe any or all of the following:
- innovative models or initiatives in primary care settings in which nurses have

played a major role in the design, implementation, or evaluation (include information on improvement measures and outcomes)
- barriers in primary care settings that nurses face in providing services or improving health outcomes
- suggestions for how nurses could be further engaged or effectively used to improve primary care

Question 3b: Presentation of Testimony on Primary Care

If you are interested in presenting your testimony on *primary care* in person at the forum on December 3 in Philadelphia, please check the box below. (Please note that there are only a limited number of 2-minute slots available, and there is no funding available to cover travel expenses to the forum.)

Question 4a: Long-Term Care

Please describe any or all of the following:
- innovative models or initiatives in long term care settings in which nurses have played a major role in the design, implementation, or evaluation (include information on improvement measures and outcomes)
- barriers in long-term care settings that nurses face in providing services or improving health outcomes
- suggestions for how nurses could be further engaged or effectively used to improve long-term care

Question 4b: Presentation of Testimony on Long-Term Care

If you are interested in presenting your testimony on *long-term care* in person at the forum on December 3 in Philadelphia, please check the box below. (Please note that there are only a limited number of 2-minute slots available, and there is no funding available to cover travel expenses to the forum.)

Question 5a: Your Vision of the Future of Nursing

Please describe your vision of the future of nursing across care settings. Your vision could include thoughts on the type of care nurses will provide, the types of settings they will be working in, how nurses will be educated and trained, how they will be paid and reimbursed, and some of the challenges nurses will be faced with.

Question 5b: Additional Comments

If you have additional thoughts about nursing in community health, public health, primary care, or long-term care settings or if you would like to share information on innovations or models of care that does not fit within the categories listed above, please use the space provided below. You may also e-mail documents or articles to support your testimony to nursing@nas.edu.

BOX A-9
Testimony Questions for the Forum on
the Future of Nursing: Education

Question 1a: What We Should Teach

What we should teach encompasses issues and recommendations related to the ideal future state of nursing curricula.

Please describe any or all of the following:

- innovative models or initiatives within nursing curricula that are being employed to better prepare and educate nurses for future challenges in a variety of care settings
- innovative funding strategies and financial incentives for both students and institutions that could be used to advance what we should teach
- barriers to implementing expanded or new curricula
- suggestions for how the nursing curricula should change to better meet the future health needs of the population

Question 1b: Presentation of Testimony on What We Should Teach

If you are interested in presenting your testimony on *what we should teach* in person at the forum on February 22 in Houston, please check the box below. (Please note that there are only a limited number of 2-minute slots available, and there is no funding available to cover travel expenses to the forum.)

Question 2a: How We Should Teach

How we should teach encompasses issues and recommendations related to method-ologies and strategies, as well as partnerships or collaboratives, that should be used for educating and training nurses in an ideal future.

Please describe any or all of the following:

- innovative models or initiatives in nursing education that are being employed to advance the way in which nurses are educated and prepared
- innovative funding strategies and financial incentives for both students and institutions that could be used to advance how we should teach
- barriers to the implementation of innovative methodologies of education and training for nurses.
- suggestions for how current education methodologies can be advanced to better meet the future health needs of the population

Question 2b: Presentation of Testimony on How We Should Teach

If you are interested in presenting your testimony on *how we should teach* in person at the forum on February 22 in Houston, please check the box below. (Please note that there are only a limited number of 2-minute slots available, and there is no funding available to cover travel expenses to the forum.)

Question 3a: Where We Should Teach

Where we should teach encompasses issues and recommendations related to various venues and locations where nurses should be educated and trained, as well as partnerships and collaboratives that could be used in nursing education in an ideal future. Please describe any or all of the following:

- innovative models or initiatives in nursing education that take advantage of a variety of venues and locations for nursing education and training/continued education
- innovative funding strategies and financial incentives for both students and institutions that could be used to advance where we should teach
- barriers to expanding nursing education beyond traditional classroom settings
- suggestions for how current education can be expanded beyond traditional classroom settings to better meet the future health needs of the population

Question 3b: Presentation of Testimony on Where We Should Teach

If you are interested in presenting your testimony on *where we should teach* in person at the forum on February 22 in Houston, please check the box below. (Please note that there are only a limited number of 2-minute slots available, and there is no funding available to cover travel expenses to the forum.)

Question 4a: Your Vision of the Future of Nursing

Please describe your vision of the future of nursing across care settings. Your vision could include thoughts on the type of care nurses will provide, the types of settings they will be working in, how nurses will be educated and trained, how they will be paid and reimbursed, and some of the challenges nurses will be faced with.

Question 4b: Additional Comments

If you have additional thoughts about the future of nursing education, or if you would like to share information on innovations or models of care that does not fit within the categories listed above, please use the space provided below. You may also e-mail documents or articles to support your testimony to nursing@nas.edu. However, please note that only the first 250 words submitted in each section of this online form will be considered for presentation of oral testimony at the Houston forum.

B

Committee Biographical Sketches

Donna E. Shalala, Ph.D., FAAN, is chair, Robert Wood Johnson Foundation (RWJF) Initiative on the Future of Nursing, at the Institute of Medicine (IOM). She is president of the University of Miami and professor of political science. Dr. Shalala has more than 30 years of experience as an accomplished scholar, teacher, and administrator in government and universities. She has also held tenured professorships in political science at Columbia University, the City University of New York (CUNY), and the University of Wisconsin-Madison. She served as president of Hunter College of CUNY from 1980 to 1987 and as chancellor of the University of Wisconsin-Madison from 1987 to 1993. In 1993, President Clinton appointed her secretary of the Department of Health and Human Services (HHS), where she served for 8 years, becoming the longest-serving HHS secretary in U.S. history. She received the Presidential Medal of Freedom, the nation's highest civilian award, in 2008, and is a member of the IOM.

Linda Burnes Bolton, Dr.P.H., R.N., FAAN, is vice chair, RWJF Initiative on the Future of Nursing, at the IOM. She serves as vice president for nursing, chief nursing officer, and director of nursing research at Cedars-Sinai Medical Center in Los Angeles, California. Dr. Burnes Bolton is a principal investigator at the Cedars-Sinai Burns and Allen Research Institute. Her research, teaching, and clinical expertise includes nursing and patient care outcomes research, performance improvement, and improvement of quality of care and cultural diversity within the health professions. Dr. Burnes Bolton served as national advisory chair for Transforming Care at the Bedside, an initiative of the Robert Wood Johnson Foundation to improve the nursing practice environment. She is a past president of the American Academy of Nursing and the National Black Nurses Association.

Michael R. Bleich, R.N., Ph.D., M.P.H., FAAN, is dean and Dr. Carol A. Lindeman Distinguished Professor for the School of Nursing and vice provost for inter-professional education and development at Oregon Health & Science University. His areas of expertise and scholarship focus on interprofessional leadership development, academic-service workforce development, strategic alignment of academic clinical enterprises, and analytics related to quality improvement to enhance practice and academic outcomes. Dr. Bleich began his health care career in 1970 and has progressed to hold administrative, education, and consultative roles in both academic and service settings. He arrived in Portland, Oregon, in August 2008, concluding a distinguished career at the University of Kansas. There, Dr. Bleich was professor and associate dean for clinical and community affairs in the School of Nursing, and concurrently served as chief executive officer of the school's faculty practice plan, KU HealthPartners, Inc. In 2006, he was appointed chair of the Department of Health Policy and Management in the School of Medicine, the first nurse to hold the role of chair.

Troyen A. Brennan, M.D., J.D., M.P.H., is executive vice president and chief medical officer of CVS Caremark Corporation, serving in these roles since November 2008. Previously, Dr. Brennan served as executive vice president and chief medical officer of Aetna, Inc., from 2006 through 2008. From 2000 through 2006, he was president and chief executive officer of Brigham and Women's Physicians Organization. He also served as professor of medicine at Harvard Medical School and as professor of law and public health at Harvard School of Public Health from 1991 to 2006. Dr. Brennan is a member of the IOM.

Robert E. Campbell, M.B.A., served as chairman of the board of trustees of the Robert Wood Johnson Foundation from July 1999 until March 2005 and was a board member until January 2009. Mr. Campbell is retired vice chairman of the board of directors of Johnson & Johnson (J&J), where he also was chairman of the Professional Sector. He joined J&J in 1955 and later served as an Air Force officer for 3 years, rejoining the company in 1959. During his career, he held numerous positions in financial and general management, including treasurer, vice president finance, and executive committee member. Mr. Campbell is chairman of the advisory board of the Cancer Institute of New Jersey and is past chairman and current trustee emeritus of the board of trustees of Fordham University. He is a member of the advisory council for the College of Science of the University of Notre Dame and an overseer of the Robert Wood Johnson Medical School.

Leah Devlin, D.D.S., M.P.H., received her dental degree and master's degree in public health administration at the University of North Carolina's (UNC) Chapel Hill campus. At UNC, she was inducted into Phi Beta Kappa and the School of Public Health's honor society. In 2008, she was recognized with the UNC Distinguished Alumni Award. Dr. Devlin began her professional career at the Wake

County Department of Health, where she served as director for 10 years. She joined the North Carolina Department of Health and Human Services in 1996 and served as state health director from 2001 to 2009. Beginning in September 2009, Dr. Devlin became Gillings Visiting Professor at the UNC Gillings School of Global Public Health. She is also past president of the North Carolina Association of Local Health Directors, past president of the North Carolina Public Health Association, and past president of the Association of State and Territorial Health Officials.

Catherine Dower, J.D., is associate director for research at the University of California, San Francisco, Center for the Health Professions. At the center, she codirects the Health Workforce Tracking Collaborative, which assesses health care workforce challenges such as maldistribution, shortages, language access, and scope-of-practice issues. For 5 years she directed the California Workforce Initiative, a comprehensive research and policy program that included studies on physician supply and distribution, nursing and allied health shortages, and safety net workforce challenges. As staff to the Pew Health Professions Commission, Ms. Dower codirected the commission's national Taskforce on Health Care Workforce Regulation and was a principal author of the commission's reports on health professions regulation. Her published work targets health professions regulation, practice models, and workforce analysis. Ms. Dower serves or has served on several boards and committees, including the National Commission for Certifying Agencies, the National Certification Commission for Acupuncture and Oriental Medicine, and the Foreign Credentialing Commission for Physical Therapy. She received her undergraduate and law degrees from the University of California at Berkeley and is licensed to practice law in the state of California.

Rosa Gonzalez-Guarda, Ph.D., M.S.N., M.P.H., R.N., CPH, is currently an assistant professor at the University of Miami School of Nursing and Health Studies. Throughout her academic and professional career, she has focused on improving the behavioral health and public health of minorities and other at-risk communities throughout the world. In the past, she has worked on various community health nursing projects, public health programs, and research targeting African Americans; Hispanic Americans; and other vulnerable populations in Europe, Latin America, and the Caribbean. Dr. Gonzalez-Guarda has been a funded fellow of the Substance Abuse and Mental Health Services Administration's Minority Fellowship Program at the American Nurses Association, the National Hispanic Science Network on Drug Abuse, and the University of Miami Graduate School. She is currently a co-investigator for two studies within a research center funded by the National Center on Minority Health and Health Disparities/National Institutes of Health referred to as El Centro (Center of Excellence for Hispanic Health Disparities Research). One of these studies explores the experiences of Hispanic men with substance abuse, violence, and risky sexual behaviors (Project VIDA—Violence, Intimate Relationships, and Drug Abuse among Latinos), while the other evaluates the effectiveness of an HIV prevention program targeting Hispanic women in the community (Project SEPA—Salud, Prevención y Auto cuidado).

David C. Goodman, M.D., M.S., is professor of pediatrics and of health policy at the Dartmouth Institute for Health Policy and Clinical Practice in Hanover, New Hampshire; director of the Center for Health Policy Research; and co–principal investigator, *Dartmouth Atlas of Health Care*. Dr. Goodman's primary research interest is geographic and hospital variation in the health workforce and its relationship to health outcomes. His research papers and editorials on this topic have been published in the *New England Journal of Medicine*, the *Journal of the American Medical Association*, *Health Affairs*, *Pediatrics*, and *The New York Times*. Dr. Goodman is also a charter member of the *Dartmouth Atlas of Health Care* working group. He currently leads *Atlas* projects examining variation in end-of-life cancer care, post–hospital discharge care, and regional hospital and physician capacity. Dr. Goodman is a member and recent member, respectively, of the editorial boards of the journals *Health Services Research* and *Pediatrics*. After joining the Dartmouth faculty in 1988, he undertook allergy and clinical immunology training. He recently stepped down as chief of the Section of Allergy and Clinical Immunology, a position he held for a number of years.

Jennie Chin Hansen, R.N., M.S., FAAN, was elected by the AARP board to serve as president for the 2008–2010 biennium. She previously chaired the board of the AARP Foundation. Ms. Hansen currently holds an appointment as senior fellow at the University of California, San Francisco's Center for the Health Professions and consults with various foundations. She transitioned to teaching in 2005 after nearly 25 years at On Lok, where she served as executive director for 11 years. On Lok, Inc., is a nonprofit family of organizations providing integrated and comprehensive community-based primary and long-term care services in San Francisco. Ms. Hansen serves in various leadership roles that include commissioner of the Medicare Payment Advisory Commission (MedPAC) and board officer of the National Academy of Social Insurance, the SCAN Foundation, and the Robert Wood Johnson Executive Nurse Fellows Program. She is also a past president of the American Society on Aging. In April 2010, she became chief executive officer of the American Geriatrics Society.

C. Martin Harris, M.D., M.B.A., is chief information officer and chairman of the Information Technology Division of Cleveland Clinic in Cleveland, Ohio. Additionally, he is executive director of eCleveland Clinic, a series of secure, Internet-based information technology–enabled clinical and connectivity programs offered to patients and medical professionals. Dr. Harris's expertise in the innovative application of health information technology to improve the contemporary medical practice model is reflected in his service for numerous national organizations, including the President's Commission on Caring for America's Returning Wounded Warriors, the Board of Regents of the National Library of Medicine, and the Board of the Healthcare Information Management Systems Society. He received his undergraduate and medical degrees from the University of Pennsylvania in Philadelphia. He completed his residency training in general internal medicine at The Hospital of the University of Pennsylvania, a Robert Wood Johnson Clinical Scholar fellowship in general internal medicine at the University of Pennsylvania School of Medicine, and a master's in business administration in healthcare management at the Wharton School of the University of Pennsylvania.

Anjli Aurora Hinman, C.N.M., F.N.P.-B.C., M.P.H., is a certified nurse midwife and family nurse practitioner, providing antepartum, intrapartum, postpartum, and gynecological services to women. She is also a volunteer at Community Advanced Practice Nurses, Inc., an organization that provides free physical, mental, and preventive health care to homeless and medically underserved women and families in the Atlanta metropolitan area. An alumna of the Emory University School of Nursing, she is past president and current alumni chair of Health Students Taking Action Together, a Georgia nonprofit run by health professional students whose mission is to create a statewide community of health professional students and engage them in education, activism, and service. Ms. Hinman is also past president of the Emory Student Nurses Association and Breakthrough to Nursing director for the Georgia Association of Nursing Students.

William D. Novelli, M.A., is a distinguished professor at the McDonough School of Business at Georgetown University. He is the former chief executive officer of AARP, whose mission is to enhance the quality of life for all as we age. Prior to joining AARP, Mr. Novelli was president of the Campaign for Tobacco-Free Kids, whose mandate is to change public policies and the social environment, limit tobacco companies' marketing and sales to children, and counter the industry and its special interests. He now serves as chairman of the board for that organization. Mr. Novelli was also executive vice president of CARE, the world's largest private relief and development organization. Earlier, he cofounded and was president of Porter Novelli, now part of the Omnicom Group, an international marketing communications corporation. Porter Novelli was founded to apply marketing to social and health issues and now is one of the world's largest public relations agencies. Mr. Novelli is a recognized leader in social marketing and social change, and has managed programs in cancer control, diet and nutrition, cardiovascular health, reproductive health, infant survival, and other areas in the United States and the developing world. His book *50+: Give Meaning and Purpose to the Best Time of Your Life* was updated in 2008. A second book (with Peter Cappelli of the Wharton School at the University of Pennsylvania), *Managing the Older Workforce*, will be published in 2010.

Liana Orsolini-Hain, Ph.D., R.N., CCRN, with almost 20 years of experience in associate degree nursing education, is a tenured instructor at City College of San Francisco. In addition, she coordinates a community college chancellor's grant developing ADN-to-BSN and ADN-to-MSN educational collaboration models. Her research and scholarly work address issues in nursing education including the factors that influence educational progression of associate degree nurses. Dr. Orsolini-Hain serves on the advisory committee to members of the board of California Institute for Nursing & Health Care (CINHC). She also co-chaired CINHC's White Paper on Nursing Education Redesign for California's committee on nursing collaborative education models. She is also an Assistant Clinical Professor (volunteer) at the University of California San Francisco department of physiological nursing, and a per diem staff nurse at the San Francisco Veterans Administration Medical Center. She is the immediate past president of California League for Nursing and has served on several professional nursing organization committees including the Association of Critical-Care Nurses.

Yolanda Partida, M.S.W., D.P.A., is director of Hablamos Juntos and assistant adjunct professor at the University of California, San Francisco, Fresno Center for Medical and Education Research in California. Hablamos Juntos (We Speak Together) is a national initiative of the Robert Wood Johnson Foundation created in 2001 to work with ten demonstrations and to develop practical solutions to language barriers in health care. Hablamos Juntos has produced a set of Universal Health Care symbols for health care signage and the More Than Words Toolkit, containing practical tools for commissioning and assessing the quality of translated materials. The Translation Quality Assessment Tool was found to have high interrater reliability in quality evaluations of materials translated from English into Spanish and Chinese. Dr. Partida has extensive experience in public/teaching and private hospital administration, public health administration, and private consulting. In these settings, she has been responsible for overseeing a variety of health care and public health programs, forming public–private partnerships, developing multiagency strategic plans, conducting feasibility studies, and preparing business case analyses.

Robert D. Reischauer, Ph.D., is president of the Urban Institute. A former director of the Congressional Budget Office (CBO) and a nationally known expert on the federal budget, Medicare, and Social Security, he began his tenure as the second president of the Urban Institute in February 2000. He had been a senior fellow of economic studies at the Brookings Institution since 1995. From 1989 to 1995, he was director of the nonpartisan CBO. Mr. Reischauer served as the Urban Institute's senior vice president from 1981 to 1986. He was the CBO's assistant director for human resources and its deputy director between 1977 and 1981. Mr. Reischauer serves on the boards of several educational and nonprofit organizations. He was a member of MedPAC from 2000 to 2009 and its vice chair from 2001 to 2008. He is a member of the IOM.

John W. Rowe, M.D., is professor in the Department of Health Policy and Management at the Columbia University Mailman School of Public Health. From 2000 until late 2006, he served as chairman and CEO of Aetna, Inc., one of the nation's leading health care and related benefits organizations. Before his tenure at Aetna, from 1998 to 2000, Dr. Rowe served as president and CEO of Mount Sinai NYU Health, one of the nation's largest academic health care organizations. From 1988 to 1998, prior to the Mount Sinai–NYU Health merger, he was president of the Mount Sinai Hospital and the Mount Sinai School of Medicine in New York City. Before joining Mount Sinai, Dr. Rowe was a professor of medicine and founding director of the Division on Aging at Harvard Medical School, as well as chief of gerontology at Boston's Beth Israel Hospital. He has authored more than 200 scientific publications, mainly on the physiology of the aging process, including a leading textbook of geriatric medicine, in addition to more recent publications on health care policy. Dr. Rowe has received many honors and awards for his research and health policy efforts regarding care of the elderly. He was director of the MacArthur Foundation Research Network on Successful Aging and is coauthor, with Robert Kahn, Ph.D., of *Successful Aging* (Pantheon, 1998). Currently, Dr. Rowe leads the MacArthur Foundation's Network on an Aging Society. In addition, he is a former member of MedPAC, has served as president of the Gerontological Society of America, and chaired the IOM's Committee on the Future Health Care Workforce for Older Americans. He is a member of the IOM.

Bruce C. Vladeck, Ph.D., is senior advisor to Nexera Consulting. He is also chairman of the board of the Medicare Rights Center, a member of the New York City Board of Health, and a director of the March of Dimes and Independence Care Systems. Dr. Vladeck is a nationally recognized expert on health care policy, health care financing, and long-term care. From 1993 through 1997, he was administrator of the Health Care Financing Administration (HCFA) within HHS. Subsequently, he was appointed by President Clinton to the National Bipartisan Commission on the Future of Medicare. Dr. Vladeck's career in health care has included 10 years as president of the United Hospital Fund of New York and senior positions at Columbia University, the New Jersey State Department of Health, the Robert Wood Johnson Foundation, and Mount Sinai Medical Center. In 2006–2007, he served as interim president of the University of Medicine and Dentistry of New Jersey. He previously chaired the IOM's Committee on Health Care for the Homeless (1991–1992). He is a member of the IOM.

C

Highlights from the Forums on the Future of Nursing

Throughout course of the Robert Wood Johnson Initiative on the Future of Nursing, at the Institute of Medicine (IOM), the Initiative hosted three public forums on the future of nursing. These forums were designed to inform the committee about the critical and varied roles that nurses play across settings and were part of a much broader information-gathering effort by the IOM committee and staff, which is discussed in greater detail in Appendix A. The forums provided an opportunity for members of the committee to hear from a range of experts, stakeholders, and members of the public and to see, first-hand, the challenges and innovations in settings where nurses provide care and are educated. The three forums were held in Los Angeles, Philadelphia, and Houston and focused on acute care, care in the community, and education, respectively.

Prior to the forums a variety of stakeholders and the public were invited to submit written testimony to the committee in areas relevant to the forums. Those submitting written testimony were asked to share their insight and describe innovative models in these areas; barriers that nurses face in delivering care or advancing the profession; how nurses could be further involved in advancing these areas; and their vision for the future of nursing. Each of the forums was webcasted live to a much larger national audience. Additionally, participants at the forum were encouraged to share their thoughts and reactions to the discussion through open microphone sessions, as well as social media tools such Facebook and Twitter.

Each of the three forums was planned with the guidance of a subgroup of the committee, which was led by a planning-group chair; Robert Reischauer chaired the planning group for the acute care forum in Los Angeles, Jennie Chin Hansen led the planning group for the care in the community forum in Philadelphia, and

Michael Bleich served as chair for the planning group for the education forum in Houston. The half-day forums were not meant to be an exhaustive examination of all settings in which nurses practice nor an exhaustive examination of the complexity of the nursing profession as a whole. Given the limited amount of time for each of the three forums, a comprehensive review of all facets and all players of each of the main forum themes was not possible. Rather, the forums were meant to inform the committee on important topics within the nursing profession and to highlight some of the key challenges, barriers, opportunities, and innovations that nurses are confronted with while working in an evolving health care system. Many of the critical challenges, barriers, opportunities, and innovations discussed at the forums overlap across settings and throughout the nursing profession and also are applicable to other health providers and individuals who work with nurses.

The following sections of this appendix offer brief summaries and highlights from each of the three forums on the future of nursing: acute care, care in the community, and education. Appendix A of this report includes the agendas for the forums, and the full text of the forum summaries are available at www.iom.edu/nursing and are also included on the CD-ROM in the back cover of this report.

ACUTE CARE

The Initiative on the Future of Nursing held its first forum on October 19, 2009, at Cedars-Sinai Medical Center in Los Angeles. This forum was designed to explore the challenges and opportunities for nurses in acute care settings and the changes needed to improve the quality, efficiency, and effectiveness of patient care. The forum focused on three topics within the context of acute care: quality and safety, technology, and interdisciplinary collaboration. Acute care settings were particularly important for the committee to examine, because well over half of all nurses work in acute care settings, where they are patients' primary, professional caregivers and the individuals most likely to intercept medical errors. However, because hospital systems and acute care settings are often complex and chaotic, many nurses spend unnecessary time hunting for supplies, filling out paperwork, and coordinating staff time and patient care, reducing the time they are able to spend with patients and delivering care.

Nearly 300 people attended the acute care forum and heard presentations and discussions with 30 experts, including welcoming remarks from Thomas Priselac, president and chief executive officer of the Cedars-Sinai Health System and chair of the Board of Directors for the American Hospital Association, and a keynote presentation from Dr. Marilyn Chow, vice president of National Patient Care Services at Kaiser Permanente in Oakland, California. During the forum, 19 individuals offered testimony for the committee's consideration. These individuals provided organizational and personal perspectives on the future of nursing in acute care settings.

Key Themes

The presentations offered the committee with insight into the important role that frontline nurses play across acute care settings, as well as the challenges and barriers that these frontline nurses face in their daily work. It was apparent from the presentations that there are a number of successful and promising innovative models being used in acute care settings across the country. However, these models are infrequently transferred widely. The discussion at the forum provided the committee with an opportunity to consider how rapidly advancing technology, interdisciplinary relationships, and changes in the way acute care is delivered will affect the nursing profession and how nurses will need to be educated to be adequately prepared for their varying roles and responsibilities.

A number of important points emerged at the forum:

- The knowledge of frontline nurses that they gather from their interactions with patients is critical to reducing medical errors and improving patient outcomes.
- Involving nurses at a variety of levels across the acute care setting in decision making and leadership benefits the patient, improves the organizations in which nurses practice, and strengthens the health care system in general.
- Increasing the time that nurses can spend at the bedside is an essential component of achieving the goal of patient-centered care.
- High-quality acute care settings require integrated systems that use technology effectively while increasing the efficiency of nurses and affording them increased time to spend with patients.
- Multidisciplinary care teams characterized by extensive and respectful collaboration among team members improve the quality, safety, and effectiveness of care.
- Many of the innovations that need to be implemented in the health care system already exist somewhere in the United States, but barriers to their dissemination keep them from being adopted more widely. As Dr. Marilyn Chow observed, "the future is here, it just isn't everywhere."

Site Visits and Solutions Session

In the morning before the forum began, individual committee members participated in a series of site visits to a variety of acute care units within Cedars-Sinai Medical Center. They spoke with nurses, other care providers, and administrators about the challenges nurses encounter in their work in acute care settings. The units that were visited within the Medical Center ranged from critical care, emergency department, and surgical units to child and maternal health and obstetrics units. Following the site visits and the forum, a group of Robert Wood

Johnson Foundation (RWJF) scholars and fellows,[1] who had attended the forum and participated in the site visits, met to consider solutions and the most promising future roles for nurses in acute care settings with respect to the subthemes of quality and safety, technology, and interdisciplinary collaboration. A summary of this session was provided to the committee for its review and consideration at the committee's subsequent meeting in November 2009.

CARE IN THE COMMUNITY

On December 3, 2009, the Initiative on the Future of Nursing held its second forum at the Community College of Philadelphia. This forum examined the challenges facing the nursing profession with regard to care in the community, including aspects of community health, public health, primary care, and long-term care. Members of the committee planning group for this forum believed that these topics were especially important to the committee's work overall; as the health care system evolves, the provision of care is increasingly occurring in nonacute settings and is increasingly focused on disease prevention, health promotion, and management of chronic illnesses. Nurses who practice in community settings are vital to ensuring access to quality care.

More than 200 forum attendees heard a series of presentations from leaders in the field, including opening remarks from Pennsylvania Governor Edward Rendell and a keynote from Mary C. Selecky, Secretary of Washington State's Department of Health (an agenda for this forum can be found in Appendix A). During the forum, committee members also heard testimony from 15 individuals representing a wide variety of organizations and personal viewpoints, as well as remarks made by a number of forum participants as part of an open-microphone session.

Key Themes

The forum presenters described a segment of best practices in the community that shed light on what is currently available and what will be required to meet the changing health needs of the diverse populations of this country. As a result of this forum, the committee was given an opportunity to consider how changing health needs in the community will affect the future of the nursing profession in terms of the way care is delivered, the settings in which care is provided, and

---

[1] RWJF works to build human capital by supporting individuals who seek to advance health and health care in America. RWJF invited alumni of 17 of its scholar, fellow, and leader programs to participate in the Forum on the Future of Nursing. The alumni came from a variety of backgrounds and disciplines, including academia, service delivery, research, policy, and health plan administration. Many of the participants were alumni of the RWJF Executive Nurse Fellows Program and the RWJF Nurse Faculty Scholars Program. Non-nurse participants included alumni of the Investigator Award Program, the RWJF Health Policy Fellows Program, and the RWJF Clinical Scholar Program.

the education requirements for the necessary skills and competencies to provide quality care.

Many important messages emerged from the presentations, discussions, and site visits, including the following:

- Budgets for public health and community health programs are being cut at a time when these programs are needed most to care for aging populations and when greater emphasis is being placed on prevention, wellness, chronic disease management, and moving care into the community.
- Nursing in the community occurs through partnerships with many other individuals and organizations, and nurses need to take a leadership role in establishing these vital partnerships. Fostering this type of collaboration could improve the continuum of care between acute and community care settings.
- Technology has the potential to transform the lives of nurses providing care in the community, as well as their patients, just as it is transforming commerce, education, communications, and entertainment for the public.
- Varying scopes of practice across states have, in some cases, prevented nurses from providing care to the fullest extent possible at the community level.
- Nurse-managed health clinics offer opportunities to expand access; provide quality, evidence-based care; and improve outcomes for individuals who may not otherwise receive needed care. These clinics also provide the necessary support to engage individuals in wellness and prevention activities.
- Nursing students need to have greater exposure to principles of community care, leadership, and care provision through changes in nursing school curricula and increased opportunities to gain experience in community care settings.
- The delivery of quality nursing care has the potential to provide value across community settings and can be achieved though effective leadership, policy, and accountability.

Site Visits and Solutions Session

Prior to the forum, several members of the IOM committee visited a number of community-based health centers across Philadelphia. The six Philadelphia sites visited by committee members and the RWJF fellows and scholars were the Living Independently for Elders (LIFE) program at the University of Pennsylvania School of Nursing, the Sayre High School School-Based Health Clinic, Community Health Center #3 of the Philadelphia Department of Health, Health

Annex, Health Connections, and the 11th Street Family Health Services of Drexel University. Concluding the day's events, RWJF fellows and scholars reviewed what they had heard at the forum and seen during the site visits to develop a set of recommendations for the committee's consideration that were relevant to the delivery of nursing care in the community; highlights from the solutions session were provided to the committee at its January 2010 meeting.

EDUCATION

On February 22, 2010, the Initiative held its final forum on the future of nursing at the University of Texas M.D. Anderson Cancer Center in Houston. This forum was designed to examine challenges and opportunities associated with nursing education. The nursing education system consists of multifaceted educational pathways with a mixture of starting points and opportunities for advancement to higher levels. This complex system is responsible for educating and training future generations of nursed that are prepared and able to meet the needs of diverse populations across the lifespan in a health care system that is constantly evolving.

This forum on the future of nursing featured welcoming remarks from Dr. John Lumpkin of RWJF and Dr. John Mendelsohn of the University of Texas M.D. Anderson Cancer Center and included three armchair discussions that were each led by a moderator from the committee. The armchair discussions focused on three broad, overlapping subjects: what to teach, how to teach, and where to teach (an agenda for this forum can be found in Appendix A). More than 300 people assembled in Houston to listen to the discussion and participate in the forum, and an additional 330 registered for the forum's live webcast. During the forum 12 participants presented formal testimony to the committee, while several more participants offered ad hoc remarks and insight during an open-microphone session that concluded the discussion at the forum.

Key Themes

The armchair discussions clearly illustrated the challenges of educating and developing a nursing workforce that can achieve the delicate balance among advancing science, translating and applying research, caring for individuals and families across all settings, and providing leadership. The committee heard about the shortcomings of the educational pipeline and infrastructure that have resulted in a deficiency in the number of nurses completing advanced degrees and moving into faculty positions, which in turn contributes to the limited the capacity of the system. Armchair discussants offered a glimpse of the future of nursing education as they described strategies, innovative models, and technologies that are being implemented across the country to expand the capacity of the education system and to better prepare nursing graduates with the competencies and skills required to confront the challenges they will encounter in practice settings throughout their careers.

Several important points emerged from the forum:

- Collaboration, communication, and systems thinking should be the new basics in nursing education.
- Nurses, particularly nurse educators, need to keep up with a rapidly changing knowledge base and new technologies throughout their careers to ensure a well-educated workforce.
- Care for older adults, increasingly occurring outside of acute care settings, will be a large and growing component of nursing in the future, and the nursing education system needs to prepare educators and practitioners for that reality.
- The nation will face serious consequences if there are inadequate numbers of nursing educators to develop a nursing workforce adequate in both number and competencies to meet the needs of diverse populations.
- Technology—such as that used in high-fidelity simulations—that fosters problem-solving and critical thinking skills in nurses will be essential for nursing education to produce sufficient numbers of competent, well-trained nurses.
- Nursing education needs to make use of resources and partnerships available in the community to prepare nurses who can serve their communities.
- Articulation agreements and education consortiums among different kinds of institutions can provide multiple entry points and continued opportunities for progression through an educational and career ladder.
- In addition to necessary skill sets, nursing education needs to provide students with the ability to mature as professionals and to continue learning throughout their careers.

Site Visits and Solutions Session

Following the forum, committee members participated in visits to one of three sites in Houston: the University of Texas Health Science Center at Houston School of Nursing, the Texas Woman's University, or the National Aeronautics and Space Administration (NASA). During the site visits, committee members had the opportunity to converse with nursing students, educators, administrators, and experts in training for quality, safety, and collaboration about some of the innovative strategies that are being used to better educate nurses. Some of the models described included use of: distance learning and accelerated doctoral programs; advanced technology in educational settings and interdisciplinary education programs; and training for quality and safety, collaboration in a team environment, and continuing education. The site visits also offered a number of demonstrations such as a physical assessment lab using retired physicians as educators, students working in high-fidelity simulation labs, and a nurse-managed clinic.

After the completion of the forum and the site visits, a group of RWJF scholars and fellows, who had attended both activities, met to discuss possible solutions and the most promising directions for the future nursing education with respect to what should be taught, how it should be taught, and where it should be taught. A summary of this session and the solutions suggested was provided to the committee for its review and consideration at the committee's subsequent meeting in April 2010.

D

APRN Consensus Model[1]

Consensus Model for APRN Regulation: Licensure, Accreditation, Certification & Education

July 7, 2008

Completed through the work of the APRN Consensus Work Group & the National Council of State Boards of Nursing APRN Advisory Committee

The APRN Consensus Work Group and the APRN Joint Dialogue Group members would like to recognize the significant contribution to the development of this report made by Jean Johnson, PhD, RN-C, FAAN, Senior Associate Dean, Health Sciences, George Washington School of Medicine and Health Sciences. Consensus could not have been reached without her experienced and dedicated facilitation of these two national, multi-organizational groups.

LIST OF ENDORSING ORGANIZATIONS

This Final Report of the APRN Consensus Work Group and the National Council of State Boards of Nursing APRN Advisory Committee has been disseminated to participating organizations. The names of endorsing organizations will be added periodically.

The following organizations have endorsed the Consensus Model for APRN Regulation: Licensure, Accreditation, Certification, and Education (July 2008).

(Posted December 2010)
N = 48

Academy of Medical-Surgical Nurses (AMSN)
Accreditation Commission for Midwifery Education (ACME)
American Academy of Nurse Practitioners (AANP)
American Academy of Nurse Practitioners Certification Program
American Association of Colleges of Nursing (AACN)
American Association of Critical-Care Nurses (AACN)
American Association of Critical-Care Nurses Certification Corporation
American Association of Legal Nurse Consultants (AALNC)
American Association of Nurse Anesthetists (AANA)
American Board of Nursing Specialties (ABNS)
American College of Nurse-Midwives (ACNM)
American College of Nurse Practitioners (ACNP)
American Holistic Nurses Association (AHNA)
American Midwifery Certification Board (AMCB)
American Nurses Association (ANA)
American Nurses Credentialing Center (ANCC)
American Psychiatric Nurses Association (APNA)
Arkansas State Board of Nursing
Association of Faculties of Pediatric Nurse Practitioners (AFPNP)
Association of Women's Health, Obstetric, and Neonatal Nurses (AWHONN)
Commission on Collegiate Nursing Education (CCNE)
Council on Accreditation of Nurse Anesthesia Educational Programs (COA)
Dermatology Nurses Association (DNA)
Dermatology Nursing Certification Board (DNCB)
Emergency Nurses Association (ENA)
Gerontological Advanced Practice Nurses Association (GAPNA)
Hospice and Palliative Nurses Association (HPNA)
The International Society of Psychiatric Nurses (ISPN)
National Association of Clinical Nurse Specialists (NACNS)
National Association of Neonatal Nurses (NANN)

National Association of Orthopedic Nurses (NAON)
National Association of Pediatric Nurse Practitioners (NAPNAP)
National Board for Certification of Hospice and Palliative Nurses (NBCHPN)
National Board on Certification & Recertification of Nurse Anesthetists (NBCRNA)
National Certification Corporation (NCC)
National Council of State Boards of Nursing (NCSBN)
National Gerontological Nursing Association (NGNA)
National League for Nursing (NLN)
National League for Nursing Accrediting Commission, Inc. (NLNAC)
National Organization of Nurse Practitioner Faculties (NONPF)
Nurse Practitioners in Women's Health (NPWH)
Nurses Organization of Veterans Affairs (NOVA)
Oncology Nursing Certification Corporation (ONCC)
Oncology Nursing Society (ONS)
Orthopedic Nurses Certification Board (ONCB)
Pediatric Nursing Certification Board (PNCB)
Wound, Ostomy and Continence Nurses Society (WOCN)
Wound, Ostomy and Continence Nursing Certification Board (WOCNCB)

INTRODUCTION

Advanced Practice Registered Nurses (APRNs) have expanded in numbers and capabilities over the past several decades with APRNs being highly valued and an integral part of the health care system. Because of the importance of APRNs in caring for the current and future health needs of patients, the education, accreditation, certification and licensure of APRNs need to be effectively aligned in order to continue to ensure patient safety while expanding patient access to APRNs.

APRNs include certified registered nurse anesthetists, certified nurse-midwives, clinical nurse specialists and certified nurse practitioners. Each has a unique history and context, but shares the commonality of being APRNs. While education, accreditation, and certification are necessary components of an overall approach to preparing an APRN for practice, the licensing boards-governed by state regulations and statutes-are the final arbiters of who is recognized to practice within a given state. Currently, there is no uniform model of regulation of APRNs across the states. Each state independently determines the APRN legal scope of practice, the roles that are recognized, the criteria for entry-into advanced practice and the certification examinations accepted for entry-level competence assessment. This has created a significant barrier for APRNs to easily move from state to state and has decreased access to care for patients.

Many nurses with advanced graduate nursing preparation practice in roles and specialties (e.g., informatics, public health, education, or administration) that are essential to advance the health of the public but do not focus on direct care to individuals and, therefore, their practice does not require regulatory recognition beyond the Registered Nurse license granted by state boards of nursing. Like the four current APRN roles, practice in these other advanced specialty nursing roles requires specialized knowledge and skills acquired through graduate-level education. Although extremely important to the nursing profession and to the delivery of safe, high quality patient care, these other advanced, graduate nursing roles, which do not focus on direct patient care, are not roles for Advanced Practice Registered Nurses (APRN) and are not the subject or focus of the Regulatory Model presented in this paper.

The model for APRN regulation is the product of substantial work conducted by the Advanced Practice Nursing Consensus Work Group and the National Council of State Boards of Nursing (NCSBN) APRN Committee. While these groups began work independent of each other, they came together through representatives of each group participating in what was labeled the APRN Joint Dialogue Group. The outcome of this work has been unanimous agreement on most of the recommendations included in this document. In a few instances, when agreement was not unanimous a 66 percent majority was used to determine the final recommendation. However, extensive dialogue and transparency in the decision-making process is reflected in each recommendation. The background of each group can be found on pages 13-16 and individual and organizational participants in each group in Appendices C-H.

This document defines APRN practice, describes the APRN regulatory model, identifies the titles to be used, defines specialty, describes the emergence of new roles and population foci, and presents strategies for implementation.

Overview of APRN Model of Regulation

The APRN Model of Regulation described will be the model of the future. It is recognized that current regulation of APRNs does not reflect all of the components described in this paper and will evolve incrementally over time. A proposed timeline for implementation is presented at the end of the paper.

In this APRN model of regulation there are four roles: certified registered nurse anesthetist (CRNA), certified nurse-midwife (CNM), clinical nurse specialist (CNS), and certified nurse practitioner (CNP). These four roles are given the title of advanced practice registered nurse (APRN). APRNs are educated in one of the four roles and in at least one of six population foci: family/individual across the lifespan, adult-gerontology, pediatrics, neonatal, women's health/gender-related or psych/mental health. APRN education programs, including degree-granting and post-graduate education programs[2], are accredited. APRN education consists of a broad-based education, including three separate graduate-level courses in advanced physiology/pathophysiology, health assessment and pharmacology as well as appropriate clinical experiences. All developing APRN education programs or tracks go through a pre-approval, pre-accreditation, or accreditation process prior to admitting students. APRN education programs must be housed within graduate programs that are nationally accredited[3] and their graduates must be eligible for national certification used for state licensure.

Individuals who have the appropriate education will sit for a certification examination to assess national competencies of the APRN core, role and at least one population focus area of practice for regulatory purposes. APRN certification programs will be accredited by a national certification accrediting body[4]. APRN certification programs will require a continued competency mechanism.

Individuals will be licensed as independent practitioners for practice at

---

[2] Degree granting programs include master's and doctoral programs. Post-graduate programs include both post-master's and post-doctoral certificate education programs.

[3] APRN education programs must be accredited by a nursing accrediting organization that is recognized by the U.S. Department of Education (USDE) and/or the Council for Higher Education Accreditation (CHEA), including the Commission on Collegiate Nursing Education (CCNE), National League for Nursing Accrediting Commission (NLNAC), Council on Accreditation of Nurse Anesthesia Educational Programs (COA), Accreditation Commission for Midwifery Education (ACME), and the National Association of Nurse Practitioners in Women's Health Council on Accreditation.

[4] The certification program should be nationally accredited by the American Board of Nursing Specialties (ABNS) or the National Commission for Certifying Agencies (NCCA).

the level of one of the four APRN roles within at least one of the six identified population foci. Education, certification, and licensure of an individual must be congruent in terms of role and population foci. APRNs may specialize but they cannot be licensed solely within a specialty area. In addition, specialties can provide depth in one's practice within the established population foci. Education and assessment strategies for specialty areas will be developed by the nursing profession, i.e., nursing organizations and special interest groups. Education for a specialty can occur concurrently with APRN education required for licensure or through post-graduate education. Competence at the specialty level will not be assessed or regulated by boards of nursing but rather by the professional organizations.

In addition, a mechanism that enhances the communication and transparency among APRN licensure, accreditation, certification and education bodies (LACE) will be developed and supported.

APRN REGULATORY MODEL

APRN Regulation includes the essential elements: licensure, accreditation, certification and education (LACE).

- Licensure is the granting of authority to practice.
- Accreditation is the formal review and approval by a recognized agency of educational degree or certification programs in nursing or nursing-related programs.
- Certification is the formal recognition of the knowledge, skills, and experience demonstrated by the achievement of standards identified by the profession.
- Education is the formal preparation of APRNs in graduate degree-granting or post-graduate certificate programs.

The APRN Regulatory Model applies to all elements of LACE. Each of these elements plays an essential part in the implementation of the model.

Definition of Advanced Practice Registered Nurse

Characteristics of the advanced practice registered nurse (APRN) were identified and several definitions of an APRN were considered, including the NCSBN and the American Nurses Association (ANA) definitions, as well as others. The characteristics identified aligned closely with these existing definitions. The definition of an APRN, delineated in this document, includes language that addresses responsibility and accountability for health promotion and the assessment, diagnosis, and management of patient problems, which includes the use and prescription of pharmacologic and non-pharmacologic interventions.

The definition of an Advanced Practice Registered Nurse (APRN) is a nurse:

1. who has completed an accredited graduate-level education program preparing him/her for one of the four recognized APRN roles;
2. who has passed a national certification examination that measures APRN, role and population-focused competencies and who maintains continued competence as evidenced by recertification in the role and population through the national certification program;
3. who has acquired advanced clinical knowledge and skills preparing him/her to provide direct care to patients, as well as a component of indirect care; however, the defining factor for all APRNs is that a significant component of the education and practice focuses on direct care of individuals;
4. whose practice builds on the competencies of registered nurses (RNs) by demonstrating a greater depth and breadth of knowledge, a greater synthesis of data, increased complexity of skills and interventions, and greater role autonomy;
5. who is educationally prepared to assume responsibility and accountability for health promotion and/or maintenance as well as the assessment, diagnosis, and management of patient problems, which includes the use and prescription of pharmacologic and non-pharmacologic interventions;
6. who has clinical experience of sufficient depth and breadth to reflect the intended license; and
7. who has obtained a license to practice as an APRN in one of the four APRN roles: certified registered nurse anesthetist (CRNA), certified nurse-midwife (CNM), clinical nurse specialist (CNS), or certified nurse practitioner (CNP).

Advanced practice registered nurses are licensed independent practitioners who are expected to practice within standards established or recognized by a licensing body. Each APRN is accountable to patients, the nursing profession, and the licensing board to comply with the requirements of the state nurse practice act and the quality of advanced nursing care rendered; for recognizing limits of knowledge and experience, planning for the management of situations beyond the APRN's expertise; and for consulting with or referring patients to other health care providers as appropriate.

All APRNs are educationally prepared to provide a scope of services across the health wellness-illness continuum to at least one population focus as defined by nationally recognized role and population-focused competencies; however, the emphasis and implementation within each APRN role varies. The services or care provided by APRNs is not defined or limited by setting but rather by patient care needs. The continuum encompasses the range of health states from homeostasis (or wellness) to a disruption in the state of health in which basic needs are not met or maintained (illness), with health problems of varying acuity occurring along the continuum that must be prevented or resolved to maintain wellness or an optimal level of functioning (WHO, 2006). Although all APRNs are educationally prepared to provide care to patients across the health wellness-illness continuum, the emphasis and how implemented within each APRN role varies.

The Certified Registered Nurse Anesthetist

The Certified Registered Nurse Anesthetist is prepared to provide the full spectrum of patients' anesthesia care and anesthesia-related care for individuals across the lifespan, whose health status may range from healthy through all recognized levels of acuity, including persons with immediate, severe, or life-threatening illnesses or injury. This care is provided in diverse settings, including hospital surgical suites and obstetrical delivery rooms; critical access hospitals; acute care; pain management centers; ambulatory surgical centers; and the offices of dentists, podiatrists, ophthalmologists, and plastic surgeons.

The Certified Nurse-Midwife

The certified nurse-midwife provides a full range of primary health care services to women throughout the lifespan, including gynecologic care, family planning services, preconception care, prenatal and postpartum care, childbirth, and care of the newborn. The practice includes treating the male partner of their female clients for sexually transmitted disease and reproductive health. This care is provided in diverse settings, which may include home, hospital, birth center, and a variety of ambulatory care settings including private offices and community and public health clinics.

The Clinical Nurse Specialist

The CNS has a unique APRN role to integrate care across the continuum and through three spheres of influence: patient, nurse, system. The three spheres are overlapping and interrelated but each sphere possesses a distinctive focus. In each of the spheres of influence, the primary goal of the CNS is continuous improvement of patient outcomes and nursing care. Key elements of CNS practice are to create environments through mentoring and system changes that empower nurses to develop caring, evidence-based practices to alleviate patient distress, facilitate ethical decision-making, and respond to diversity. The CNS is responsible and accountable for diagnosis and treatment of health/illness states, disease management, health promotion, and prevention of illness and risk behaviors among individuals, families, groups, and communities.

The Certified Nurse Practitioner

For the certified nurse practitioner (CNP), care along the wellness-illness continuum is a dynamic process in which direct primary and acute care is provided across settings. CNPs are members of the health delivery system, practicing autonomously in areas as diverse as family practice, pediatrics, internal medicine, geriatrics, and women's health care. CNPs are prepared to diagnose and treat patients with undifferentiated symptoms as well as those with established diagnoses. Both primary and acute care CNPs provide initial, ongoing, and comprehensive care, includes taking comprehensive histories, providing physical examinations and other health assessment and screening activities, and diagnosing, treating, and managing patients with acute and chronic illnesses and diseases. This includes ordering, performing, supervising, and interpreting laboratory and imaging studies; prescribing medication and durable medical equipment; and making appropriate referrals for patients and families. Clinical CNP care includes health promotion, disease prevention, health education, and counseling as well as the diagnosis and management of acute and chronic diseases. Certified nurse practitioners are prepared to practice as primary care CNPs and acute care CNPs, which have separate national consensus-based competencies and separate certification processes.

Titling

The title Advanced Practice Registered Nurse (APRN) is the licensing title to be used for the subset of nurses prepared with advanced, graduate-level nursing knowledge to provide direct patient care in four roles: certified registered nurse anesthetist, certified nurse-midwife, clinical nurse specialist, and certified nurse practitioner.[5] This title, APRN, is a legally protected title. Licensure and scope of practice are based on graduate education in one of the four roles and in a defined population.

Verification of licensure, whether hard copy or electronic, will indicate the role and population for which the APRN has been licensed.

At a minimum, an individual must legally represent themselves, including in a legal signature, as an APRN and by the role. He/she may indicate the population as well. No one, except those who are licensed to practice as an APRN, may use the APRN title or any of the APRN role titles. An individual also may add the specialty title in which they are professionally recognized in addition to the legal title of APRN and role.

---

[5] Nurses with advanced graduate nursing preparation practicing in roles and specialties that do not provide direct care to individuals and, therefore, whose practice does not require regulatory recognition beyond the Registered Nurse license granted by state boards of nursing may not use any term or title which may confuse the public, including advanced practice nurse or advanced practice registered nurse. The term "advanced public health nursing" however, may be used to identify nurses practicing in this advanced specialty area of nursing.

APRN REGULATORY MODEL

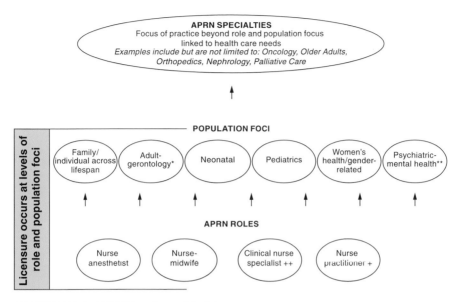

FIGURE D-1 APRN Regulatory Model

Under this APRN Regulatory Model, there are four roles: certified registered nurse anes-thetist (CRNA), certified nurse-midwife (CNM), clinical nurse specialist (CNS), and certified nurse practitioner (CNP). These four roles are given the title of advanced practice registered nurse (APRN). APRNs are educated in one of the four roles and in at least one of six population foci: family/individual across the lifespan, adult-gerontology, neonatal, pediatrics, women's health/gender-related or psych/mental health. Individuals will be licensed as independent practitioners for practice at the level of one of the four APRN roles within at least one of the six identified population foci. Education, certification, and licensure of an individual must be congruent in terms of role and population foci. APRNs may specialize but they can not be licensed solely within a specialty area. Specialties can provide depth in one's practice within the established population foci.

NOTES:

* The population focus, adult-gerontology, encompasses the young adult to the older adult, including the frail elderly. APRNs educated and certified in the adult-gerontol-ogy population are educated and certified across both areas of practice and will be titled Adult-Gerontology CNP or CNS. In addition, all APRNs in any of the four roles providing care to the adult population, e.g., family or gender specific, must be prepared to meet the growing needs of the older adult population. Therefore, the education program should include didactic and clinical education experiences necessary to prepare APRNs with these enhanced skills and knowledge.

** The population focus, psychiatric/mental health, encompasses education and practice across the lifespan.

+The certified nurse practitioner (CNP) is prepared with the acute care CNP competen-cies and/or the primary care CNP competencies. At this point in time the acute care and primary care CNP delineation applies only to the pediatric and adult-gerontology CNP population foci. Scope of practice of the primary care or acute care CNP is not setting specific but is based on patient care needs. Programs may prepare individuals across both the primary care and acute care CNP competencies. If programs prepare graduates across both sets of roles, the graduate must be prepared with the consensus-based competencies for both roles and must successfully obtain certification in both the acute and the primary care CNP roles. CNP certification in the acute care or primary care roles must match the educational preparation for CNPs in these roles.

++ The Clinical Nurse Specialist (CNS) is educated and assessed through national certification processes across the continuum from wellness through acute care.

Broad-Based APRN Education

For entry into APRN practice and for regulatory purposes, APRN education must:

- be formal education with a graduate degree or post-graduate certificate (either post-master's or post-doctoral) that is awarded by an academic institution and accredited by a nursing or nursing-related accrediting organization recognized by the U.S. Department of Education (USDE) and/or the Council for Higher Education Accreditation (CHEA);
- be awarded pre-approval, pre-accreditation, or accreditation status prior to admitting students;
- be comprehensive and at the graduate level;
- prepare the graduate to practice in one of the four identified APRN roles;
- prepare the graduate with the core competencies for one of the APRN roles across at least one of the six population foci;
- include at a minimum, three separate comprehensive graduate-level courses (the APRN Core) in:
  - Advanced physiology/pathophysiology, including general principles that apply across the lifespan;
  - Advanced health assessment, which includes assessment of all human systems, advanced assessment techniques, concepts and approaches; and
  - Advanced pharmacology, which includes pharmacodynamics, pharmacokinetics and pharmacotherapeutics of all broad categories of agents.
- Additional content, specific to the role and population, in these three APRN core areas should be integrated throughout the other role and population didactic and clinical courses;
- Provide a basic understanding of the principles for decision making in the identified role;

- Prepare the graduate to assume responsibility and accountability for health promotion and/or maintenance as well as the assessment, diagnosis, and management of patient problems, which includes the use and prescription of pharmacologic and non-pharmacologic interventions; and
- Ensure clinical and didactic coursework is comprehensive and sufficient to prepare the graduate to practice in the APRN role and population focus.

Preparation in a specialty area of practice is optional but if included must build on the APRN role/population-focus competencies. Clinical and didactic coursework must be comprehensive and sufficient to prepare the graduate to obtain certification for licensure in and to practice in the APRN role and population focus.

As part of the accreditation process, all APRN education programs must undergo a pre-approval, pre-accreditation, or accreditation process prior to admitting students. The purpose of the pre-approval process is twofold: 1) to ensure that students graduating from the program will be able to meet the education criteria necessary for national certification in the role and population-focus and if successfully certified, are eligible for licensure to practice in the APRN role/population-focus; and 2) to ensure that programs will meet all educational standards prior to starting the program. The pre-approval, pre-accreditation or accreditation processes may vary across APRN roles.

APRN Specialties

Preparation in a specialty area of practice is optional, but if included must build on the APRN role/population-focused competencies. Specialty practice represents a much more focused area of preparation and practice than does the APRN role/population focus level. Specialty practice may focus on specific patient populations beyond those identified or health care needs such as oncology, palliative care, substance abuse, or nephrology. The criteria for defining an APRN specialty is built upon the ANA (2004) Criteria for Recognition as a Nursing Specialty (see Appendix B). APRN specialty education and practice build upon and are in addition to the education and practice of the APRN role and population focus. For example, a family CNP could specialize in elder care or nephrology; an Adult-Gerontology CNS could specialize in palliative care; a CRNA could specialize in pain management; or a CNM could specialize in care of the post-menopausal woman. State licensing boards will not regulate the APRN at the level of specialties in this APRN Regulatory Model. Professional certification in the specialty area of practice is strongly recommended.

An APRN specialty

- preparation cannot replace educational preparation in the role or one of the six population foci;
- preparation can not expand one's scope of practice beyond the role or population focus
- addresses a subset of the population-focus;
- title may not be used in lieu of the licensing title, which includes the role or role/population; and
- is developed, recognized, and monitored by the profession.

New specialties emerge based on health needs of the population. APRN specialties develop to provide added value to the role practice as well as providing flexibility within the profession to meet these emerging needs of patients. Specialties also may cross several or all APRN roles. A specialty evolves out of an APRN role/population focus and indicates that an APRN has additional knowledge and expertise in a more discrete area of specialty practice. Competency in the specialty areas could be acquired either by educational preparation or experience and assessed in a variety of ways through professional credentialing mechanisms (e.g., portfolios, examinations, etc.).

Education programs may concurrently prepare individuals in a specialty providing they meet all of the other requirements for APRN education programs, including preparation in the APRN core, role, and population core competencies. In addition, for licensure purposes, one exam must assess the APRN core, role, and population-focused competencies. For example, a nurse anesthetist would write one certification examination, which tests the APRN core, CRNA role, and population-focused competencies, administered by the Council on Certification for Nurse Anesthetist; or a primary care family nurse practitioner would write one certification examination, which tests the APRN core, CNP role, and family population-focused competencies, administered by ANCC or AANP. Specialty competencies must be assessed separately. In summary, education programs preparing individuals with this additional knowledge in a specialty, if used for entry into advanced practice registered nursing and for regulatory purposes, must also prepare individuals in one of the four nationally recognized APRN roles and in one of the six population foci. Individuals must be recognized and credentialed in one of the four APRN roles within at least one population foci. APRNs are licensed at the role/population focus level and not at the specialty level. However, if not intended for entry-level preparation in one of the four roles/population foci and not for regulatory purposes, education programs, using a variety of formats and methodologies, may provide licensed APRNs with the additional knowledge, skills, and abilities, to become professionally certified in the specialty area of APRN practice.

Emergence of New APRN Roles and Population-Foci

As nursing practice evolves and health care needs of the population change, new APRN roles or population-foci may evolve over time. An APRN role would encompass a unique or significantly differentiated set of competencies from any of the other APRN roles. In addition, the scope of practice within the role or population focus is not entirely subsumed within one of the other roles. Careful consideration of new APRN roles or population-foci is in the best interest of the profession.

For licensure, there must be clear guidance for national recognition of a new APRN role or population-focus. A new role or population focus should be discussed and vetted through the national licensure, accreditation, certification, education communication structure: LACE. An essential part of being recognized as a role or population-focus is that educational standards and practice competencies must exist, be consistent, and must be nationally recognized by the profession. Characteristics of the process to be used to develop nationally recognized core competencies, and education and practice standards for a newly emerging role or population-focus are:

1. national in scope
2. inclusive
3. transparent
4. accountable
5. initiated by nursing
6. consistent with national standards for licensure, accreditation, certification and education
7. evidence-based
8. consistent with regulatory principles.

To be recognized, an APRN role must meet the following criteria:

- nationally recognized education standards and core competencies for programs preparing individuals in the role;
- education programs, including graduate degree granting (master's, doctoral) and post-graduate certificate programs, are accredited by a nursing or nursing-related accrediting organization that is recognized by the U.S. Department of Education (USDE) and/or the Council for Higher Education Accreditation (CHEA); and
- professional nursing certification program that is psychometrically sound, legally defensible, and which meets nationally recognized accreditation standards for certification programs.[6]

---

[6] The professional certification program should be nationally accredited by the American Board of Nursing Specialties (ABNS) or the National Commission for Certifying Agencies (NCCA).

IMPLEMENTATION STRATEGIES FOR
APRN REGULATORY MODEL

In order to accomplish the above model, the four prongs of regulation: licensure, accreditation, certification, and education (LACE) must work together. Expectations for licensure, accreditation, certification, and education are listed below:

Foundational Requirements for Licensure

Boards of nursing will:

1. license APRNs in the categories of Certified Registered Nurse Anesthetist, Certified Nurse-Midwife, Clinical Nurse Specialist or Certified Nurse Practitioner within a specific population focus;
2. be solely responsible for licensing Advanced Practice Registered Nurses[7];
3. only license graduates of accredited graduate programs that prepare graduates with the APRN core, role and population competencies;
4. require successful completion of a national certification examination that assesses APRN core, role and population competencies for APRN licensure.
5. not issue a temporary license;
6. only license an APRN when education and certification are congruent;
7. license APRNs as independent practitioners with no regulatory requirements for collaboration, direction or supervision;
8. allow for mutual recognition of advanced practice registered nursing through the APRN Compact;
9. have at least one APRN representative position on the board and utilize an APRN advisory committee that includes representatives of all four APRN roles; and,
10. institute a grandfathering[8] clause that will exempt those APRNs already practicing in the state from new eligibility requirements.

---

[7] Except in states where state boards of nurse-midwifery or midwifery regulate nurse-midwives or nurse-midwives and midwives jointly.

[8] Grandfathering is a provision in a new law exempting those already in or a part of the existing system that is being regulated. When states adopt new eligibility requirements for APRNs, currently practicing APRNs will be permitted to continue practicing within the state(s) of their current licensure.

However, if an APRN applies for licensure by endorsement in another state, the APRN would be eligible for licensure if s/he demonstrates that the following criteria have been met:

- current, active practice in the advanced role and population focus area,
- current active, national certification or recertification, as applicable, in the advanced role and population focus area,

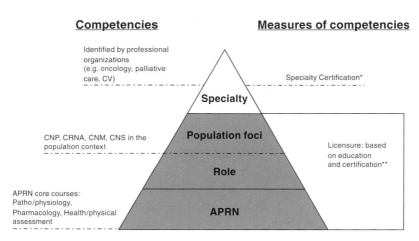

FIGURE D-2 Relationship Among Educational Competencies, Licensure, & Certification in the Role/Population Foci and Education and Credentialing in a Specialty
NOTES:
*Certification for specialty may include exam, portfolio, peer review, etc.
**Certification for licensure will be psychometrically sound and legally defensible examination by an accredited certifying program.

Foundational Requirements for Accreditation of Education Programs

Accreditors will:

1. be responsible for evaluating APRN education programs including graduate degree-granting and post-graduate certificate programs;[9]
2. through their established accreditation standards and process, assess APRN education programs in light of the APRN core, role core, and population core competencies;
3. assess developing APRN education programs and tracks by reviewing them using established accreditation standards and granting pre-approval, pre-accreditation, or accreditation prior to student enrollment;

- compliance with the APRN educational requirements of the state in which the APRN is applying for licensure that were in effect at the time the APRN completed his/her APRN education program, and
- compliance with all other criteria set forth by the state in which the APRN is applying for licensure (e.g. recent CE, RN licensure).

Once the model has been adopted and implemented (date to be determined by the state boards of nursing. See proposed timeline on page 14-15.) all new graduates applying for APRN licensure must meet the requirements outlined in this regulatory model.

[9] Degree-granting programs include both master's and doctoral programs. Post-graduate certificate programs include post-master's and post-doctoral education programs.

4. include an APRN on the visiting team when an APRN program/track is being reviewed; and

5. monitor APRN educational programs throughout the accreditation period by reviewing them using established accreditation standards and processes.

Foundational Requirements for Certification

Certification programs providing APRN certification used for licensure will:

1. follow established certification testing and psychometrically sound, legally defensible standards for APRN examinations for licensure (see appendix A for the NCSBN Criteria for APRN Certification Programs);

2. assess the APRN core and role competencies across at least one population focus of practice;

3. assess specialty competencies, if appropriate, separately from the APRN core, role and population-focused competencies;

4. be accredited by a national certification accreditation body;[10]

5. enforce congruence (role and population focus) between the education program and the type of certification examination;

6. provide a mechanism to ensure ongoing competence and maintenance of certification;

7. participate in ongoing relationships which make their processes transparent to boards of nursing;

8. participate in a mutually agreeable mechanism to ensure communication with boards of nursing and schools of nursing.

Foundational Requirements for Education

APRN education programs/tracks leading to APRN licensure, including graduate degree-granting and post-graduate certificate programs will:

1. follow established educational standards and ensure attainment of the APRN core, role core and population core competencies;[11,12]

---

[10] The certification program should be nationally accredited by the American Board of Nursing Specialties (ABNS) or the National Commission for Certifying Agencies (NCCA).

[11] The APRN core competencies for all APRN nursing education programs located in schools of nursing are delineated in the American Association of Colleges of Nursing (1996) *The Essentials of Master's Education for Advanced Practice Nursing Education* or the AACN (2006) *The Essentials of Doctoral Education for Advanced Nursing Practice*. The APRN core competencies for nurse anesthesia and nurse-midwifery education programs located outside of a school of nursing are delineated by the accrediting organizations for their respective roles i.e., Council on Accreditation of Nurse Anesthesia Educational Programs (COA), Accreditation Commission for Midwifery Education (ACME).

[12] APRN programs outside of schools of nursing must prepare graduates with the APRN core which includes three separate graduate-level courses in pathophysiology/physiology, health assessment, and pharmacology.

2. be accredited by a nursing accrediting organization that is recognized by the U.S. Department of Education (USDE) and/or the Council for Higher Education Accreditation (CHEA);[13]
3. be pre-approved, pre-accredited, or accredited prior to the acceptance of students, including all developing APRN education programs and tracks;
4. ensure that graduates of the program are eligible for national certification and state licensure; and
5. ensure that official documentation (e.g., transcript) specifies the role and population focus of the graduate.

Communication Strategies

A formal communication mechanism, LACE, which includes those regulatory organizations that represent APRN licensure, accreditation, certification, and education entities would be created. The purpose of LACE would be to provide a formal, ongoing communication mechanism that provides for transparent and aligned communication among the identified entities. The collaborative efforts between the APRN Consensus Group and the NCSBN APRN Advisory Panel, through the APRN Joint Dialogue Group have illustrated the ongoing level of communication necessary among these groups to ensure that all APRN stakeholders are involved. Several strategies including equal representation on an integrated board with face-to-face meetings, audio and teleconferencing, pass-protected access to agency web sites, and regular reporting mechanisms have been recommended. These strategies will build trust and enhance information sharing. Examples of issues to be addressed by the group would be: guaranteeing appropriate representation of APRN roles among accreditation site visitors, documentation of program completion by education institutions, notification of examination outcomes to educators and regulators, notification of disciplinary action toward licensees by boards of nursing.

Creating the LACE Structure and Processes

Several principles should guide the formulation of a structure including: 1) all four entities of LACE should have representation; 2) the total should allow effective discussion of and response to issues and; 3) the structure should not be duplicative of existing structures such as the Alliance for APRN Credentialing. Consideration should be given to evolving the existing Alliance structure to meet the needs of LACE. Guidance from an organizational consultant will be useful in

---

[13] APRN education programs must be accredited by a nursing accrediting organization that is recognized by the U.S. Department of Education (USDE) and/or the Council for Higher Education Accreditation (CHEA), including the Commission on Collegiate Nursing Education (CCNE), National League for Nursing Accrediting Commission (NLNAC), Council on Accreditation of Nurse Anesthesia Educational Programs (COA), Accreditation Commission for Midwifery Education (ACME), and the National Association of Nurse Practitioners in Women's Health Council on Accreditation.

forming a permanent structure that will endure and support the work that needs to continue. The new structure will support fair decision-making among all relevant stakeholders. In addition, the new structure will be in place as soon as possible.

The LACE organizational structure should include representation of:

- State licensing boards, including at least one compact and one non-compact state;
- Accrediting bodies that accredit education programs of the four APRN roles;
- Certifying bodies that offer APRN certification used for regulatory purposes; and,
- Education organizations that set standards for APRN education.

Timeline for Implementation of Regulatory Model

Implementation of the recommendations for an APRN Regulatory Model will occur incrementally. Due to the interdependence of licensure, accreditation, certification, and education, certain recommendations will be implemented sequentially. However, recognizing that this model was developed through a consensus process with participation of APRN certifiers, accreditors, public regulators, educators, and employers, it is expected that the recommendations and model delineated will inform decisions made by each of these entities as the APRN community moves to fully implement the APRN Regulatory Model. A target date for full implementation of the Regulatory Model and all embedded recommendations is the Year 2015.

HISTORICAL BACKGROUND

NCSBN APRN Committee (previously APRN Advisory Panel)

NCSBN became involved with advanced practice nursing when boards of nursing began using the results of APRN certification examinations as one of the requirements for APRN licensure. During the 1993 NCSBN annual meeting, delegates adopted a position paper on the licensure of advanced nursing practice which included model legislation language and model administrative rules for advanced nursing practice. NCSBN core competencies for certified nurse practitioners were adopted the following year.

In 1995, NCSBN was directed by the Delegate Assembly to work with APRN certifiers to make certification examinations suitable for regulatory purposes. Since then, much effort has been made toward that purpose. During the mid and late 90's, the APRN certifiers agreed to undergo accreditation and provide additional information to boards of nursing to ensure that their examinations were psychometrically sound and legally defensible (NCSBN, 1998).

During the early 2000s, the APRN Advisory Panel developed criteria for ARPN certification programs and for accreditations agencies. In January 2002, the board of directors approved the criteria and process for a new review process for APRN certification programs. The criteria represented required elements of certification programs that would result in a legally defensible examination suitable for the regulation of advanced practice nurses. Subsequently, the APRN Advisory Panel has worked with certification programs to improve the legal defensibility of APRN certification examinations and to promote communication with all APRN stakeholders regarding APRN regulatory issues such as with the establishment of the annual NCSBN APRN Roundtable in the mid 1990's. In 2002, the Advisory Panel also developed a position paper describing APRN regulatory issues of concern.

In 2003, the APRN Advisory Panel began a draft APRN vision paper in an attempt to resolve APRN regulatory concerns such as the proliferation of APRN subspecialty areas. The purpose of the APRN Vision Paper was to provide direction to boards of nursing regarding APRN regulation for the next 8-10 years by identifying an ideal future APRN regulatory model. Eight recommendations were made. The draft vision paper was completed in 2006. After reviewing the draft APRN vision paper at their February 2006 board meeting, the board of directors directed that the paper be disseminated to boards of nursing and APRN stakeholders for feedback. The Vision paper also was discussed during the 2006 APRN Roundtable. The large response from boards of nursing and APRN stakeholders was varied. The APRN Advisory Panel spent the remaining part of 2006, reviewing and discussing the feedback with APRN stakeholders. (See Appendix C for the list of APRN Advisory Panel members who worked on the draft APRN Vision Paper and Appendix D for the list of organizations represented at the 2006 APRN Roundtable where the draft vision paper was presented.)

APRN Consensus Group

In March 2004, the American Association of Colleges of Nursing (AACN) and the National Organization of Nurse Practitioner Faculties (NONPF) submitted a proposal to the Alliance for Nursing Accreditation, now named Alliance for APRN Credentialing[14] (hereafter referred to as "the APRN Alliance") to establish a process to develop a consensus[15] statement on the credentialing of advanced

---

[14] At its March 2006 meeting, the Alliance for Nursing Accreditation voted to change its name to the Alliance for APRN Credentialing which more accurately reflects its membership.

[15] The goal of the APRN Work Group was unanimous agreement on all issues and recommendations. However, this was recognized as an unrealistic expectation and may delay the process; therefore, consensus was defined as a two thirds majority agreement by those members of the Work Group present at the table as organizational representatives with each participating organization having one vote.

practice nurses (APNs).[16] The APRN Alliance[17], created in 1997, was convened by AACN to regularly discuss issues related to nursing education, practice, and credentialing. A number of differing views on how APN practice is defined, what constitutes specialization versus subspecialization, and the appropriate credentialing requirements that would authorize practice had emerged over the past several years.

An invitation to participate in a national APN consensus process was sent to 50 organizations that were identified as having an interest in advanced practice nursing (see Appendix F). Thirty-two organizations participated in the APN Consensus Conference in Washington, D.C. June 2004. The focus of the one-day meeting was to initiate an in-depth examination of issues related to APN definition, specialization, sub-specialization, and regulation, which includes accreditation, education, certification, and licensure[18]. Based on recommendations generated in the June 2004 APN Consensus Conference, the Alliance formed a smaller work group made up of designees from 23 organizations with broad representation of APN certification, licensure, education, accreditation, and practice. The charge to the work group was to develop a statement that addresses the issues, delineated during the APN Consensus Conference with the goal of envisioning a future model for APNs. The Alliance APN Consensus Work Group (hereafter referred to as "the Work Group") convened for 16 days of intensive discussion between October 2004 and July 2007 (see Appendix H for a list of organizations represented on the APN Work Group).

In December 2004, the American Nurses Association (ANA) and AACN co-hosted an APN stakeholder meeting to address those issues identified at the June 2004 APN Consensus meeting. Attendees agreed to ask the APN Work Group to continue to craft a consensus statement that would include recommendations regarding APN regulation, specialization, and subspecialization. It also was agreed that organizations in attendance who had not participated in the June 2004 APN Consensus meeting would be included in the APN Consensus Group and that this

---

[16] The term advanced practice nurse (APN) was initially used by the Work Group and is used in this section of the report to accurately reflect the background discussion. However, the Work group reached consensus that the term advanced practice registered nurse (APRN) should be adopted for use in subsequent discussions and documents.

[17] Organizational members of the Alliance for APRN Credentialing : American Academy of Nurse Practitioners Certification Program, American Association of Colleges of Nursing, American Association of Critical-Care Nurses Certification Corporation, Council on Accreditation of Nurse Anesthesia Educational Programs, American College of Nurse-Midwives, American Nurses Credentialing Center, Association of Faculties of Pediatric Nurse Practitioners, Inc., Commission on Collegiate Nursing Education, National Association of Clinical Nurse Specialists, National Association of Nurse Practitioners in Women's Health, Council on Accreditation, Pediatric Nursing Certification Board, The National Certification Corporation for the Obstetric Gynecologic and Neonatal Nursing Specialties, National Council of State Boards of Nursing, National Organization of Nurse Practitioner Faculties

[18] The term regulation refers to the four prongs of regulation: licensure, accreditation, certification and education.

larger group would reconvene at a future date to discuss the recommendations of the APN Work Group.

Following the December 2004 APN Consensus meeting, the Work Group continued to work diligently to reach consensus on the issues surrounding APRN education, practice, accreditation, certification, and licensure, and to create a future consensus-based model for APRN regulation. Subsequent APRN Consensus Group meetings were held in September 2005 and June 2006. All organizations who participated in the APRN Consensus Group are listed in Appendix G.

APRN Joint Dialogue Group

In April, 2006, the APRN Advisory Panel met with the APRN Consensus Work Group to discuss APRN issues described in the NCSBN draft vision paper. The APRN Consensus Work Group requested and was provided with feedback from the APRN Advisory Panel regarding the APRN Consensus Group Report. Both groups agreed to continue to dialogue.

As the APRN Advisory Panel and APRN Consensus Work Group continued their work in parallel fashion, concerns regarding the need for each group's work not to conflict with the other were expressed. A subgroup of seven people from the APRN Consensus Work Group and seven individuals from the APRN Advisory Panel were convened in January, 2007. The group called itself the APRN Joint Dialogue Group (see Appendix E) and the agenda consisted of discussing areas of agreement and disagreement between the two groups. The goal of the subgroup meetings was anticipated to be two papers that did not conflict, but rather complemented each other. However, as the APRN Joint Dialogue Group continued to meet, much progress was made regarding areas of agreement; it was determined that rather than two papers being disseminated, one joint paper would be developed, which reflected the work of both groups. This document is the product of the work of the APRN Joint Dialogue Group and through the consensus-based work of the APRN Consensus Work Group and the NCSBN APRN Advisory Committee.

Assumptions Underlying the Work of the Joint Dialogue Group

The consensus-based recommendations that have emerged from the extensive dialogue and consensus-based processes delineated in this report are based on the following assumptions:

- Recommendations must address current issues facing the advanced practice registered nurse (APRN) community but should be future oriented.
- The ultimate goal of licensure, accreditation, certification, and education is to promote patient safety and public protection.

- The recognition that this document was developed with the participation of APRN certifiers, accreditors, public regulators, educators, and employers. The intention is that the document will allow for informed decisions made by each of these entities as they address APRN issues.

CONCLUSION

The recommendations offered in this paper present an APRN regulatory model as a collaborative effort among APRN educators, accreditors, certifiers, and licensure bodies. The essential elements of APRN regulation are identified as licensure, accreditation, certification, and education. The recommendations reflect a need and desire to collaborate among regulatory bodies to achieve a sound model and continued communication with the goal of increasing the clarity and uniformity of APRN regulation.

The goals of the consensus processes were to:

- strive for harmony and common understanding in the APRN regulatory community that would continue to promote quality APRN education and practice;
- develop a vision for APRN regulation, including education, accreditation, certification, and licensure;
- establish a set of standards that protect the public, improve mobility, and improve access to safe, quality APRN care; and
- produce a written statement that reflects consensus on APRN regulatory issues.

In summary, this report includes: a definition of the APRN Regulatory Model, including a definition of the Advanced Practice Registered Nurse; a definition of broad-based APRN education; a model for regulation that ensures APRN education and certification as a valid and reliable process, that is based on nationally recognized and accepted standards; uniform recommendations for licensing bodies across states; a process and characteristics for recognizing a new APRN role; and a definition of an APRN specialty that allows for the profession to meet future patient and nursing needs.

The work of the Joint Dialogue Group in conjunction with all organizations representing APRN licensure, accreditation, certification, and education to advance a regulatory model is an ongoing collaborative process that is fluid and dynamic. As health care evolves and new standards and needs emerge, the APRN Regulatory Model will advance accordingly to allow APRNs to care for patients in a safe environment to the full potential of their nursing knowledge and skill.

REFERENCES

American Association of Colleges of Nursing. (1996). *The Essentials of Master's Education for Advanced Practice Nursing Education.* Washington, DC: Author.

American Association of Colleges of Nursing. (2004). *Position Statement on the Practice Doctorate in Nursing.* Washington, DC: Author. Accessed at http://www.aacn.nche.edu/DNP/DNPPositionStatement.htm.

American Association of Colleges of Nursing. (2006). *The Essentials of Doctoral Education for Advanced Nursing Practice.* Washington, DC: Author.

American College of Nurse-Midwives (2002). Core Competencies for Basic Midwifery Practice. Accessed at http://www.midwife.org/display.cfm?id=137.

American Educational Research Association, American Psychological Association and National Council on Measurement in Education (2002). "Professional and Occupational Licensure and Certification: Standards for Educational and Psychological Testing, Washington, DC: American Psychological Association, Inc.

American Nurses Association. (2004). *Nursing: Scope and Standards of Practice.* Washington, DC: Author.

Association of Women's Health, Obstetric and Neonatal Nurses & National Association of Nurse Practitioners Women's Health (2002). *The Women's Health Nurse Practitioner: Guidelines for Practice and Education, 5th edition.* Washington, DC: Author.

Atkinson, Dale J. (2000). Legal issues in Licensure Policy. In Schoon, Craig, & Smith I. Lion (eds.) *The Licensure and Certification Mission: Legal, Social, and Political Foundations. Professional Examination Service.* New York.

Bauer, Jeffrey. (1998). *Not What the Doctor Ordered: How to End the Medical Monopoly in the Pursuit of Managed Care 2nd ed.* McGraw-Hill Companies: New York.

Citizen Advocacy Center (2004). *Maintaining and Improving Health Professional Competence; Roadway to Continuing Competency Assurance.*

Council on Accreditation of Nurse Anesthesia Educational Programs. (2004). *Standards for Accreditation of Nurse Anesthesia Educational Programs.* Chicago: Author.

Finocchio, L.J., Dower, C.M., Blick N.T., Gragnola, C.M., & The Taskforce on Health Care Workforce Regulation. (1998). *Strengthening Consumer Protection: Priorities for Health Care Workforce Regulation.* San Francisco, CA: Pew Health Professions Commission.

Hamric, Ann B. & Hanson, Charlene (2003). Educating Advanced Practice Nurses for Practice Reality. *Journal of Professional Nursing, 19,* No 5 (September-October) 262-268.

Hanson, C. & Hamric, Ann. (2003). Reflections on the continuing Evolution of Advanced Practice Nursing. *Nursing Outlook. 51.* No. 5 (September/October) 203-211.

Institute of Medicine (2003). *Health Professions Education: A Bridge to Quality.* Board on Health Care Services.

Kaplan, Louise, & Brown, Marie-Annette (2004). Prescriptive Authority and Barriers to NP Practice. *The Nurse Practitioner, 29,* No. 33, 28-35.

Marion, Lucy, et al. (2003). The Practice Doctorate in Nursing: Future or Fringe. *Topics in Advanced Practice Nursing eJournal 3*(2).2003 @ 2003 Medscape.

National Association of Clinical Nurse Specialists (2003). *Statement on Clinical Nurse Specialist Practice.*

National Council of State Boards of Nursing (1993). *Regulation of Advanced Practice Nursing: 1993 National Council of State Boards of Nursing Position Paper.* Chicago: Author.

National Council of State Boards of Nursing (1997). *The National Council of State Boards of Nursing Position Paper on Approval and Accreditation: Definition and Usage.* Chicago: Author.

National Council of State Boards of Nursing (1998). *Using Nurse Practitioner Certification for State Nursing Regulation: A Historical Perspective.* Chicago: Author.

National Council of State Boards of Nursing (2001). *Advanced Practice Registered Nurse Compact.* Chicago: Author.

National Council of State Boards of Nursing (2002). *Regulation of Advanced Practice Nursing: 2002 National Council of State Boards of Nursing Position Paper.* Chicago: Author.

National Council of State Boards of Nursing (2002). *Uniform Advanced Practice Registered Nurse Licensure/Authority to Practice Requirements.* Chicago: Author.

National Council of State Boards of Nursing. (2002). *Regulation of Advanced Practice Nursing.* Printed from http://www.ncsbn.org. Chicago, IL: Author.

National Organization of Nurse Practitioner Faculties. (2000). *Domains and Competencies of Nurse Practitioner Practice.* Washington, DC: Author.

National Panel for Acute Care Nurse Practitioner Competencies. (2004). *Acute Care Nurse Practitioner Competencies.* Washington, DC: NONPF

National Panel for Psychiatric-Mental Health NP Competencies. (2003). *Psychiatric-Mental Health Nurse Practitioner Competencies.* Washington, DC: NONPF

National Task Force on Quality Nurse Practitioner Education. (2002). *Criteria for Evaluation of Nurse Practitioner Programs.* Washington, DC: NONPF

Pew Health Professions Commission (1995). *Critical Challenges: Revitalizing The Health Professions for the Twenty-First Century.* National Academies Press, Washington, D.C.

Safriet, Barbara J. "Health Care Dollars & Regulatory Sense: The Role of Advanced Practice Nursing", *Yale Journal on Regulation*, Vol., No. 2, 447.

World Health Organization. (2006). *WHO Health Promotion Glossary: new terms. Health Promotion International Advance Access.* Oxford University Press: Author. Can be accessed at http://www.who.int/healthpromotion/about/HP%20Glossay%20in%20HPI.pdf.

APPENDIX A

NCSBN Criteria for Evaluating Certification Programs

Criteria	Elaboration
I. The program is national in the scope of its credentialing.	A. The advanced nursing practice category and standards of practice have been identified by national organizations.
	B. Credentialing services are available to nurses throughout the United States and its territories.
	C. There is a provision for public representation on the certification board.
	D. A nursing specialty organization that establishes standards for the nursing specialty exists.
	E. A tested body of knowledge related to the advanced practice nursing specialty exists.
	F. The certification board is an entity with organizational autonomy.
II. Conditions for taking the examination are consistent with acceptable standards of the testing community.	A. Applicants do not have to belong to an affiliated professional organization in order to apply for certification offered by the certification program.
	B. Eligibility criteria rationally related to competence to practice safely.
	C. Published criteria are enforced.
	D. In compliance with the American Disabilities Act.

	E. Sample application(s) are available.
	1) Certification requirements included
	2) Application procedures include:
	  • procedures for ensuring match between education and clinical experience, and APRN specialty being certified,
	  • procedures for validating information provided by candidate,
	  • procedures for handling omissions and discrepancies
	3) Professional staff responsible for credential review and admission decisions.
	4) Examination should be administered frequently enough to be accessible but not so frequently as to over-expose items.

	F. Periodic review of eligibility criteria and application procedures to ensure that they are fair and equitable.

Criteria	Elaboration

III. Educational requirements are consistent with the requirements of the advanced practice specialty.	A. Current U.S. registered nurse licensure is required.
	B. Graduation from a graduate advanced practice education program meets the following requirements:
	   1) Education program offered by an accredited college or university offers a graduate degree with a concentration in the advanced nursing practice specialty the individual is seeking
	   2) If post-masters certificate programs are offered, they must be offered through institutions meeting criteria B.1.
	   3) Both direct and indirect clinical supervision must be congruent with current national specialty organizations and nursing accreditation guidelines
	   4) The curriculum includes, but is not limited to:
	     • biological, behavioral, medical, and nursing sciences relevant to practice as an APRN in the specified category;
	     • legal, ethical, and professional responsibilities of the APRN; and
	     • supervised clinical practice relevant to the specialty of APRN
	   1) The curriculum meets the following criteria:
	     • Curriculum is consistent with competencies of the specific areas of practice
	     • Instructional track/major has a minimum of 500 supervised clinical hours overall
	     • The supervised clinical experience is directly related to the knowledge and role of the specialty and category
	C. All individuals, without exception, seeking a national certification must complete a formal didactic and clinical advanced practice program meeting the above criteria.

IV. The standard methodologies used are acceptable to the testing community such as incumbent job analysis study, logical job analysis studies.	A. Exam content based on a job/task analysis. B. Job analysis studies are conducted at least every five years. C. The results of the job analysis study are published and available to the public. D. There is evidence of the content validity of the job analysis study.

V. The examination represents entry-level practice in the advanced nursing practice category.	A. Entry-level practice in the advanced practice specialty is described including the following:
	   1) Process
	   2) Frequency
	   3) Qualifications of the group making the determination
	   4) Geographic representation
	   5) Professional or regulatory organizations involved in the reviews

Criteria	**Elaboration**
VI. The examination represents the knowledge, skills, and abilities essential for the delivery of safe and effective advanced nursing care to the clients.	A. The job analysis includes activities representing knowledge, skills, and abilities necessary for competent performance. B. The examination reflects the results of the job analysis study. C. Knowledge, skills, and abilities, which are critical to public safety, are identified. D. The examination content is oriented to educational curriculum practice requirements and accepted standards of care.
VII. Examination items are reviewed for content validity, cultural bias, and correct scoring using an established mechanism, both before use and periodically.	A. Each item is associated with a single cell of the test plan. B. Items are reviewed for currency before each use at least every three years. C. Items are reviewed by members of under-represented gender and ethnicities who are active in the field being certified. Reviewers have been trained to distinguish irrelevant cultural dependencies from knowledge necessary to safe and effective practice. Process for identifying and processing flagged items is identified. D. A statistical bias analysis is performed on all items. E. All items are subjected to an "unscored" use for data collection purposes before their first use as a "scored" item. F. A process to detect and eliminate bias from the test is in place. G. Reuse guidelines for items on an exam form are identified. H. Item writing and review is done by qualified individuals who represent specialties, population subgroups, etc.
VIII. Examinations are evaluated for psychometric performance.	A. Reference groups used for comparative analysis are defined.
IX. The passing standard is established using acceptable psychometric methods, and is re-evaluated periodically.	A. Passing standard is criterion-referenced.

X. Examination security is maintained through established procedures.	A. Protocols are established to maintain security related to:
	  1) Item development (e.g., item writers and confidentiality, how often items are re-used)
	  2) Maintenance of question pool
	  3) Printing and production process
	  4) Storage and transportation of examination is secure
	  5) Administration of examination (e.g., who administers, who checks administrators)
	  6) Ancillary materials (e.g., test keys, scrap materials)
	  7) Scoring of examination
	  8) Occurrence of a crisis (e.g., exam is compromised, etc.)

Criteria	**Elaboration**

XI. Certification is issued based upon passing the examination and meeting all other certification requirements.	A. Certification process is described, including the following:
	  1) Criteria for certification decisions are identified
	  2) The verification that passing exam results and all other requirements are met
	  3) Procedures are in place for appealing decisions
	B. There is due process for situations such as nurses denied access to the examination or nurses who have had their certification revoked.
	C. A mechanism is in place for communicating with candidate.
	D. Confidentiality of nonpublic candidate data is maintained.

XII. A retake policy is in place.	A. Failing candidates permitted to be reexamined at a future date. B. Failing candidates informed of procedures for retakes. C. Test for repeating examinees should be equivalent to the test for first time candidates. D. Repeating examinees should be expected to meet the same test performance standards as first time examinees. E. Failing candidates are given information on content areas of deficiency. F. Repeating examinees are not exposed to the same items when taking the exam previously.

XIII. Certification maintenance program, which includes review of qualifications and continued competence, is in place.	A. Certification maintenance requirements are specified (e.g., continuing education, practice, examination, etc.).
	B. Certification maintenance procedures include:
	  1) Procedures for ensuring match between continued competency measures and APRN specialty
	  2) Procedures for validating information provided by candidates
	  3) Procedures for issuing re-certification
	C. Professional staff oversee credential review.
	D. Certification maintenance is required a minimum of every 5 years.

XIV. Mechanisms are in place for communication to boards of nursing for timely verification of an individual's certification status, changes in certification status, and changes in the certification program, including qualifications, test plan and scope of practice.	A. Communication mechanisms address:
	  1) Permission obtained from candidates to share information regarding the certification process
	  2) Procedures to provide verification of certification to Boards of Nursing
	  3) Procedures for notifying Boards of Nursing regarding changes of certification status
	  4) Procedures for notification of changes in certification programs (qualifications, test plan or scope of practice) to Boards of Nursing

Criteria	**Elaboration**

XV. An evaluation process is in place to provide quality assurance in its certification program.	A. Internal review panels are used to establish quality assurance procedures.
	  1) Composition of these groups (by title or area of expertise) is described
	  2) Procedures are reviewed
	  3) Frequency of review
	B. Procedures are in place to ensure adherence to established QA policy and procedures.

Revised 11-6-01

APPENDIX B

American Nurses Association
Congress on Nursing Practice and Economics
2004
Recognition as a Nursing Specialty

The process of recognizing an area of practice as a nursing specialty allows the profession to formally identify subset areas of focused practice. A clear description of that nursing practice assists the larger community of nurses, healthcare consumers, and others to gain familiarity and understanding of the nursing specialty. Therefore, the document requesting ANA recognition must clearly and fully address each of the fourteen specialty recognition criteria. The inclusion of additional materials to support the discussion and promote understanding of the criteria is acceptable. A scope of practice statement must accompany the submission requesting recognition as a nursing specialty.

Criteria for Recognition as a Nursing Specialty

The following criteria are used by the Congress on Nursing Practice and Economics in the review and decision-making processes to recognize an area of practice as a nursing specialty:

A nursing specialty:

1. Defines itself as nursing.
2. Adheres to the overall licensure requirements of the profession.
3. Subscribes to the overall purposes and functions of nursing.
4. Is clearly defined.
5. Is practiced nationally or internationally.
6. Includes a substantial number of nurses who devote most of their practice to the specialty.
7. Can identify a need and demand for itself.
8. Has a well derived knowledge base particular to the practice of the nursing specialty.
9. Is concerned with phenomena of the discipline of nursing.
10. Defines competencies for the area of nursing specialty practice.
11. Has existing mechanisms for supporting, reviewing and disseminating research to support its knowledge base.
12. Has defined educational criteria for specialty preparation or graduate degree.
13. Has continuing education programs or continuing competence mechanisms for nurses in the specialty.
14. Is organized and represented by a national specialty association or branch of a parent organization.

APPENDIX C

NCSBN APRN Committee Members, 2003 -2008

2003

- Katherine Thomas, Executive Director, Texas Board of Nurse Examiners
- Patty Brown, Board Staff, Kansas State Board of Nursing
- Kim Powell, Board President, Montana Board of Nursing
- Charlene Hanson, Consultant
- Georgia Manning, Arkansas State Board of Nursing
- Deborah Bohannon-Johnson, Board President, North Dakota Board of Nursing
- Jane Garvin, Board President, Maryland Board of Nursing
- Janet Younger, Board President, Virginia Board of Nursing
- Nancy Chornick, NCSBN

2004

- Katherine Thomas, Executive Director, Texas Board of Nurse Examiners
- Patty Brown, Board Staff, Kansas State Board of Nursing
- Kim Powell, Board President, Montana Board of Nursing
- Charlene Hanson, Consultant
- Janet Younger, Board President, Virginia Board of Nursing
- Polly Johnson, Board Representative, North Carolina Board of Nursing
- Laura Poe, Member, Utah State Board of Nursing
- Georgia Manning, Arkansas State Board of Nursing
- Jane Garvin RN, Board President, Maryland Board of Nursing
- Ann Forbes, Board Staff, North Carolina Board of Nursing
- Nancy Chornick, NCSBN

2005

- Katherine Thomas, Executive Director, Texas Board of Nurse Examiners
- Patty Brown, Board Staff, Kansas State Board of Nursing
- Charlene Hanson, Consultant
- Janet Younger, Board President, Virginia Board of Nursing
- Polly Johnson, Board Representative, North Carolina Board of Nursing
- Laura Poe, Member, Utah State Board of Nursing
- Marcia Hobbs, Board Member, Kentucky Board of Nursing
- Randall Hudspeth, Board Member, Idaho Board of Nursing
- Ann Forbes, Board Staff, North Carolina Board of Nursing

- Cristiana Rosa, Board Member, Rhode Island Board of Nurse
- Kim Powell, Board President, Montana Board of Nursing
- Nancy Chornick, NCSBN

2006

- Katherine Thomas, Executive Director, Texas Board of Nurse Examiners
- Patty Brown, Board Staff, Kansas State Board of Nursing
- Charlene Hanson, Consultant
- Janet Younger, Board President, Virginia Board of Nursing
- Laura Poe, Member, Utah State Board of Nursing
- Marcia Hobbs, Board Member, Kentucky Board of Nursing
- Randall Hudspeth, Board Member, Idaho Board of Nursing
- Cristiana Rosa, Board Member, Rhode Island Board of Nurse
- James Luther Raper, Board Member, Alabama Board of Nursing
- Linda Rice, Board Member, Vermont Board of Nursing
- Cathy Williamson, Board Member, Mississippi Board of Nursing
- Ann Forbes, Board Staff, North Carolina Board of Nursing
- Polly Johnson, Board Representative, North Carolina Board of Nursing
- Sheila N. Kaiser, Board Vice-Chair, Massachusetts Board of Registration in Nursing
- Nancy Chornick, NCSBN

2007

- Faith Fields, Board Liaison, Arkansas State Board of Nursing
- Katherine Thomas, Executive Director, Texas Board of Nurse Examiners
- Ann L. O'Sullivan, Board Member, Pennsylvania Board of Nursing
- Patty Brown, Board Staff, Kansas State Board of Nursing
- Charlene Hanson, Consultant
- Laura Poe, Member, Utah State Board of Nursing
- John C. Preston, Board Member, Tennessee Board of Nursing
- Randall Hudspeth, Board Member, Idaho Board of Nursing
- Cristiana Rosa, Board Member, Rhode Island Board of Nurse
- James Luther Raper, Board Member, Alabama Board of Nursing
- Linda Rice, Board Member, Vermont Board of Nursing
- Cathy Williamson, Board Member, Mississippi Board of Nursing
- Janet Younger, Board President, Virginia Board of Nursing
- Marcia Hobbs, Board Member, Kentucky Board of Nursing
- Nancy Chornick, NCSBN

2008

- Doreen K. Begley, Board Member, Nevada State Board of Nursing
- Ann L. O'Sullivan, Board Member, Pennsylvania Board of Nursing
- Patty Brown, Board Staff, Kansas State Board of Nursing
- Charlene Hanson, Consultant
- Laura Poe, Member, Utah State Board of Nursing
- John C. Preston, Board Member, Tennessee Board of Nursing
- Randall Hudspeth, Board Member, Idaho Board of Nursing
- Cristiana Rosa, Board Member, Rhode Island Board of Nurse
- James Luther Raper, Board Member, Alabama Board of Nursing
- Linda Rice, Board Member, Vermont Board of Nursing
- Cathy Williamson, Board Member, Mississippi Board of Nursing
- Tracy Klein, Member Staff, Oregon State Board of Nursing
- Darlene Byrd, Board Member, Arkansas State Board of Nursing
- Nancy Chornick, NCSBN

APPENDIX D

2006 NCSBN APRN Roundtable Organization Attendance List

Alabama Board of Nursing
American Academy of Nurse Practitioners
American Academy of Nurse Practitioners National Certification
    Program, Inc
American Association of Colleges of Nursing
American Association of Critical-Care Nurses
American Association of Nurse Anesthetists
American Association of Psychiatric Nurses
American Board of Nursing Specialties
American College of Nurse-Midwives
American College of Nurse Practitioners
American Holistic Nurses' Certification Corporation
American Midwifery Certification Board
American Nurses Association
American Nurses Credentialing Center
American Organization of Nurses Executives
Association of Women's Health, Obstetric and Neonatal Nurses
Board of Certification for Emergency Nursing
Council on Accreditation of Nurse Anesthesia Educational Programs
Emergency Nurses Association
George Washington School of Medicine
Idaho Board of Nursing
Kansas Board of Nursing
Kentucky Board of Nursing
Massachusetts Board of Nursing
Mississippi Board of Nursing
National Association of Clinical Nurse Specialists
National Association of Nurse Practitioners in Women's Health
National Association of Pediatric Nurse Practitioners
National Board for Certification of Hospice & Palliative Nurses
National Certification Corporation for the Obstetric, Gynecologic and
    Neonatal Nursing Specialties
National League for Nursing Accrediting Commission
North Carolina Board of Nursing
Oncology Nursing Certification Corporation
Pediatric Nursing Certification Board
Rhode Island Board of Nursing
Texas Board of Nurse Examiners
Utah Board of Nursing

Vermont Board of Nursing
Wound, Ostomy and Continence Nursing Certification Board

2007 APRN Roundtable Attendance List

ABNS Accreditation Council
Alabama Board of Nursing
American Academy of Nurse Practitioners
American Academy of Nurse Practitioners National Certification
    Program, Inc
American Association of Colleges of Nursing
American Association of Critical-Care Nurses
American Association of Nurse Anesthetists
American College of Nurse-Midwives
American College of Nurse Practitioners
American Midwifery Certification Board
American Nurses Credentialing Center - Certification Services
American Organization of Nurse Executives
Arkansas State Board of Nursing
Association of Women's Health, Obstetric and Neonatal Nurses
Board of Certification for Emergency Nursing
Colorado Board of Nursing
Commission on Collegiate Nursing Education
Council on Accreditation of Nurse Anesthesia Educational Programs
Council on Certification of Nurse Anesthetists and Council on
    Recertification of Nurse Anesthetists
Emergency Nurses Association
Idaho Board of Nursing
Illinois State Board of Nursing
Kansas Board of Nursing
Kentucky Board of Nursing
Loyola University Chicago Niehoff School of Nursing
Minnesota Board of Nursing
Mississippi Board of Nursing
National Association of Clinical Nurse Specialists
National Association of Pediatric Nurse Practitioners
National Certification Corporation for the Obstetric, Gynecologic and
    Neonatal Nursing Specialties
National League for Nursing Accrediting Commission
National Organization of Nurse Practitioner Faculties
Oncology Nursing Certification Corporation
Pediatric Nursing Certification Board
Pennsylvania Board of Nursing

Rhode Island Board of Nursing
Rush University College of Nursing
South Dakota Board of Nursing
Tennessee Board of Nursing
Texas Board of Nurse Examiners
Vermont Board of Nursing

APPENDIX E

APRN Joint Dialogue Group
Organizations represented at the Joint Dialogue Group Meetings

American Academy of Nurse Practitioners Certification Program
American Association of Colleges of Nursing
American Association of Nurse Anesthetists
American College of Nurse-Midwives
American Nurses Association
American Organization of Nurse Executives
Compact Administrators
National Association of Clinical Nurse Specialists
National Council of State Boards of Nursing
National League for Nursing Accrediting Commission
National Organization of Nurse Practitioner Faculties
NCSBN APRN Advisory Committee Representatives (5)

APPENDIX F

Organizations invited to APN Consensus Conference
June 2004

Accreditation Commission for Midwifery Education
American Academy of Nurse Practitioners
American Academy of Nurse Practitioners Certification Program
American Academy of Nursing
American Association of Critical Care Nurses
American Association of Critical Care Nurses Certification Program
American Association of Nurse Anesthetists
American Association of Occupational Health Nurses
American Board of Nursing Specialties
American College of Nurse-Midwives
American College of Nurse Practitioners
American Nurses Association
American Nurses Credentialing Center
American Organization of Nurse Executives
American Psychiatric Nurses Association
Association of Faculties of Pediatric Nurse Practitioners
Association of Rehabilitation Nurses
Association of Women's Health, Obstetric and Neonatal Nurses
Certification Board Perioperative Nursing
Commission on Collegiate Nursing Education
Council on Accreditation of Nurse Anesthesia Educational Programs
Division of Nursing, DHHS, HRSA
Emergency Nurses Association
Hospice and Palliative Nurses Association
International Nurses Society on Addictions
International Society of Psychiatric-Mental Health Nurses
NANDA International
National Association of Clinical Nurse Specialists
National Association of Neonatal Nurses
National Association of Nurse Practitioners in Women's Health
National Association of Nurse Practitioners in Women's Health, Council on
    Accreditation
National Association of Pediatric Nurse Practitioners
National Association of School Nurses
National Board for Certification of Hospice and Palliative Nurses
National Certification Corporation for the Obstetric, Gynecologic and Neonatal
    Nursing Specialties
National Conference of Gerontological Nurse Practitioners

National Council of State Boards of Nursing
National Gerontological Nursing Association
National League for Nursing
National League for Nursing Accrediting Commission
National Organization of Nurse Practitioner Faculties
Nurse Licensure Compact Administrators/State of Utah Department of
    Commerce/Division of Occupational & Professional Licensing
Nurses Organization of Veterans Affairs
Oncology Nursing Certification Corporation
Oncology Nursing Society
Pediatric Nursing Certification Board
Sigma Theta Tau, International
Society of Pediatric Nurses
Wound Ostomy & Continence Nurses Society
Wound Ostomy Continence Nursing Certification Board

APPENDIX G

Organizations participating in APRN consensus process

Academy of Medical-Surgical Nurses
Accreditation Commission for Midwifery Education
American Academy of Nurse Practitioners
American Academy of Nurse Practitioners Certification Program
American Association of Colleges of Nursing
American Association of Critical Care Nurses Certification
American Association of Neuroscience Nurses
American Association of Nurse Anesthetists
American Association of Occupational Health Nurses
American Board for Occupational Health Nurses
American Board of Nursing Specialties
American College of Nurse-Midwives
American College of Nurse-Midwives Division of Accreditation
American College of Nurse Practitioners
American Holistic Nurses Association
American Nephrology Nurses Association
American Nurses Association
American Nurses Credentialing Center
American Organization of Nurse Executives
American Psychiatric Nurses Association
American Society for Pain Management Nursing
American Society of PeriAnesthesia Nurses
Association of Community Health Nursing Educators
Association of Faculties of Pediatric Nurse Practitioners
Association of Nurses in AIDS Care
Association of PeriOperative Registered Nurses
Association of Rehabilitation Nurses
Association of State and Territorial Directors of nursing
Association of Women's Health, Obstetric and Neonatal Nurses
Board of Certification for Emergency Nursing
Commission on Collegiate Nursing Education
Commission on Graduates of Foreign Nursing Schools
Council on Accreditation of Nurse Anesthesia Educational Programs
Department of Health
Dermatology Nurses Association
District of Columbia Board of Nursing
Division of Nursing, DHHS, HRSA
Emergency Nurses Association
George Washington University

Health Resources and Services Administration
Infusion Nurses Society
International Nurses Society on Addictions
International Society of Psychiatric-Mental Health Nurses
Kentucky Board of Nursing
National Association of Clinical Nurse Specialists
National Association of Neonatal Nurses
National Association of Nurse Practitioners in Women's Health, Council on
    Accreditation
National Association of Orthopedic Nurses
National Association of Pediatric Nurse Practitioners
National Association of School of Nurses
National Certification Corporation for the Obstetric, Gynecologic, and Neonatal
    Nursing Specialties
National Conference of Gerontological Nurse Practitioners
National Council of State Boards of Nursing
National League for Nursing
National League for Nursing Accrediting Commission
National Organization of Nurse Practitioner Faculties
Nephrology Nursing Certification Commission
North American Nursing Diagnosis Association International
Nurses Organization of Veterans Affairs
Oncology Nursing Certification Corporation
Oncology Nursing Society
Pediatric Nursing Certification Board
Pennsylvania State Board of Nursing
Public Health Nursing Section of the American Public Health Association.
Rehabilitation Nursing Certification Board
Society for Vascular Nursing
Texas Nurses Association
Texas State Board of Nursing
Utah State Board of Nursing
Women's Health, Obstetric & Neonatal Nurses
Wound, Ostomy, & Continence Nurses Society
Wound, Ostomy, & Continence Nursing Certification

APPENDIX H

APRN Consensus Process Work Group
Organizations Represented at the Work Group Meetings

Jan Towers, American Academy of Nurse Practitioners Certification Program
Joan Stanley, American Association of Colleges of Nursing
Carol Hartigan, American Association of Critical Care Nurses Certification
    Corporation
Leo LeBel, American Association of Nurse Anesthetists
Bonnie Niebuhr, American Board of Nursing Specialties
Peter Johnson & Elaine Germano, American College of Nurse-Midwives
Mary Jean Schumann, American Nurses Association
Mary Smolenski, American Nurses Credentialing Center
M.T. Meadows, American Organization of Nurse Executives
Edna Hamera & Sandra Talley, American Psychiatric Nurses Association
Elizabeth Hawkins-Walsh, Association of Faculties of Pediatric Nurse
    Practitioners
Jennifer Butlin, Commission on Collegiate Nursing Education
Laura Poe, APRN Compact Administrators
Betty Horton, Council on Accreditation of Nurse Anesthesia Educational
    Programs
Kelly Goudreau, National Association of Clinical Nurse Specialists
Fran Way, National Association of Nurse Practitioners in Women's Health,
    Council on Accreditation
Mimi Bennett, National Certification Corporation for the Obstetric,
    Gynecologic, and Neonatal Nursing Specialties
Kathy Apple, National Council of State Boards of Nursing
Grace Newsome & Sharon Tanner, National League for Nursing Accrediting
    Commission
Kitty Werner & Ann O'Sullivan, National Organization of Nurse Practitioner
    Faculties
Cyndi Miller-Murphy, Oncology Nursing Certification Corporation
Janet Wyatt, Pediatric Nursing Certification Board
Carol Calianno, Wound, Ostomy and Continence Nursing Certification Board
Irene Sandvold, DHHS, HRSA, Division of Nursing *(observer)*

ADDENDUM

Example of a National Consensus-Building Process to Develop Nationally Recognized Education Standards and Role/Specialty Competencies

The national consensus-based process described here was originally designed, with funding by the Department of Health and Human Services, Health Resources and Services Administration, Bureau of Health Professions, Division of Nursing, to develop and validate national consensus-based primary care nurse practitioner competencies in five specialty areas. The process was developed with consultation from a nationally recognized expert in higher education assessment. The process subsequently has been used and validated for the development of similar sets of competencies for other areas of nursing practice, including competencies for mass casualty education for all nurses and competencies for acute care nurse practitioners and psych/mental health nurse practitioners.

This process for developing nationally recognized educational standards, nationally recognized role competencies and nationally recognized specialty competencies is an iterative, step wise process. The steps are:

Step 1: At the request of the organization(s) representing the role or specialty, a neutral group or groups convenes and facilitates a national panel of all stakeholder organizations as defined in step 2.

Step 2: To ensure broad representation, invitations to participate should be extended to one representative of each of the recognized nursing accrediting organizations, certifiers within the role and specialty, groups whose primary mission is graduate education and who have established educational criteria for the identified role and specialty, and groups with competencies and standards for education programs that prepare individuals in the role and specialty.

Step 3: Organizational representatives serving on the national consensus panel bring and share role delineation studies, competencies for practice and education, scopes and standards of practice, and standards for education programs.

Step 4: Agreement is reached among the panel members

Step 5: Panel members take the draft to their individual boards for feedback.

Step 6: That feedback is returned to the panel. This is an iterative process until agreement is reached.

Step 7: Validation is sought from a larger group of stakeholders including organizations and individuals. This is known as the Validation Panel.

Step 8: Feedback from the Validation Panel is returned to National Panel to prepare the final document.

Step 9: Final document is sent to boards represented on the National Panel and the Validation Panel for endorsement.

The final document demonstrates national consensus through consideration of broad input from key stakeholders. The document is then widely disseminated.

E

Undergraduate Nursing Education

According to the findings of the 2008 National Sample Survey of registered nurses (RNs), just over 3 million licensed RNs live in the United States; nearly 85 percent of these women and men are actively working in the nursing profession. Nearly 450,000 RNs are estimated to have received their first U.S. license between 2004 and 2008 (HRSA, 2010). The current nursing workforce includes a high proportion of nurses working in the later years of their careers, soon to retire, and a high proportion of nurses at the onset of their careers. Midcareer nurses, the group most needed to fill the roles of those leaving the workforce, are the lowest in number. Therefore, the knowledge, experience, and mentoring that senior nurses can provide could potentially be lost (Bleich et al., 2009). Table E-1 shows the demographic and educational distribution of the current nursing workforce.

Nursing is unique among the health care professions in the United States in that it offers multiple educational pathways leading to an entry-level license to practice. For the past four decades, nursing students have been able to pursue three different educational paths: the diploma in nursing, the associate's degree in nursing (ADN), and the bachelor's of science in nursing (BSN). More recently, an accelerated, second-degree bachelor's program for students who possess a baccalaureate degree in another field has become a popular option.

DIPLOMA IN NURSING

For many years, the most common choice of nursing students was the diploma program at a hospital-based school. Generally lasting 3 years and providing limited liberal arts content, diploma programs trace their origin to the work of Florence Nightingale and her colleagues in the 19th century. In many ways,

TABLE E-1 Demographic and Educational Characteristics of Registered Nurses, by Age

	Under Age 50	Age 50 or Older	Total
Estimated total population	1,694,088	1,369,074	3,063,162
Race/ethnicity			
White, non-Hispanic	80.0	87.2	83.2
Nonwhite or Hispanic	20.0	12.8	16.8
Gender			
Male	7.7	5.3	6.6
Female	92.3	94.7	93.4
Initial nursing education			
Diploma	9.0	34.5	20.4
Associate's	48.5	41.6	45.4
Bachelor's or higher	42.5	23.9	34.2
Highest nursing or nursing-related education			
Diploma	6.6	23.0	13.9
Associate's	40.0	31.2	36.1
Bachelor's	43.1	28.9	36.8
Graduate	10.3	16.8	13.2

SOURCE: HRSA, 2010.

diploma programs are similar to apprenticeship programs for physicians in the 1800s before the widespread development of medical schools (Gebbie, 2009). As nursing gained a stronger theoretical foundation and other types of nursing programs increased in number, the number of diploma programs declined remarkably throughout the 20th century except in a few states, such as New Jersey, Ohio, and Pennsylvania. One advantage of the diploma program is that there are guaranteed clinical spaces for those accepted into the program, something ADN and BSN programs cannot offer. The number of all working nurses who began their nursing education in diploma schools fell from 63.7 percent in 1980 to 20.4 percent in 2008; the number of new diploma graduates dropped to 3.1 percent of all graduates in the 2005–2008 graduation cohort (HRSA, 2010).

ASSOCIATE'S DEGREE IN NURSING

At present, the most common way to become an RN is to pursue an ADN at a community college. The proportion of nurses in the United States whose initial education was an ADN increased from 42.9 percent in 2004 to 45.4 percent in 2008 (HRSA, 2010). ADN programs in nursing were launched in the mid–20th century in response to the nursing shortage that followed World War II (Lynaugh, 2008; Lynaugh and Brush, 1996). Generally speaking, the ADN remains less expensive than a BSN because of the cost structure of the community college system and the shorter program duration. Once conceived as a 2-year program, the ADN is seen as taking less time than a BSN, but this situation has changed over the years (Orsolini-Hain, 2008). In most non–health care disciplines, the associate's degree takes 2 years to complete. In nursing, however, surveys have found that it takes students 3–4 years to complete an ADN program because of the need to fulfill prerequisites and the lack of adequate faculty, which lead to long waiting lists for many programs and classes (Orsolini-Hain, 2008). The ADN curriculum often combines intense science and clinical coursework into a condensed time frame, posing additional challenges to completing the program in 2 years.

BACHELOR'S OF SCIENCE IN NURSING

The BSN is a 4-year degree, typically offered at a university; the first university-based schools of nursing were founded in the early 20th century (Lynaugh, 2008; Lynaugh and Brush, 1996). BSN programs emphasize liberal arts, advanced sciences, and nursing coursework across a wide range of settings, along with leadership development and exposure to community and public health competencies. As of 2008, 34.2 percent of RNs throughout the United States had started with a BSN, up from 31.5 percent in 2004 (HRSA, 2010). Beginning in the latter part of the 20th century, an accelerated option for a BSN or MSN became available to applicants who had already completed a bachelor's degree in a different field. Also known as fast-track or second-degree programs, these programs have added substantially to the growing number of baccalaureate graduates (AACN, 2010).

Most BSN students complete their degrees in 4 years. Accelerated programs that offer the BSN to students who have already completed a bachelor's degree are typically completed in 11–18 months, with intense coursework and professional formation accelerated based on previous collegiate and life experience (AACN, 2010).

For much of the 20th century, following the release of a significant 1965 position paper of the American Nurses Association, nursing leaders and educators tried to standardize nursing education and make the BSN the minimum entry-level requirement for nursing practice. Four states were targeted for early implementation (Smith, 2010). Only one of them—North Dakota—fully followed through on that recommendation by establishing the BSN as the minimum degree in nursing in 1987 (Smith, 2010). In 2003, however, the state legislature, at the urging of hospitals and long-term-care stakeholders, passed a law that allowed nurses with an ADN to practice (Boldt, 2003). Nationwide, market forces and the needs of individual employers generally determine whether a BSN is required for entry into practice.

LICENSED PRACTICAL NURSES

In addition to the RNs, who receive a diploma, associate, or baccalaureate degree in nursing, another undergraduate-level degree offered is the licensed practical/vocational degree in nursing. Licensed practical/vocational nurses (LPNs/LVNs) are especially important because of their contributions to care in long-term care facilities and nursing homes.

Historically, LPN/LVN programs have fluctuated based on need. The first training program for licensed practical/vocational nurses (LPNs/LVNs) dates back to the late 19th century. These programs increased in number following the nursing shortage of World War I, and the passage of the Smith Hughes Act, and again following the nursing shortage of World War II, when LPNs/LVNs were in demand to assist RNs in civilian hospitals (lpntraining.org, 2010), which were short-staffed as a result of war efforts. LPNs/LVNs also found employment in long-term-care facilities and nursing homes.

LPN/LVN receives a diploma after completion of a 12-month program. The LPN/LVN is not educated for independent decision making for complex care but obtains basic training in anatomy and physiology, nutrition, and nursing techniques. With additional study, these nurses can perform supplemental nursing tasks that are useful to patients and nursing home residents and can contribute to clinical documentation and team performance. Some LPNs/LVNs also supervise nursing attendants and direct care workers in long-term care settings.

CONCLUSION

The fact that each educational pathway (i.e., diploma, ADN, and BSN) leads to the same licensure exam (the NCLEX-RN; see Chapter 4) makes it difficult to argue that a graduate with a BSN is more competent to perform entry-level tasks than one who has a diploma or an ADN. Statistics from the National Council of State Boards of Nursing show little difference in the pass rates of BSN, ADN, and diploma graduates, which is to be expected because the exam tests the minimum standards for safe practice. In 2009, 89.49 percent of 52,241 BSN candidates passed the NCLEX-RN exam, compared with 87.61 percent of 78,665 ADN candidates and 90.75 percent of 3,677 diploma candidates (NCSBN, 2010).

REFERENCES

AACN (American Association of Colleges of Nursing). 2010. *Accelerated baccalaureate and master's degrees in nursing: Fact sheet.* http://www.aacn.nche.edu/Media/FactSheets/AcceleratedProg. htm (accessed July 2, 2010).

Bleich, M. R., B. L. Cleary, K. Davis, B. J. Hatcher, P. O. Hewlett, and K. S. Hill. 2009. Mitigating knowledge loss: A strategic imperative for nurse leaders. *Journal of Nursing Administration* 39(4):160-164.

Boldt, M. 2003. Legislature approves relaxed education standards for nurses. *The Associated Press State & Local Wire*, April 16.

Gebbie, K. M. 2009. 20th-century reports on nursing and nursing education: What difference did they make? *Nurse Outlook* 57(2):84-92.

HRSA (Health Resources and Services Administration). 2010. *The registered nurse population: Findings from the 2008 National Sample Survey of Registered Nurses.* HRSA.

lpntraining.org. 2010. *The history of practical nursing.* http://www.lpntraining.org/the-history-of-practical-nursing.html (accessed September 9, 2010).

Lynaugh, J. E. 2008. Kate Hurd-Mead lecture. Nursing the great society: The impact of the Nurse Training Act of 1964. *Nursing History Review* 16:13-28.

Lynaugh, J. E., and B. L. Brush. 1996. *American nursing: From hospitals to health systems.* Cambridge, MA and Oxford, U.K.: Blackwell Press.

NCSBN (National Council of State Boards of Nursing). 2010. *Nurse licensure and NCLEX examination statistics.* https://www.ncsbn.org/1236.htm (accessed August 20, 2010).

Orsolini-Hain, L. 2008. An interpretive phenomenological study on the influences on associate degree prepared nurses to return to school to earn a higher degree in nursing, Department of Nursing, University of California, San Francisco.

Smith, T. G. 2010. A policy perspective on the entry into practice issue. *OJIN: The Online Journal of Issues in Nursing* 15(1).

Appendixes F–J are not printed in this report
but can be found on the CD-ROM in the back of this book.

Index*

---

*Pages 375-642 are not printed in this report but can be found on the CD-ROM in the back of this book.